Bruce — all best wishes —

Chris ..

The History of Moorfields Eye Hospital

Volume III

Forty Years On

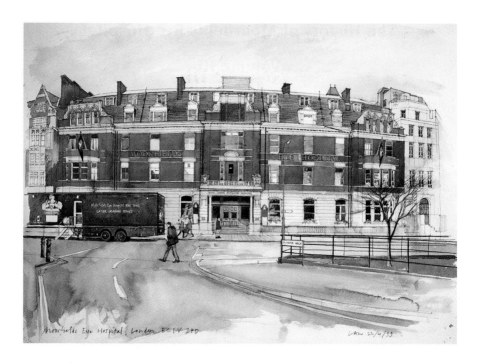

Frontispiece: Moorfields through the eyes of a patient. This fine painting was commissioned as part of the celebrations in 1999 to mark 100 years since the move to the new building on City Road (then titled the Royal London Ophthalmic Hospital). The artist, a patient of the Hospital (it is simply signed 'Law'), has included the mobile unit in the picture, although it was never in fact parked in front of the Hospital.

The reproduction of this painting as a frontispiece was generously funded by the Moorfields Surgeons Association.

The History of Moorfields Eye Hospital

Volume III

Forty Years On

Peter K Leaver FRCS FRCOphth

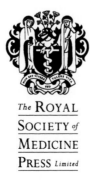

The ROYAL
SOCIETY *of*
MEDICINE
PRESS *Limited*

© 2004 Royal Society of Medicine Press Ltd

Published by the Royal Society of Medicine Press Ltd
1 Wimpole Street, London W1G 0AE, UK
Tel: +44 (0) 20 7290 2921
Fax: +44 (0) 20 7290 2929
Email: publishing@rsm.ac.uk
Website: www.rsmpress.co.uk

British Library Cataloguing in Publication Data
A catalogue record for this book is available from the British Library

ISBN 1–85315–580–2

Distribution in Europe and Rest of World:
Marston Book Services Ltd
PO Box 269
Abingdon
Oxon OX14 4YN, UK
Tel: +44 (0) 1235 465500
Fax: +44 (0) 1235 465555

Distribution in the USA and Canada:
Royal Society of Medicine Press Ltd
c/o Jamco Distribution Inc
1401 Lakeway Drive
Lewisville, TX 75057, USA
Tel: +1 800 538 1287
Fax: +1 972 353 1303
Email: jamco@majors.com

Distribution in Australia and New Zealand:
Elsevier Australia
30–52 Smidmore Street
Marrickville
NSW 2204
Australia
Tel: +61 2 9517 8999
Fax: +61 2 9517 2249
Email: service@elsevier.com.au

Design and typeset by Phoenix Photosetting, Chatham, Kent, UK
Printed and bound by Krips b.v., Meppel, The Netherlands

Contents

❧❧❧

To

Barrie R Jones

who led the way

Foreword

Why write a history of a hospital? A common reason is to describe the good works of the many who contribute to the building and operation of what are invariably complicated institutions. A more important reason is to do with the role of institutions in society. Institutions are important to the communities they serve. Moorfields Eye Hospital is an institution that has not merely survived but flourished for 200 years and is known and influential all over the world, wherever ophthalmology is practised. Institutions that have been influential for so long deserve examination, particularly when they continue to grow and thrive. What is it about them that leads to their success? This is best determined by critical analysis of their history.

The history of an organization, the decisions that it has taken and the direction it has moved, depends largely on its inherent character. Defining the character of an organization is more complex than determining the character of an individual – there are questionnaires to help with the latter. Although an increasing amount is written and studied in the field of organizational behaviour, there is no universally acceptable formula with which to examine the soul of an institution. Nevertheless it is important to do so if the successes are to be replicated within the wider community. The exercise is essentially descriptive and often best done by recording the history and examining the underlying mechanics of what has transpired.

Moorfields Eye Hospital is an effective institution that has been influential over a prolonged period of time. It will celebrate its bicentenary in 2005. For two centuries it has directly served the London community on an everyday basis, provided consultative care on a national level and beyond, and through extensive teaching programs and research, played an important leadership role at a global level for the eye care professions. Perhaps not surprisingly in view of its long history, the circumstances under which the Hospital has operated have changed dramatically over the years.

Originally established to relieve the pressure on general hospitals from the sequelae of Egyptian ophthalmia, Moorfields played the role of a charitable dispenser of eye care until the introduction of the National Health Service in 1948, when it became an instrument for delivering a government health service. Since then it has been subjected to increasing demands, controls and politicization, particularly in the last 40 years. The miracle has been that not only has the Hospital survived the rapidly changing requirements placed on it, but it has thrived and prospered and is today stronger than at any time in its long and distinguished history. This book documents what has happened over the last 40 years and explores the various forces and influences that have mapped and directed its course.

The book deals with a paradox. The last 40 years have been the most turbulent in the history of the Hospital – and the most progressive. Despite escalating demands imposed on the organization, it has gone from strength to strength and grown impressively. This progression reflects one of the most obvious traits in the Moorfields character – the ability to adapt to prevailing conditions and to see opportunity where others might see only constraint. Moorfields has continually reinvented itself throughout its history, particularly in the last 40 years. Over this period the scope of its operations has increased impressively, the range of services and the number of patients has increased dramatically, and what could have been described in the past as a cloistered ivory tower has now transmuted into an institution without walls, one that operates well beyond its headquarters and provides extensive services across London and beyond. The story of the last 40 years is a case study in how an organization can cope with frequent changes in Government policy, conflicting demands for service, and prodigious advances in science and clinical practice.

The ability of Moorfields not only to adapt to prevailing conditions but also to prosper when conditions are not particularly encouraging is a striking feature of the organization. This is not attributable to any individual, or group, or anything in the formal element of its organizational structure of governance. It is more related to the inherent character and culture of the place. The strong culture is particularly noticeable to those who are transplanted into the Hospital from outside.

When I arrived at Moorfields in the early 1970s I found all the technical prowess and clinical acumen that I expected. But there was more. It was a remarkably welcoming place and very encouraging to foreigners – and there were many foreigners there – one of them in the top job. This willingness to include people from all over the world no doubt accounts for the high standing of the Moorfields name internationally. We all returned home with only good things to say about the place. Not that the foreigners were the only ones talking it up. The Moorfields staff hold a view that theirs is 'the best hospital in the country and probably the world'. Whether this view is justified is beside the point. It is held with the conviction of a religious tenet, and holds people together in the same way others are held together by unchallengeable religious beliefs. The cohesion of the Moorfields staff – professional and others – has seriously contributed to the way the organization has been able to adapt to changing circumstances throughout its history and particularly during the last few decades.

To describe the history of the last 40 years for Moorfields is particularly challenging. Unlike the previous two volumes of the history, which dealt with the first 160 years of the Hospital, this book deals with many contemporary issues and personalities. Most of the people mentioned in the book are alive and many are still working. Unlike many history books, this one is written about people who are around to comment and challenge. Dealing with such contemporary and continuing issues, perhaps the work would be better described as anthropology rather than history. However it is described, writing about current issues offers challenges.

Peter Leaver is uniquely qualified to take on this difficult task. After 30 years as a retinal surgeon he is unable to say no when requested to deal with what others may consider an impossible task. This is fortunate because he has been remarkably successful in drawing together the various elements in the story and capturing not only the sequence of events accurately, but also the spirit of the place and the times. Perhaps this is not surprising bearing in mind that he has been an important member of the Moorfields staff for most of the 40 years that he has written about here. He began his association with the Hospital in 1967 and worked in both the City Road and High Holborn branches – and lived to tell the tale. Showing uncharacteristic modesty for a Moorfields man, he makes little of his own considerable contribution to the development of ophthalmology at Moorfields in playing a central role in the development of vitreoretinal surgery – an important part of the modern Moorfields story.

For those of us who have been associated with Moorfields over the last 40 years, Peter Leaver has provided a valuable memento of an important time in our lives. More than this, he has provided an accurate, but no doubt disputable, account of the day-to-day history of the institution, and a fearless account of the forces that have brought about a remarkable period of achievement, and most importantly a reason to be confident, but not complacent, about its future.

Professor Douglas Coster AO
Adelaide, January 2004

Preface

Moorfields is more than just the largest and busiest eye hospital in the Western world; it seems to have a personality of its own that inspires unusual affection and loyalty in patients and staff alike. The two previous volumes recording its history, by Treacher Collins (1929) and Frank Law (1975), bear testimony to this. Although it is only 30 years since the publication of Volume II, the enormous changes in technology, culture and economics that have influenced Moorfields in recent years are rooted firmly in circumstances and events that had their origins in the 1950s and 1960s. It is for this reason that the present account overlaps to some extent with its predecessor. The appointment of Barrie Jones to the first Chair of Clinical Ophthalmology in 1963 was an event of seminal importance; it was he who really did lead Moorfields forward, towards the position it enjoys today.

The Hospital has grown and changed enormously during the last 40 years, consolidating its position on one site in the City Road and becoming an independent NHS Trust, while opportunities for collaborative work with the Institute of Ophthalmology have been greatly improved by the transfer of the latter to the same island site. What is more, a fundamental change in the way in which Moorfields functions took place during the 1970s with the introduction of micro-surgery and subspecialization, and in the 1990s with the development of day-surgery and of an outreach programme in the wider community. These alone were worth recording, but there have been a great many other important changes during this vital period in its history.

This book is designed to satisfy the curiosity of anyone who wants to know what makes Moorfields tick. The text is divided into four parts. The first is a general, rolling account of the past 40 or so years and how changes in medicine – technological, socio-economic and political – have altered the Hospital's course. I have tried to make it readable and understandable to anyone who is interested, no matter what their background, job or station in life; they might be a visitor, a patient or a member of the public who takes a notion to find out more about this remarkable institution. The second part is necessarily more technical and detailed, exploring as it does each of the clinical and clinical support services in greater depth. The third part discusses issues of education and research. Finally, the fourth part deals (pragmatically) with matters of management, administration, finance, and the fabric and infrastructure of the Hospital. I imagine that few, if any, would want to read the book right through in one go, but rather they might read Part 1 and then dip into other bits that excite their own particular interests. As I dislike having to refer back and forth all the time, thereby losing the thread of the narrative, I have tried to make each section as free-standing as possible.

The text is written in a broadly narrative style that, while sticking closely to accuracy of facts and dates, is nevertheless my own. Where I have chosen to tell stories, either directly attributable or apocryphal, or to quote directly from those I have interviewed, these appear in *italics*. Perceptions of events are not only mine, but those of the many members of staff, both past and present, who gave up their time to talk to me. These perceptions may not always accord fully with those of others, but I have been at pains to talk to a great many people, over 150 in fact, to reach a reasonable consensus. To them I extend my heartfelt thanks for their time and willingness to talk to me at length. It would be self-defeating to attempt to mention them all by name, so I will not attempt to do so (a list of those who kindly agreed to be interviewed appears elsewhere), but one or two deserve special mention.

John Atwill, House Governor from 1976 to 1993, has been a formidable source of information and a more than willing mentor and helper in other ways. His sharp mind and accurate recall of events, some more than 20 years ago, has been especially helpful, and he has also been responsible for researching many of the photographs. For the production of the latter and for technical advice about the design of the book's dust jacket, cover and pictorial layout, I am deeply indebted to Kulwant Sehmi, Richard Poynter, Richard Leung and other members of the Hospital's Imaging Department. Sehmi especially has been more than generous with his time and patient expertise. Ann Hughes, formerly Director of Nursing Services and now Divisional Director of Nursing, has been unsparing with her encyclopaedic knowledge of the Hospital and recall of events past while Roslyn Emblin, formerly Chief Nurse and Deputy Chief Executive, was equally generous with historical documents from her personal archive. Rolf Blach, consultant surgeon from 1968 to 1995, and Dean of the Medical School from 1985 to 1991, has been especially helpful and encouraging. Lastly,

Debbie Heatlie and her staff in the Joint Library have been kind, courteous, informative and patient with me at all times.

The essential facts I have researched from a wide range of sources, notably from Hospital and Institute reports, the previous two volumes of the History of Moorfields, government white papers and reports, and the relentless pursuit of colleagues past and present. In January 2003 I travelled to New Zealand to interview Professor Barrie Jones at his home in Tauranga. He gave me seven hours of invaluable discourse, for which I am truly grateful. More than any man alive, he was responsible for the Hospital's continuing strength of purpose and vitality, and it is for that reason that this volume is dedicated to him. My trip to the Antipodes was generously supported by the Moorfields Surgeons Association, and to its members I owe my sincere thanks.

In order to iron out any misconceptions and weigh against possible bias, Hugh Peppiatt, distinguished lawyer and former Chairman of the Board of Governors (later Directors) of Moorfields, has kindly read through the manuscript and suggested modifications where appropriate. He also suggested a number of helpful improvements to the grammar, syntax, and sense of the text. This was an onerous task and one that he undertook with greater skill and care than I could possibly have expected. I am very grateful to him for doing it. In the final analysis, however, the buck stops with me and I am happy that the story I have penned is faithful to the truth. In more than 30 years of service I have had ample opportunity to observe the Hospital's many facets from every angle. In the end, however, history comes down to perceptions, and needless to say my own are influenced by personal characteristics, my politics – more pink than blue – my passionate belief in the Hospital's importance, and an unquenchable optimism for its future.

One notable omission that may attract predictable criticism is the absence in this account of any description of research work itself. This is something over which I agonized but briefly: while the importance of research and the manner of its production is extensively covered, I did not feel that I could do any justice to its content; in the first instance I am not personally equipped to undertake the task, and in the second I believe it warrants a separate account in its own right – perhaps a 'History of the Institute of Ophthalmology', written by someone with the necessary credentials. It would be a Herculean task, but one that would surely be its own reward.

Mention of Herculean tasks brings me to my two most loyal, conscientious and uncomplaining helpers: Brenda Aveyard, my Personal Assistant, and my wife Jane. Without the unstinting labours of the former (she set up the 150 or so interviews and then transcribed more than 2500 pages of text from the audio-tapes alone), and the unfailing patience and good humour of both, it is certain this book would not have seen the light of day, nor the author kept his sanity; to both of them I owe my heartfelt gratitude. I must also thank the Royal Society of Medicine Press, especially Alison Campbell, Managing Editor, and her assistant Shirley Mukisa, for all they have done to make the task easier, and the House Governor, Medical Director and Board of Directors of Moorfields Eye Hospital NHS Trust for their unfailing encouragement. Last and perhaps most importantly of all, my thanks are due to the Moorfields Special Trustees, without whose financial support we could not have gone to press. To spend one's retirement talking to friends and colleagues old and new can give nothing but enjoyment, so the writing of this history, although hard work, has been both a privilege and a pleasure.

Peter Leaver
London, January 2004

List of Illustrations

❧

Acknowledgements

Interviews were kindly given by the following, many of whom offered the author generous hospitality, and to all of whom he extends his warmest thanks:

James Acheson, Lettie Apilado, Geoffrey Arden, John Atwill, GW (Bill) Aylward, John Bach, Ian Balmer, Grainne Barron, Tony Beltrami, Brian Benson, Alan Bird, Rolf Blach, Brian Blackgrove, Jill Bloom, Elizabeth Boultbee, Thomas Boyd-Carpenter, Roger Buckley, Caroline Carr, Anthony Chignell, Patricia Clarke (by telephone), Richard Collin, Robert Cooling, Douglas Coster, Barry Crane, Louise Culham, Carol Cunningham, Rhodri Daniel, John Dart, Parul Desai, Mary Digby, Jonathan Dowler, Ian Duguid, Christopher Earl, Roslyn Emblin, Patti Evans, Peter Fells, Timothy Ffytche, Alec Finch, Sarah Fisher, Lorimer Fison, Wendy Franks, David Galton, Alec Garner, David (Ted) Garway-Heath, Kenneth Gold, Desmond Greaves, Zdenek Gregor, AMH (Peter) Hamilton, Maureen Hamilton-Smith (by telephone), Marion Handscombe, John Harry, Debbie Heatlie, David Hill, Roger Hitchings, Chris Hogg, Graham Holder, Patrick Holmes-Sellors, Jackie Howe, Ann Hughes, John Hungerford, Philip Hykin, David Hyman, Elaine Iannou, Barrie Jay, Gordon Johnson, Barrie R Jones, Barry Jones, Peng Lee Khaw, Ian Knott, Eva Kohner, Alan Lacey, Frank Larkin, John Lee, Ricky Lee (by telephone), Leila Lessoff, Susan Lightman, Alex Lines (by telephone), Jonathan Lord, Katherine Lowe, Philip Luthert, Susan Lydiard, Patricia Maddison, Alan Marjoram, Ronald Marsh, John Marshall, Ian McDonald, Anne McIntyre, David McLoed, Christine Miles, Michael Miller, Darwin Minassian, Tony Moore, Joyce Morrin, Ivan Moseley, Ian Murdoch, Norman Musgrove, Clive Nickolds, Graham Nunn, Amanda O'Keefe, Sarah Parker, Hugh Peppiatt, Cyril Peskett, Brian Pickard, Gordon Plant, Suzanne Powrie, Eilish Quinn, Marie Restori, David Rhys-Tyler, Noel Rice, Sybil Ritten, Geoffrey Rose, Michael Sanders, John Scott, Kulwant Sehmi, Sally Sherman, Adam Sillito, Janet Silver, Barry Smith, Jean Smith, Redmond Smith, Sri Srikantha, Arthur Steele, Julian Stevens, Paul Sullivan, Patrick Trevor-Roper, Mala Viswalingam, Peter Watson, Richard Welham, Hugh Williams, Tony Willoughby, Barry Winnard, John Winstanley, Richard Wormald, John Wright, Peter Wright.

PART 1

A General Account

CHAPTER 1

Moorfields past and present: 1963–2003

The Hospital's origins

Moorfields Eye Hospital NHS Trust in the year 2003 is a place very different from that depicted in previous accounts of its history. The Hospital that we know today has its origins in three London eye hospitals founded in the 19th Century: the Royal London Ophthalmic, the Central London Ophthalmic and the Royal Westminster Ophthalmic. Each of the three hospitals had undergone gradual migration and metamorphosis. The Royal London Ophthalmic, founded in 1805 by John Cunningham Saunders, began life in Charterhouse Square as the London Dispensary for Curing Diseases of the Eye and Ear, and subsequently moved and changed its name twice before ending up in 1899 in City Road (**Figure 1**, Plate 1, top). The Central London Ophthalmic opened its doors in 1834 in Russell Square, moving to Gray's Inn Road and finally in 1913 to Judd Street, near Kings Cross railway station. In 1816 a renowned army surgeon, George James Guthrie, founded The Royal Westminster Ophthalmic Hospital, with premises in Marylebone Street, whence it moved via Warwick Street and Chandos Street, to High Holborn (formerly Broad Street) in 1928 (**Figure 1**, Plate 1, bottom).

In 1946 the three hospitals were amalgamated by Act of Parliament into 'The Moorfields, Westminster and Central Eye Hospital'. Then, with the launch of the National Health Service (NHS) in 1948, the combined Hospital lost its charitable status and the newly appointed Board of Governors decided to close the Central branch to provide accommodation for Sir Stewart Duke-Elder's new Institute of Ophthalmology. This left the City Road and High Holborn branches to function separately but under joint governance, the Institute becoming, de facto, a member of the British Postgraduate Medical Federation, a school of London University.

The name 'Moorfields' was acquired as a result of the relocation in

1821 of John Saunders' London Dispensary for Curing Diseases of the Eye and Ear from Charterhouse Square to a new purpose-built hospital on a piece of former moorland (moor fields) lying just to the north of the old City wall, access to which was gained through the Moor Gate. Because of its location, this new eye hospital, although now called the London Ophthalmic Infirmary, soon acquired the soubriquet 'Moorfields'. Even when it finally moved to its present site on City Road in 1899, however, it was titled The Royal London Ophthalmic Hospital and not Moorfields. It was not until many years later (1956) that, by order of the Minister of Health, the two clinical branches of the Hospital (in City Road and High Holborn) were together officially given the title 'Moorfields Eye Hospital'.

During the latter two decades of the 20th Century, the three stems from which the modern Moorfields grew finally came together. In 1988 the High Holborn branch was closed and merged with the hospital on City Road, and in 1991 the Institute moved to the same island of land (bounded by City Road, Peerless Street and Bath Street) occupied by

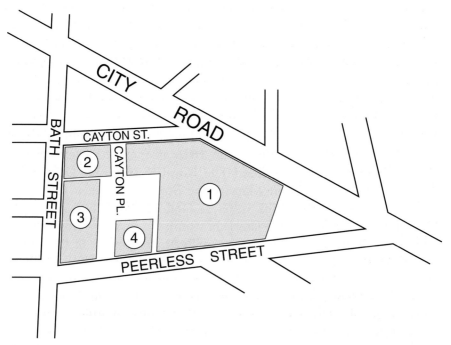

Figure 2   Plan of the 'island site', bordered by City Road, Peerless Street, Bath Street and Cayton Street, on which now stand Moorfields Eye Hospital and the Institute of Ophthalmology. (The proposed International Children's Eye Centre will be built on the site in Peerless Street at present occupied by Fryer House.) 1, Hospital Building (1899); 2, Dean's and Pathology Departments (1973); 3, New Institute of Ophthalmology (1991); 4, Fryer House (1985).

the redeveloped hospital so formed (**Figure 2**). The transformation of Moorfields into an independent NHS Trust in April 1994 heralded the final chapter and was a far cry from those early pioneering steps along the path to specialist ophthalmic practice.

The rising tide of change

A veritable tempest of change has swept through medicine during the past 40 years. Indeed, to paraphrase the NHS historian Geoffrey Rivett, 'more has happened than in all the centuries back to Hippocrates'. Ophthalmology has been no exception, the first waves of real significance beginning to lap at the feet of Moorfields during the late 1950s and early 1960s. The successful bid by Sir Stewart Duke-Elder in 1963 to establish a Professorial Chair in Ophthalmology was destined to unleash a cascade of events that would engulf and overturn the established order and thereafter gradually change the face of ophthalmology throughout the UK.

By all accounts, the creation of the Institute of Ophthalmology in 1948, although of enormous importance to the future of ophthalmology, had, up until the establishment of the Chair of Clinical Ophthalmology, only a marginal influence on the life of the Hospital. The Institute was geographically separate from both branches, and research played only a small part, if any, in daily practice. Except perhaps for Henry Stallard's pioneering advances in surgical technique and treatment of retinoblastoma, some seminal work on juvenile glaucoma by Arthur Lister, and the introduction to the UK of modern retinal reattachment surgery by Lorimer Fison, life for those on the staff at Moorfields continued in the comfortable security afforded by confidence in long-established surgical skills practised by generations of distinguished surgeons before them. This was all about to change.

As has been documented in Volume II of this *History* (pp. 213–214), the appointment of the new Professor was not a straightforward affair, with half promises and divided loyalties (a result of overweening patronage perhaps), leaving a bitter taste, but the end result was the emergence of the most important figure in ophthalmology since Duke-Elder ('the Duke') himself. Sir Stewart was a towering figure on the world stage of medicine and the first to establish ophthalmology as a recognized scientific discipline in its own right. While many others had made huge contributions to the understanding and treatment of eye disease, he alone had brought together the knowledge and expertise of the developing world of ophthalmology and melded it into a cohesive science, firstly in his *Textbook* and then in the 15 volumes of the *System of Ophthalmology*. His outgoing personality, clear vision and incredible energy, coupled with intellectual prowess, acknowledged worldwide, enabled him to bring together leaders in all fields, culminating in the foundation of the Institute of Ophthalmology.

Thus, at the outset of the 1960s, the stage was set for ophthalmology to move into the realms of scientific respectability. There was for the first time a treasure-trove of scientific knowledge, ready to be plundered by the clinical community, in the search for understanding of and new treatments for all kinds of eye diseases. Duke-Elder, as Director of the Institute, although he was by this time no longer on the consultant staff of either branch of Moorfields, realized the benefits and opportunities that would follow in the wake of close collaboration between the Institute and Hospital. The creation of a Chair of Clinical Ophthalmology brought this dream closer to reality, and the appointment of Barrie Russell Jones to the post made its successful realization a certainty.

Possessed of a powerful intellect, Barrie Jones (**Figure 3**, Plate 2) also had drive and great personal charm, allied with proven clinical ability. He was an excellent surgeon. A New Zealander, he had come to England and trained 'on the House' at Moorfields, before moving on to become a Senior Lecturer at the Institute and an honorary member of the consultant staff, before his appointment as Professor of Clinical Ophthalmology in 1963. Whatever the manner of this appointment and the controversy surrounding it, there is no doubt that it was an event that was destined to revolutionize Moorfields and set in motion changes in its culture and practice, which were to have lasting effects on its future.

Barrie Jones arrived in England in 1951, with the intention of getting advanced training at Moorfields before returning to New Zealand to succeed Rowland Wilson as Professor in Dunedin. The unique culture of privilege prevailing in the upper echelons of London's medical world at that time meant that UK graduates applying for training posts at Moorfields were seriously disadvantaged if they had not received an 'approved', usually public school, education. As far as 'colonials' were concerned, however, there was no such discrimination and they were accepted at face value, so that, after obtaining the Diploma of Ophthalmology, Barrie Jones found himself at a considerable advantage and had little difficulty in securing his appointment to 'the House' at City Road. Once there, however, he found that the name Jones was not particularly helpful in distinguishing him from other trainees, especially the Welshmen among them.

This perceived drawback was soon solved for him by serendipity when, being late for a ward-round one day, the consultant, Mr 'Uncle' Robert

Davenport, the most senior and influential member of the consultant staff and Dean of the Institute, asked 'where is Jones?' which met with the response from his chief assistant 'do you mean Barrie Jones, Sir?' thus earning him a sobriquet which would last in perpetuity.

After finishing his residency in 1956, he obtained a part-time post as a senior registrar at the London Hospital, together with appointments as a clinical assistant to Terry Perkins at City Road and as a lecturer at the Institute of Ophthalmology, where he pursued his interests in microbiology and diseases of the anterior segment, happy to leave glaucoma and the rest of ocular pathology to Perkins (already the University Reader in Ophthalmology), and others. His outstanding talents soon attracted the attention of Duke-Elder and of Clifford Seath, the all-powerful Secretary of the Institute, both of whom were impressed, and of Norman Ashton (see Part 3), Head of Pathology and the Institute's rising star, who was less so. Working in Ashton's laboratory, he became aware that Ashton was not only intellectually head and shoulders above almost everyone except for 'the Duke' himself, but also wielded great power, which he guarded closely. This he protected by forbidding anyone working in his department to visit other laboratories without his express permission, a rule that Barrie Jones chose to ignore, much to Ashton's chagrin.

He made it clear that he was not to be thwarted (Ashton allegedly describing him as 'like an oak tree growing up through concrete') and persuaded Duke-Elder of the importance of his intended microbiological studies of the conjunctiva and cornea. 'The Duke', in his capacity as Hospitaller of the Order of St John of Jerusalem, had at his disposal considerable funds donated by the British Petroleum company for the purpose of supporting ophthalmological work overseas, and decided to use these to support Barrie Jones. He was thereby able to set up his own laboratory, independent of Ashton's. From then on, the combination of busy clinical posts and ever increasing research took over his life, his intentions of obtaining a PhD degree and returning to New Zealand soon melting away in the sea of opportunity available to him in London. Two years later the Medical Research Council added their support, providing for the continued independence of his laboratory. The die was cast.

Maintaining a presence at the Institute, with laboratories there in addition to space at the Hospital, Barrie Jones forged links between the two institutions, which have never, before or since, been stronger, his appointment to the University Chair of Clinical Ophthalmology setting the seal on this happy and productive relationship. It is no exaggeration to say that within the space of 10 years he had transformed Moorfields from an institution with a formidable reputation as a hospital of the old school, but with a dwindling influence on the world outside it, to a centre of excellence equipped to compete successfully with any eye unit throughout the world. That is not to say that he did not need and have the support of many of those around him, in particular his contemporaries on the consultant staff. His ability to identify the clinical problems that mattered most, organize and direct the research to solve them, and bridge the gap between academe and practical medicine was, however, unique, while his charm and acknowledged clinical skills, matched with relentless determination, made him a formidable champion of change and progress.

> *Not that his dedicated pursuit of the truth was always appreciated by either his colleagues or his patients: called upon to give a second opinion about a case of ocular melanosis, he took nearly an hour to examine the patient and then wrote a whole page in the patient's notes. A senior colleague then came along, pulled down the eyelids, took one look, said 'they look alright', wrote a single line, and left the room. Upon which the patient was heard to comment 'Now you can tell **he's** an expert'!*

Not only was Barrie Jones gifted in the fundamentals of scientific and clinical skills, but he also possessed the ability to raise funds to support his research, and to encourage others to do likewise. The Professorial Unit was soon able to employ a number of lecturers and senior lecturers, these individuals obtaining grants and awards enabling them to pursue their research and obtain equipment, as well as to travel widely and exchange new ideas with colleagues, both at home and abroad.

While some degree of subspecialization within ophthalmology had been recognized and encouraged previously, old habits died hard. Apart from retinal detachment surgery, which had established itself as a unique case following Jules Gonin's seminal work in the 1920s and 1930s, consultant appointments to the Moorfields staff up until the late 1960s were still made on the basis of general skills allied with (usually) a special interest. Even Lorimer Fison, appointed as retinal surgeon to succeed C Dee Shapland in 1963 (see Part 2), was expected to undertake his share of general work. Indeed it was to be another 30 years before Moorfields would finally abrogate this general principle entirely. Most surgeons of the time, having grown up in the days of voluntarily funded hospitals, were still steeped in the traditions of independent practice and paternalism, guarding their practices fiercely and reluctant to compromise their general knowledge and skills in the interests of super-specialization.

The new culture introduced by Barrie Jones brought about a fundamental change in thinking throughout the Hospital. Incorporation of the Professorial Unit (officially titled the Department of Clinical Ophthalmology), with its own beds, into the hospital building, and the subsequent use of this facility to concentrate on identifying areas of special interest and developing new treatment methods, was a major innovation, while his outstanding abilities as a researcher and teacher attracted a host of bright and ambitious young ophthalmologists. In addition to his other attributes, Barrie Jones proved to have the capacity not only to identify and inspire but also to direct a corps of especially able surgeons into developing subspecialties of their own. As a consequence, new consultant positions were awarded to his protégés, a number of whom were encouraged to compete with one another for such appointments at Moorfields, thereby assuring that the successful candidates not only were of the highest quality, but in addition were loyal not only to the Hospital but also to the Professorial Unit and its Director, several of them remaining members of the academic department as honorary senior lecturers, long after their appointment as consultants.

The sudden and unexpected death in 1968 of Arthur George Leigh, with whom Barrie Jones had forged a close and fruitful relationship in the management of corneal disease, led to the first of a new style of consultant appointment. Rolf Blach was appointed to serve on the staff of Moorfields, without what had previously been customary – a joint appointment at a London undergraduate teaching hospital. Even so, his interests (in diseases of the retina) were not the same as those of his predecessor, his appointment, as the most talented candidate, at that time over-riding any consideration of priorities that the Hospital might have with respect to expertise in a particular subspecialty.

A succession of other important appointments to the consultant staff soon followed, however, covering corneal and external disease, orbital and lacrimal surgery, and strabismus and ocular motility, fields in which Barrie Jones had persuaded his colleagues that there was a special need for greater expertise or wider representation. The new breed of consultants were committed to evidence-based medicine. They had frequently pioneered the most recent advances in their chosen fields, and continued to undertake clinical research and push forward the frontiers of knowledge, even as they undertook their routine duties at the Hospital, sometimes remaining on the Professorial Unit in an honorary academic capacity. In other instances, appointments were made to substantive academic posts, with honorary consultant status granted by the Hospital. As a result of the Professor's influence, they were all committed to the use of the operating microscope, and the Hospital was soon obliged to provide ceiling-mounted microscopes in all the theatres in which microsurgery routinely took place, as well as mobile instruments for more occasional use (**Figure 4**, Plate 3).

As the Professorial Unit grew, both physically and in its sphere of influence, so the Hospital relied increasingly on it to maintain momentum in the pursuit of excellence. At no time in its history has the Institute been more closely allied with the Hospital, in pursuing similar objectives, than it was during the 1970s. This was a situation that may have been made all the more readily achievable by virtue of Francis Cumberlege's joint position as Chairman of both the Hospital's Board of Governors and the Committee of Management of the Institute, although, as we shall see later (see Part 3), this was not a view shared by all concerned.

Sadly, the common ground uniting the two institutions was not to stand the test of time. Developments, both political and personal, were to establish a very different relationship between Hospital and Institute after Barrie Jones retired from the Chair of Clinical Ophthalmology. This notwithstanding, it is still true to say that the interdependent nature of the two institutions is of crucial importance to the viability of both, and their close physical proximity, sharing laboratory space and personnel, is fundamental to the strength of that relationship.

Perhaps most crucial to the progress of ophthalmology and the reputation of Moorfields has been the influence of the Department of Clinical Ophthalmology on the teaching and training of the resident staff and their attitude to research. The development of academic interests and the teaching of highly specialized skills in the treatment of infections, trauma, tumours and other disorders of the anterior segment, ocular adnexae and orbit, during the 1960s and 1970s, soon led to the dissemination of increasingly high standards of ophthalmic care throughout the country.

> *Not that this was always pain-free for Barrie Jones' students. The present author well remembers an occasion when, after waiting for some 45 minutes for the professor to emerge from a cataract operation, he peered into the theatre only to see it shrouded in complete darkness. 'What are they doing?' he whispered to a nurse. 'The Professor is examining the vitreous face' came the somewhat baffling and unexpected reply.*

So great did the demands on Barrie Jones' time become that he took to stopping off, on his journey from home, and sitting in the waiting room at London Bridge Station (he lived in South London), where no-one could reach him (there were no mobile phones at that time), and working on his papers, sometimes for several hours. Furthermore, the extent and breadth of his activities and involvement in all aspects of clinical research inevitably had an impact on his ability to keep a grip on more mundane matters, so that in time his reputation as the archetypal 'absent-minded professor' became legendary. Several good examples of this were recounted to the present author during research for this *History*, one of which is worth recounting here.

*Arriving at Heathrow airport (a much less hectic and impersonal place in those days than it is today), he explained to the check-in staff that he had a serious problem: he had forgotten his ticket. Familiar as they were with this frequent traveller, they were quite unfazed by this news and said: 'Never mind, Professor, just tell us where you are supposed to be going and we will re-issue you with a ticket here and now'. 'That is just my problem,' he replied 'I don't know where I **am** supposed to be going'.*

Training in microsurgical techniques became an essential part of the curriculum for the Residents, especially at the City Road branch, where they spent time in the Professorial Unit during their residency. Similar opportunities were offered to a number of other trainee ophthalmologists, after their residencies at Moorfields or elsewhere, either as lecturers or so-called Visiting Fellows, a concept hitherto unknown, but one that subsequently became the norm at Moorfields and throughout the UK.

Brief reference has already been made to the Retinal Unit and its unique place as the first truly specialized unit at the Hospital, even before the advent of the Clinical Academic Department. The concept of successful surgical repair of retinal detachment, introduced by Jules Gonin in the early part of the 20th Century, reached Moorfields in 1929, the first retinal reattachment operation being performed there by Sir William Lister. He was assisted by C Dee Shapland, subsequently appointed to the consultant staff at University College Hospital and Moorfields, who went on to become the doyen of retinal surgery in the UK. Duke-Elder set up a retinal detachment research laboratory at the Institute in 1954, and it was here that the young Lorimer Fison honed his skills (see Part 2). In 1959 the Hospital agreed to provide Shapland with operating facilities, beds and resources, at the Highgate Annexe, to facilitate what was, at that time, long and complicated surgery, often requiring protracted in-patient care. Now, recently returned from the USA armed with the newly developed head-mounted binocular indirect ophthalmoscope, Fison joined Shapland there and began to transform retinal reattachment surgery into its modern form, thereby generating the first true subspecialty at Moorfields.

Paradoxically perhaps, although the emphasis on academic and advanced microsurgical skills was considerably less (the importance of

interests outside medicine was heavily emphasized) at the High
Holborn branch of the Hospital, many of the ablest and most
influential ophthalmologists of the next generation (including a
majority of the first UK professors and three of the first Presidents of
the Royal College of Ophthalmologists) trained there. Whether this was
as a result of random statistical clustering, of the emphasis on broad
academic interests and varied abilities in the appointments process, or
of allowing trainee ophthalmologists time to stop and think for themselves is hard to judge. Nevertheless, during the 1960s and even into
the early 1970s, the High Holborn branch kept its reputation as the
more relaxed institution while City Road retained its place as the
powerhouse of the Hospital. Meanwhile, High Holborn, undoubtedly
regarded with great affection and loyalty as the embodiment of a
superior life-style, for doctors and patients alike, and hugely supportive
of its alumni, functioned more in the old-fashioned style of a passing
age.

> *Indeed this perceived difference was brought sharply into focus when the
> Residents at High Holborn allegedly reported a series of eye injuries caused
> by champagne corks, while shortly afterwards those at City Road did the
> same for exploding beer bottles.*

Clinical developments in the 1970s

The 1970s was a golden age of discovery. Barrie Jones himself led the
world in the treatment of external ocular disease. Noel Rice and Peter
Wright taught the latest advances in its management. John Wright
became an unchallenged expert in orbital tumours and Peter Fells in
disorders of ocular movements, thyroid eye disease and orbital trauma,
while Peter Watson established a global reputation in the management
of inflammatory conditions involving the sclera and adnexal tissues. In
1969 Alan Bird (see Part 2), fresh from finishing his residency at the
High Holborn branch of the Hospital, returned from a year's
Fellowship at the Bascom Palmer Eye Institute in Miami, to start a
Retinal Diagnostic Service at City Road. This led on to the development of the Medical Retinal Service, which became in the course of
time, the busiest service in the hospital, while Bird was to have an influence on Moorfields' academic reputation second only to that of Barrie
Jones himself.

Inspired by work in the Medical Professorial Unit at the Royal
Postgraduate Medical School at the Hammersmith Hospital, led by
Professor Russell Fraser, Dr Colin Dollery (later Professor Sir Colin)
and Dr Graham Joplin, a joint project was set up with the academic

department at Moorfields, involving Rolf Blach, Hung Cheng, Eva Kohner and later Peter Hamilton, to investigate the nature and management of diabetic eye disease. This led to the establishment of a prospective randomized controlled clinical trial, 'a first' for ophthalmology in this country or abroad. Other clinical trials soon followed, investigating the natural history and results of treatment in age-related macular degeneration, optic neuritis, retinal vein thrombosis, macroaneurysms and many other disorders of the posterior segment.

Nor was the Surgical Retinal Unit at Moorfields slow to take up new challenges, the introduction of closed intraocular microsurgery for vitreoretinal disease in 1971, following the pioneering work of Robert Machemer in the USA, leading to an entirely new approach to surgery of the posterior segment. Prior to this, retinal reattachment surgery had not incorporated microsurgical techniques, the operative method comprising accurate localization of retinal tears with binocular indirect ophthalmoscopy and a surgical approach confined to the outside of the eye. Now, however, with the development of closed vitrectomy via the pars plana and the acquisition of vitrectomy instruments, microsurgery was to become an essential component of modern retinal surgery (**Figure 5**, Plate 3). As luck would have it, plans to relocate the Retinal Unit from the Highgate Annexe, which had no microsurgical facilities, to new premises at City Road (Stallard Ward), where microsurgery could be undertaken, were already well advanced. Closed vitrectomy began at the City Road branch of the Hospital in July 1974, and soon developed into a busy and rapidly expanding service (see Part 2).

While the face of clinical ophthalmology and research was undergoing such a radical makeover at Moorfields and the Institute during the 1960s and early 1970s, little in the way of major change in the conduct of the NHS as a whole impinged on Moorfields. The postgraduate teaching hospitals remained independent of the undergraduate schools and were answerable only to the Department of Health (strictly speaking the Department of Health and Social Security, DHSS) and to the Secretary of State. Moorfields did not have to dance to the tune of a Regional Health Authority, nor to any other body outside the direct chain of command from the Department. Its budget was set and agreed annually with Whitehall mandarins and it was free, within the constraints so imposed, to act much as it liked. Even the Todd Report on Medical Education in 1968, which recommended the alliance of the postgraduate teaching hospitals with undergraduate teaching institutions (in Moorfields' case with Barts Medical College and the London Hospital), was largely ignored by the government and came to nothing.

Reorganization of the NHS

In 1974 all this was set to change. The Health Service Act of 1973 signalled a sea change in the conduct of socialized medicine throughout the country. Long before the advent of what became widely known as 'Thatcherism', and the 'internal market' (the mantra of those who prized free enterprise above all else – often at the expense of the weak and disadvantaged), politicians had had cause to be uneasy about their lack of control over the running of the hospital service. Aside from the undergraduate teaching hospitals and the specialist postgraduate teaching hospitals, the administration of hospital medicine had, since the inception of the NHS, been the responsibility of Regional Health Authorities through their Hospital Management Committees. Effective political control, at a local level, was minimal. In 1974 political control was imposed. The Hospital Management Committees were abolished and replaced by Area Health Authorities (AHAs) and District Health Authorities (DHAs), and the London undergraduate teaching hospitals were incorporated into AHAs (Teaching): AHA(T).

The postgraduate teaching hospitals were, however, allowed to retain their special status (much to the chagrin of the AHAs(T)), with direct control over their budgets and access to the DHSS, as before. Furthermore, they were permitted to maintain their Boards of Governors and keep their endowment funds – factors that would have great significance for Moorfields when, at a much later date, it came to apply for independent status as a NHS Trust. Thus, at a time of momentous change in the structure of the NHS, Moorfields escaped virtually unscathed and was able to continue as before, with direct access to the DHSS and with its vital endowment funds intact.

Even though in Moorfields' case much was undoubtedly due to the political nous and influence exerted by the Chairman of the Board of Governors, Francis Cumberlege (**Figure 6**), aided and abetted by statistics supplied to him by the House Governor and Treasurer, it is difficult to fully understand the rationale behind this surprising reprieve, except to surmise that Whitehall had 'shot its bolt' by the time it became aware of the Special Health Authorities (SHAs) and could not face another round of negotiations with (and possible recriminations from) the medical establishment.

Indeed, some credence can be offered in support of this view by the story attributed to Francis Cumberlege, and related to him by a friend in high places, that a senior civil servant in the DHSS, when asked what was to

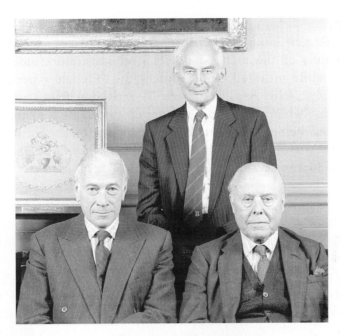

Figure 6 In 1992, soon after his retirement, Francis Cumberlege organized a lunch for his predecessor and successor as Chairman of the Board of Governors. Pictured here are the three Chairmen, spanning the years from 1956 to 1994, when the Hospital became a NHS Trust. *From left to right:* Mr Hugh Peppiatt (1991–1994), Mr Francis Cumberlege (1968–1991) and Mr Christopher Malim (1956–1968). In April 1994 the Board of Governors was disbanded and its place taken by a Board of Directors (Hugh Peppiatt continuing as its Chairman until 1997).

become of the specialist postgraduate teaching hospitals in the reorganized NHS, replied that he 'didn't know what they were, and even if he did, he wouldn't know what to do with them'.

It is sometimes difficult to identify for certain the architects of fundamental change. Certainly, in Moorfields' case, the appointment of Cumberlege as Chairman of the Board of Governors in 1968 was an event of seminal importance, especially as he was already Chairman of the London Hospital Board and thereby later to become the Chairman of the City and East London AHA(T) when the NHS Act came into force in April 1974. His parallel Chairmanship of the Moorfields Board during this entire period of change, through to 1990, brought wisdom and experience gained at the highest level, combined with a sensitivity and sense of balance, which were to prove invaluable. His contribution was enhanced by other Board members, including Lawrence Green, a formidable City financier, and Reg Fryer, a London councillor and committed socialist, as well as by senior members of the consultant staff, notably Desmond Greaves, Barrie Jones and Lorimer Fison.

Perhaps the defining moment of this period, however, was the arrival in 1976 of a new House Governor, a man with few of the reservations or inhibitions of the archetypal NHS administrator (indeed, some might say quite unsuited, temperamentally, to a senior post in NHS management). John Atwill (**Figure** 7) arrived with a career in the British army behind him and a reputation for plain speaking, forward thinking and being a fearless champion of the truth. He was not to disappoint. After the sure and steady hand of Arthur Gray and the short and unproductive tenure of GDE Wooding-Jones, John Atwill had an

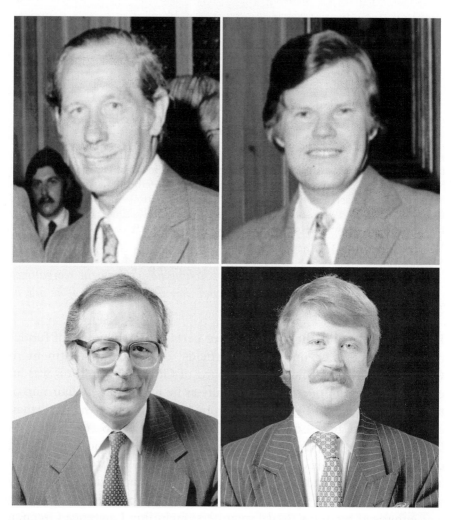

Figure 7 The four House Governors (now officially titled Chief Executives) of Moorfields Eye Hospital, spanning the years 1964 to the present day: (*top left*) Arthur Gray (1964–1974); (*top right*) GDE Wooding-Jones (1974–1976); (*bottom left*) John Atwill (1976 to 1993); (*bottom right*) Ian Balmer (1993 to the present).

empty sheet before him. His previous post at the London Hospital had convinced both him and Francis Cumberlege that they could work happily together, and this indeed proved to be the case.

While several of its fellow SHAs breathed a sigh of relief at emerging unscathed from the consequences of the 1973 Act, and thereafter continued regardless on their way as before, Moorfields was fortunate to have at its heart a core of individuals with vision and foresight who, with two such percipient leaders, were able to see how stormy might be the seas ahead if Moorfields did not take steps to alter course and proceed with care. Although the SHAs had escaped radical modifications to their operations during the 1974 reorganization, it had not escaped the notice of the Chairman, the new House Governor and their Board that Moorfields needed to take a long hard look into the future if turbulence was to be avoided.

In 1975 there had been a near disaster, when extreme Left wing members of the National Union of Public Employees (NUPE, now Unison) chose to target the Hospital to demonstrate their view (supported by the then Secretary of State, Barbara Castle) that pay-beds should not be allowed in NHS hospitals. The end result of this confrontation was a victory, of sorts, for both sides – Francis Cumberlege and Reg Fryer managed to convince the Board and Medical Committee of the wisdom of keeping the Hospital running, in spite of this threat to freedom of action, whilst the consultants, led by Lorimer Fison and Redmond Smith, took their private patients away from Moorfields and undertook their surgery elsewhere.

In this context it is interesting to observe the great difference in culture that prevailed, so short a time ago, compared with today's, as illustrated by this seemingly trivial upheaval in the Hospital's life.

Redmond Smith (see Part 2) was the Chairman of the Medical Committee at the time and as such became, however unwillingly, the mouthpiece for the consultant body's anger and frustration at the threat that the action of left-wing activists posed to their professional freedom. Lorimer Fison and other surgeons at the City Road branch of the Hospital with flourishing private practices were, understandably, determined to thwart the trade union action by taking their private patients and operating on them elsewhere. They therefore proposed setting up an association of Moorfields surgeons, independent of the Hospital, resourced by its membership to provide operating equipment, and thereby able to provide facilities for its members and their patients, at any private hospital willing to host a private eye unit. Should future industrial unrest threaten to disrupt the operation of this unit, the association could (theoretically) up sticks and move, with all its equipment, elsewhere. There was widespread support for this idea amongst the surgeons at City Road, and operating microscopes, slit-lamps and a full range of surgical instruments were purchased. Thus was the Moorfields Surgeons Association (MSA) formed.

It should not be assumed, however, that there was unanimity among the consultants. In particular, those at the High Holborn branch were far from convinced that a breakaway organization was in their best interests and were reluctant to join the Association (inevitably fuelling the antipathy that already existed between medical staff at the two branches). Furthermore, Redmond Smith and Lorimer Fison were ill-advised enough to announce their intentions to the Press. A surgeon from outside the group, with malice aforethought, immediately informed the General Medical Council, who threatened to take action against them, on the grounds that they were, by their actions, guilty of advertising. This was something that today would be considered perfectly reasonable behaviour and against which action by the GMC would be unthinkable, but which at that time was anathema to the profession. In the event, the GMC thought better of pursuing the matter and the MSA was formed and became a highly successful venture (see Part 4).

Fate also lent a friendly hand, when it transpired that a general practitioner, Dr Arthur Levin, had just founded a private hospital in St John's Wood and was looking for 'business'. The prospect of a ready-made eye unit, staffed by many of the country's most eminent ophthalmologists, who were even happy to supply their own equipment, was a gift-horse whose mouth needed no inspection. So began a long association between the Wellington Hospital and the Moorfields surgeons, lasting some 20 years, while another hospital to bid successfully for the MSA's custom was the Clementine Churchill. (Ironically, therefore, left-wing dogma in the end spawned not just one but two flourishing private eye units.)

Within three weeks of his arrival, John Atwill was assailed by officers from MI5, who arrived to tell him that Moorfields was playing host to two cells of an International Socialist organization and demanded to know what he was going to do about it. Fortunately for him (even more so for Moorfields), his experience in the armed forces and in NHS administration enabled him, with the help of Reg Fryer and Sally Sherman, both influential socialists and members of the Board of Governors, to defuse the situation. Furthermore, it gave him the opportunity to introduce modern disciplinary practices and employment procedures that were to stand the Hospital in good stead for the future.

By the second half of the 1970s, it had become abundantly clear that it was time for Moorfields to move on. Although the government of the day had accepted, in 1974, that the specialist postgraduate teaching hospitals should retain their privileged position vis-à-vis political control and central funding, there was little reason to suppose that this would go on for ever. Moorfields had always prided itself on its unique position as a provider of tertiary care services to eye units throughout the UK and beyond (tertiary care being defined as that provided to patients who were referred by one specialist to another). Such care, relying as it did on expensive facilities such as prolonged hospitalization, sophisticated investigations, and specialist care and nursing, placed a great strain on budgetary resources. It was obvious to Atwill that this would in the future need to be subsidized by the provision of cheaper and more plentiful primary and secondary care.

Furthermore, it was apparent, as the 1970s drew to a close, that a specialist eye hospital, duplicating all of its facilities on two sites, with more than 300 beds and two separate sets of 'state-of-the-art' operating theatres, situated within a stone's throw of two large teaching hospitals with their own eye units (Barts and the London), would be a prime target for a Secretary of State looking to curry favour with the Chancellor of the Exchequer by introducing efficiency savings. The Todd Report had already indicated the desirability of all the London postgraduate teaching hospitals being allied with undergraduate teaching hospitals and their schools. With the likelihood of a Conservative government led by Margaret Thatcher, the threat to rationalize the situation by subsuming Moorfields and the Institute into Barts Medical College and the London Hospital remained as real as ever. When the Conservatives finally came to power in 1979, it was clear that battle would be joined with any institution that could not clearly demonstrate value for money.

Between the years 1975 and 1977, discussions within the Hospital and between Hospital and Institute had led to the conclusion that all of the clinical and research activities of the two should be concentrated on the 'island site', bounded by City Road, Peerless Street Bath Street and Cayton Street (see **Figure 2**, p. 4). As early as 1972, the Pathology and Dean's Departments of the Institute had moved to new premises on a portion of this land, bordering the western end of the City Road branch, but these were far too small to accommodate the bulk of the Institute's activities. The new scheme envisaged the future closure of both the High Holborn branch of the Hospital and the Institute building in Judd Street, with expansion and redevelopment of City Road and the provision of new buildings for the Institute adjacent to the redeveloped hospital there.

Thus, when Atwill arrived to take up his post as House Governor in October 1976, the stage was already set for radical alterations to both the activities and the fabric of the Hospital. Not only was there no doubt in Atwill's mind that a change in direction was needed but in addition the Board of Governors, with the support of the consultant body, endorsed the proposed changes. In this respect there were two especially favourable factors. First, both Cumberlege and Atwill not only shared a common ideal but also understood the importance of gaining the confidence and support of the medical staff, before initiating any changes. Secondly, Desmond Greaves was appointed to the Chair of the Medical Committee: he was an outstanding chairman, who worked tirelessly to ensure that the consultants were kept informed and were encouraged to take an active role in the future development of the Hospital. Two obstacles remained, however: first the determined opposition of the High Holborn consultants to the amalgamation of the two branches of the Hospital, and secondly, the serious ill-health of the hospital architect.

At first glance, it is difficult to account for the antagonism between the High Holborn and City Road consultants. Looking more closely, however, it is apparent that until the emergence of Barrie Jones, Lorimer Fison and the new generation of consultants and their influence at City Road, High Holborn, although much smaller, was the stronger and more cohesive unit of the two. At City Road, major figures, in particular Harold Ridley and Henry Stallard, were at daggers drawn. In contrast, at Holborn, not only were the surgeons (**Figure 8**) friendly with one another, but several of them were also amongst the most prestigious and respected figures in ophthalmology of the day. Frederick Ridley was the doyen of therapeutic contact lenses and Keith Lyle that of strabismus and neuro-ophthalmology, Stephen Miller had distinguished himself in glaucoma and James Hudson in retinal detachment surgery, while Patrick Trevor-Roper wielded enormous influence. Several of them commanded large private practices in the capital with enormous social and professional kudos, while Miller soon became Surgeon Oculist to the Queen and received a knighthood. It was small wonder then that the City Road surgeons felt disadvantaged and were in the mood to exert their might. And little wonder either that the High Holborn men were in no mood to kowtow.

Perhaps mistakenly, the Board had previously appointed (and entered into a binding contract with) an official hospital architect, an individual with excellent credentials but whose health was now steadily deteriorating due to a progressive (and ultimately fatal) disease. Because the Hospital was locked into a contract with this one individual, it was not possible to seek other architectural advice, even in the event that, as was now the case, he was incapacitated. As a result of

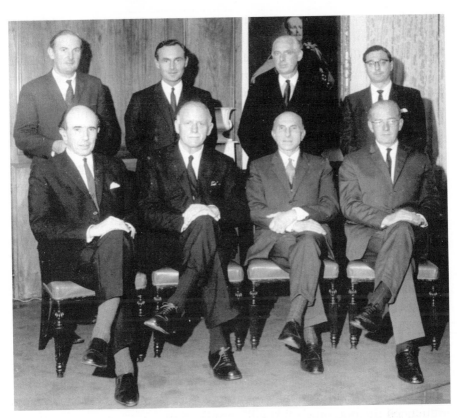

Figure 8 The High Holborn consultant surgeons (probably taken on the occasion of Frederick Ridley's retirement, in 1968). *Seated, left to right:* Mr James Hudson, Mr Frederick Ridley, Mr Keith Lyle and Mr (later Sir) Stephen Miller. *Standing, left to right:* Mr Patrick Trevor-Roper, Mr Ian Duguid, Mr Kenneth Wybar and Mr Montague Ruben.

these two factors, commencement of work on the massive project of amalgamating the two branches of the Hospital was considerably delayed, the rebuilding and transfer having to wait until after the retirement of the most senior consultant surgeons at the High Holborn branch and the sad demise of the architect.

The wisdom of appointing John Atwill to the post of House Governor soon became apparent. His previous career had, for a senior NHS manager, been somewhat unorthodox. The only son of an army officer, he left school at 16, after a contretemps with his father (and 'the establishment' in general), and travelled alone around Europe, funding himself by doing any unskilled jobs he could find, before finally deciding to join the Army himself. This he did, by enlisting in the ranks and serving for a time as a private soldier (and enduring the privations and indignities of that position), before attending the Royal Military Academy, Sandhurst to train as an officer. He was subsequently commissioned in the Royal Army Service Corps (RASC), where he learnt the skills of management, organization and supply, but most importantly how to manage people. Never one to tolerate bureaucracy and dogma for a prolonged period, he left the army and entered NHS management, becoming Hospital Secretary at St Thomas' Hospital and subsequently Operations Manager at the London (now Royal London) Hospital. (In between, in order to finance his belated professional studies, he had done a number of jobs, acquiring, amongst other things, his Heavy Goods Vehicle driving licence.) Here then was a man with a wider than usual experience of life and a broader than average view of the world, possessed of great conviction and the determination to undertake any worthwhile project and see it through.

Francis Cumberlege, the Chairman of the Board, was also possessed of exceptional qualities: an able politician, clear thinker and, above all, a good listener, who would spend little time in his office but a great part of it wandering around the Hospital talking to patients and staff alike. As Chairman of the City and Hackney Health Authority, he had had the opportunity to observe Atwill's abilities at first hand and also to take advice from his associates at the London Hospital, in particular the Chairman of that hospital's Board, a factor that is likely to have influenced the outcome of Atwill's application.

Whatever the case, Moorfields was fortunate to acquire a chief executive with the ability to think laterally, as well as the capacity to see the way forward with clarity and to translate theory into practice. From the day of Atwill's appointment, he and Francis Cumberlege worked happily together, with the unqualified support of the Board of Governors and Medical Committee, towards successful redevelopment of the Hospital on the island site and its regeneration as a modern, community-orientated organization.

Redevelopment of the Hospital

The campaign to reshape Moorfields was run along military lines. This was perhaps unsurprising, since most of the leading lights involved in its pursuit had served in the Armed Forces, some with distinction in the heat of battle: Francis Cumberlege in the Royal Corps of Signals (he had been one of a distinguished group of Signals officers in very advanced forward observation posts in the Second World War, with direct links to Army Headquarters and to Field Marshall Montgomery's Staff), Lawrence Green (Chairman of the Finance Committee) in the Royal Marines and John Atwill in the RASC, while

Reg Fryer, a key member of the Board, was one of the few beach-masters to have survived the 1944 D-Day landings. The Board decided to back Atwill in his recommendation to appoint a firm of consulting engineers to undertake a feasibility study, a move that took the DHSS by surprise and with which they were at odds. As the DHSS knew nothing of feasibility studies and refused to pay for such a thing, the Board of Governors did so out of endowment funds and were subsequently hauled over the coals for doing so. Nevertheless, the study was crucial in demonstrating beyond any reasonable doubt that amalgamation was practical, both structurally and operationally, if the DHSS would agree to the financial implications.

It was finally agreed that the redevelopment of the Hospital at City Road would be financed by the DHSS, within a budgetary framework based on the market value of the High Holborn site when the rebuilding was finished, and a deal was finally struck when the Hospital agreed to work within a £17m capital figure. The Board of Governors also promised to reduce the future annual running costs of the redeveloped hospital by £360 000 (a very significant saving in the context of monetary values at that time).

The redevelopment was undertaken in a series of stages, each of which had to be agreed with the DHSS before the go-ahead could be given to commence work. A Planning Committee was formed, with a number of working parties under its jurisdiction, each with a consultant ophthalmologist member, to address different aspects of the project. The introduction in 1981 of annual spending reviews made this process extremely difficult, because of the delay in agreeing finance for each stage of the development before it was given the go-ahead, and it was therefore necessary for the projected costs to be underwritten from endowment funds in order to keep the project running to schedule. In this respect, it was particularly valuable to have at the head of the Planning Committee the Chairman of the Finance Committee and later of the Special Trustees, Lawrence Green, investment manager of one of the largest pension funds in the City of London and an exceptionally able financier.

The Planning Committee was supported by a dedicated team of planning officers, and was also fortunate to have as its mentor an outstandingly imaginative and able successor to the previous architect, in Mr Harry Locke Smith, a partner in Watkins Gray International. He took the project to his heart and even lived in the Hospital for a period of three whole weeks in order to see for himself exactly how it functioned. His sudden and tragically early death from cancer in August 1983 was felt deeply by everyone concerned, but fortunately for

Moorfields he had by then already completed the task of redesigning it. Some small indication of the debt that the Hospital owed to him can be gauged by the fact that his widow and children were invited to attend a ceremony held in his memory in October 1985, when a plaque was unveiled in the hospital foyer, to commemorate his services (**Figures 9 and 10**, Plate 4).

The redevelopment programme went ahead relentlessly and reasonably smoothly, throughout the 1980s, in spite of profound changes in the sociopolitical climate. In 1982, three years after the Conservative Party was returned to power, a further reorganization of the NHS took place. As a result of this, the smaller and weaker of the specialist postgraduate teaching hospitals bowed to the inevitable and were subsumed into undergraduate teaching hospitals, while the six larger ones, including Moorfields, were allowed to retain their special status, but were now designated Special Health Authorities.

These SHAs continued to have direct access to the DHSS and were permitted to keep their endowment funds, but were required to appoint trustees, approved by the Secretary of State, to administer them. The Chairman of the Finance Committee, Lawrence Green, took over as Chairman of the Special Trustees, with Francis Cumberlege as his deputy and Reg Fryer, Desmond Greaves and David Hyman (a stockbroker) as members (see Part 4). The Governing Body was now required to have a broader representation, including a member drawn from a Community Health Council, a lay body representing the interests of the public. The statutory Annual Review required by the DHSS demanded an account of the way in which the previous year's financial allocation had been spent, as well as a clearly presented plan for the year ahead. As mentioned previously, this would have made implementation of complex planning arrangements for the redevelopment of the Hospital difficult, had it not been for the support of the Special Trustees, who stepped in to bridge the gap between application to the DHSS for approval of spending plans and the actual provision of funds.

Although the 1982 reorganization's direct effect on Moorfields was small, its hidden agenda was plain – increased control from above, leading to wider involvement of outside bodies in patient care, and greater accountability to the State. Several things, seemingly trivial at the time, but which were to have a profound influence on events in the future, happened right away. North East Thames Regional Health Authority identified a clear role for Moorfields in its Strategic Plan, and with the closure of the Bethnal Green Hospital in 1983, asked the Hospital to accommodate its ophthalmic in-patients. At about this time too, the London Borough of Newham became concerned at the quality of service its ophthalmic patients were getting from the London Hospital's eye department. Rather than be seen to be 'poaching' patients from other hospitals and Health Authorities, by taking their patients to Moorfields, the Hospital took the step of offering to provide a service for the beleaguered units concerned, within their own environs. Thus, as early as the beginning of the 1980s, Moorfields took its first tentative steps towards an outreach programme.

The new model

Looking back at this period in its history with the benefit of hindsight, one is struck by the uncanny convergence of events and inspiration that steered the Hospital through stormy seas and enabled it to negotiate the often unpredictable currents influencing the re-emergent Health Service. Two critical decisions made earlier by the Board were to alter entirely the way in which the Hospital would function in the brave new world of involvement and accountability: first, to amalgamate the two branches of the Hospital and expand and develop the central hub on one site, and secondly, to look outwards, towards involvement in the provision of high-quality eye care within the London Boroughs themselves. Hand in hand with these aims, and crucial to their successful achievement, was the new emphasis on provision of 'primary care', backed up by top-quality specialist services.

It was foreseen that in the long term it would not be sufficient just to run large general ophthalmic clinics staffed by general ophthalmologists, specialist clinics being there just to provide expertise in the most complicated cases. Henceforth, general ophthalmology would need to be provided at the level of primary care. Primary-care clinics had to be developed, wherein highly trained ophthalmologists (and later nurse-practitioners) could act as gatekeepers to the specialist clinics and screen-out sight-threatening eye disorders from conditions of a more trivial nature. A total revision and redirection of the existing workforce was required, in order to convert it from an army of generalists to a team of specialists. This was for some a harrowing, if necessary, transformation. Many of the long-established members of the medical staff had been trained and brought up in the broad traditions of the previous system, with knowledge and skills based on a wide understanding of ocular pathology and treatment, but without specialist, in-depth expertise in any particular area. Their general knowledge alone, however comprehensive and wide-ranging, was not sufficient to satisfy the new requirements.

Unsurprisingly, these momentous changes took time to evolve. At the beginning of the 1980s, the redevelopment project was barely under way, while the medical staffing of the Hospital was still far from adequate to meet future demands. Provision of highly specialized services on a grand scale required, first of all, expansion of the medical workforce, by the appointment of specially trained experts in all fields at consultant level. Fortunately, the ground for this had already been laid by Barrie Jones in the Professorial Unit and Lorimer Fison in the Retinal Unit, and there was a cohort of up and coming ophthalmologists ready to accept the challenge. In the late 1970s and early 1980s, therefore, retiring consultant general ophthalmologists began to be replaced by strabismologists, oculoplastic surgeons, glaucoma experts, and so forth throughout all the subspecialties of ophthalmic practice.

The Clinical Academic Department

Although the 1980s were not quite such a hotbed of therapeutic advance as the 1970s, there was nevertheless a great deal of change in other aspects of medical practice. A defining event was the abrupt decline in Barrie Jones's health. In 1979 he was aware that all was far from well, and sought medical advice. His blood pressure was found to be very high – so much so that it was recommended that he take immediate leave for at least three months. This he did and made a remarkable and full recovery, returning in 1980 to his post as Clinical Professor. As not infrequently happens in life, however, he found, somewhat to his surprise (and possibly dismay), that in his absence things had moved on. Douglas Coster, a brilliant young ophthalmologist from Australia, was firmly and competently forging ahead with external disease, Richard Collin had oculoplastics by the throat, and the academic department appeared to be running smoothly without him. His previously unchallenged position as the leader of research and innovative microsurgery was now open to question – and he was the first to question it. After giving it due consideration, he decided to do what few other men would have had the courage or vision to do, namely resign from the Chair of Clinical Ophthalmology and achieve his life's ambition, the founding of a Department of Preventive Ophthalmology.

Barrie Jones's reputation, standing and connections were more than sufficient to enable him to raise the necessary funds and persuade the Hospital and Institute to provide him with backing and space, and in 1981 the new department, the International Centre for Eye Health (located in the Cayton Street building), was opened by Her Royal Highness Princess Alexandra, with Professor Barrie Jones relocating there as its Head (see Part 3). This left the Chair of Clinical Ophthalmology vacant. Coster, for personal reasons, chose to return to Adelaide as Professor there and, in spite of several overtures to other suitable candidates from the UK and abroad, it proved impossible to fill the post.

It would be inappropriate to discuss here the whys and wherefores of this unsatisfactory situation, but suffice it to say that the Chair remained vacant for a period of three years, before Barrie Jay was finally prevailed upon to move from his position as Dean to take it over. The Clinical Academic Department was henceforward to undergo radical change, not only in its structure and function, but also in its influence on the activities of the Hospital (see Part 3). Never again was its position vis-à-vis Moorfields to be so directly powerful, although many of those whose careers had been nurtured in its environment were to provide the thrust and guidance which would guarantee the Hospital's future development.

Clinical developments in the 1980s

The foundations laid by Barrie Jones during the 1960s and 1970s stood the test of time: innovation and progress in surgery of the anterior segment, orbit and adnexal tissues continued throughout the 1980s, led by Noel Rice, Peter Watson, Arthur Steele, John Wright and Richard Collin, while the torch for external disease and infections was carried at Moorfields by Peter Wright (and later by John Dart). New and better treatments of viral, fungal and other infections of the cornea, and for dry eyes, graft rejection and other disorders of the anterior segment, were matched by advances in orbital surgery and oculoplastics, while innovations in cataract and refractive surgery brought methods and materials that were helpful to surgeons operating on the cornea and tissues of the external eye.

In cataract surgery, the 1980s saw the development of intraocular lens implantation at Moorfields – from an experimental method undergoing clinical trials under the auspices of Arthur Steele in the late 1970s, to widely and rapidly increasing acceptance throughout the Hospital. Early lens implants, designed by Binkhorst and others in Europe to complement intracapsular cataract extraction, soon gave way to capsular-supported varieties, and extracapsular extraction came back into fashion. Steele, a superb surgeon and an outstanding teacher, worked hard, as did John Wright, to overcome the prejudice against intraocular lens implantation prevailing amongst some of the more senior consultant staff (born of a deep-seated reluctance to promulgate the use of intraocular lens implants after the early foray into the field, by Harold Ridley in the 1950s). Within a few years, the removal of all but the most complicated of cataracts was being undertaken by this method – a forward step of great importance, since Moorfields had hitherto lagged dangerously behind in this important field. Further-more, the change to extracapsular surgery and the use of viscoelastic materials so simplified the procedure and encouraged early recovery that length of stay in the Hospital fell rapidly, from seven days at the beginning of the decade to two by its end.

The range of drugs for treating chronic simple glaucoma expanded, laser trabeculoplasty came in, and surgery using drainage tubes (first devised by Molteno) and silicone plates was introduced for the treat-ment of refractory cases of advanced chronic disease. With the retire-ment of Sir Stephen Miller from High Holborn and, shortly thereafter, that of Redmond Smith from City Road, Roger Hitchings' appointment to the Moorfields consultant staff in 1980 and the publication of the article reporting his Early Treatment Trial further strengthened the glau-coma services. Hitchings brought new scientific expertise, allied with surgical skills and experience in the development and use of silicone implants and tubes, heralding the advent of many new drugs and surgical developments for the management of intractable glaucoma. These were gradually to transform this difficult and previously often unrewarding discipline.

Both the surgical and medical retinal services expanded hugely during the 1980s, with the widespread acceptance of new treatments. In 1977 the increasing importance of closed vitrectomy, bringing with it the facility for successfully treating a wide variety of hitherto untreat-able disorders of the posterior segment of the eye, together with the introduction of ultrasonic diagnostic methods, led to the appointment of David McLeod. Later, with the retirement of James Hudson from the High Holborn branch and of Lorimer Fison from City Road, no less than three further consultant vitreoretinal surgeons were appointed, effectively doubling the complement of retinal surgeons at the Hospital. Because all the new appointees undertook little else but vitreoretinal surgery, the volume of work in this rapidly advancing field increased exponentially throughout the decade. More and more, vitrectomy methods were combined with the use of intraocular air, gases and silicone oil in the treatment of complicated retinal detach-ments, as well as in previously untreatable conditions such as advanced diabetic eye disease. Many cases formerly beyond the scope of treat-ment were now amenable to surgical intervention, while only a very few were irredeemable.

Reference has already been made to the huge expansion of the medical retinal service, consequent upon the new-found ability to diag-nose and treat diabetic retinopathy, other vascular occlusive diseases of the retina, age-related degenerations and assorted retinal pathology of all kinds, using fluorescein fundus photography and laser photo-coagulation. A steady increase in the number of referrals and of Alan Bird's worldwide reputation (now with a personal Professorial Chair) fuelled the expansion of the medical retinal department, and attracted ever-increasing numbers of visiting ophthalmologists from throughout the UK and abroad. Indeed, by the end of this decade, the Retinal Diagnostic Department was bursting at the seams, in its makeshift premises on the second floor, and more than justified the provision of a brand new clinical space, on the newly developed lower ground floor, when this was finally opened.

Zdenek Gregor, appointed a consultant in 1982 shared interests, as did Rolf Blach, in both medical and surgical aspects of retinal disease. In the same year John Hungerford took over the Ocular Oncology Service jointly operated by Moorfields and St Bartholomew's Hospital, originally the brainchild of Henry Stallard, undertaking the treatment of children with retinoblastoma and adults with intraocular tumours. The appointment of Susan Lightman towards the end of the decade signalled a new era in the management of disorders of the uveal tract, bringing hope to children with Still's disease and adults with Behçet's disease, while her knowledge of immunological disease was an invaluable asset to the Hospital in dealing with the upsurge of HIV-related eye disorders.

Richard Collin's 1983 appointment as the first consultant oculoplastic surgeon at Moorfields heralded a new era in the treatment of orbital and adnexal disease. Like so many other innovations, his appointment followed a carefully planned course, devised some years earlier by Barrie Jones, who, finding himself without his previous candidate for the post (Arthur Steele, who was being groomed to do oculoplastics, was required to switch to anterior segment surgery on the sudden and unanticipated retirement of Derek Ainslie in 1975), sent Collin off to do a Fellowship in the USA instead. Collin had already served a lengthy apprenticeship, including time with Roger Beare and Jack Mustardé in the UK and Crowell Beard in the USA, before returning to the Professorial Unit at Moorfields. His knowledge of the anatomy of the lids and adnexae was unparalleled, and he was soon to write a best-selling book on oculoplastic surgery, as well as transforming its practice at the Hospital. It was not long before the oculoplastic service became too busy for one person, and further surgeons were appointed.

Orbital surgery remained the province of John Wright alone during the 1980s, his reputation drawing a steady stream of Fellows from all over the globe. The collaboration between him and the radiologists (especially Glyn Lloyd), as well as the neurologists and pathologists, with weekly clinical meetings, was highly successful. Meanwhile, Peter Fells ran the Thyroid Clinic in close association with his medical colleague, Nick Lawton, and the otolaryngologist to the Hospital, Brian Pickard, with both of whom he established a happy and unique working relationship.

Fells also remained senior surgeon in strabismus and paediatrics at City Road, but was joined in 1983 by John Lee, who was initially appointed, on the retirement of Kenneth Wybar, to the High Holborn branch of the Hospital. Lee returned from a Fellowship in the USA, bringing with him special knowledge and expertise that he had acquired there in the use of botulinum toxin. He started the 'Botox' clinic and promoted the development of botulinum toxin to treat strabismus and for essential blepharospasm, as well as the use of adjustable sutures in adult squints. Both he and Fells reached the highest levels of achievement in the subspecialty, ensuring that Moorfields remained throughout the decade the most prestigious centre for tertiary referrals.

Meanwhile, in the field of ophthalmic neurology, Christopher Earl, who had served as neurologist to the High Holborn branch for 20 years, remained a towering figure, while at City Road Ralph Ross-Russell and Ian McDonald were unchallenged in their fields. McDonald was soon to be accorded the Chair at the Institute of Neurology and pursued his pioneering work on multiple sclerosis, while Ross-Russell became an acknowledged world authority on retinal vascular occlusive disease.

Redevelopment and the growth of medical management

Meanwhile, the Planning Committee, chaired by Lawrence Green, with Francis Cumberlege as his deputy, spawned the development of several outstanding medical managers, who learned the tools of their trade in the subcommittees and working parties generated by its wide remit. Notable among these management tyros were Arthur Steele and John Wright, who respectively supervised the reorganization of the in-patient and out-patient services, while the appointment to the consultant staff, and subsequently to the post of Chairman of the Out-Patient Working Party, of Bob Cooling saw the emergence of a future leader. The Medical Committee, ably chaired by Desmond Greaves, kept the medical staff informed, while the House Committees of the two branches of the Hospital did the same for the non-medical staff and were well served by Reg Fryer, Jean Smith and others.

Nor were our political masters inactive during this period. It had long been Margaret Thatcher's aim to introduce properly structured management into the NHS. In 1983 she asked Roy Griffiths, Chief General Manager of Sainsbury's supermarkets, to conduct an enquiry into management practices in the NHS. His report the following year indicated (to no-one's surprise) that these were unsatisfactory, few members of the workforce having any clear idea who, if anyone, was ultimately responsible for what. Griffiths could see no reason why running the Health Service should be any different from running a supermarket, where all members of the staff were accountable to more senior members, in a vertical line of management. This was in stark contrast to the existing NHS model, in which management, if any, consisted of teams operating in a horizontal format. Put in its simplest terms, the Griffiths Report recommended that administration should give way to management.

The report carried in its wake a huge expansion in the management tier throughout the service, but sadly led to little, if any, improvement in efficiency. Its failure to do so stemmed from the fundamentally flawed assumption that the NHS, a non-profit organization, where cost-cutting efficiencies tend to lead to more work without commensurate financial rewards, was in some way comparable to a successful business operation, based on market forces and profit margins. The new managers, with few exceptions, were not always of the very highest calibre, NHS staff with little aptitude or training often being redeployed as managers, while posts in the NHS attracted less than the going rate of pay for the same job in the private sector. Any savings they achieved were not seen to benefit directly either staff or patients, while the strain their employment placed on already tight budgets was enormous, provoking resentment amongst both. Nevertheless, the new culture of line management and greater accountability was not entirely without benefit, some doctors, nurses and paramedical staff with potential management skills being attracted into this aspect of the Health Service, most notable amongst them, so far as Moorfields was concerned, Bob Cooling, later to become its first Medical Director. Furthermore, the creation of a better management infrastructure paid dividends that were not always obvious, sometimes being obscured by unrelated pressures and economies.

In reality, John Atwill and his team had pre-empted Griffiths with some far-sighted appointments to management posts from within the existing workforce. In any event, Atwill was firmly opposed to the new style of management imposed by the Griffiths Report's recommendations, believing that if changes were to be implemented successfully, there should be participation in the decision-making process at all levels. Furthermore, as early as 1982, with the retirement of Marion

Tickner (a matron of the old school), the Board had signalled the urgent need for change, by appointing (against intense opposition from the then nursing hierarchy), a non-ophthalmic-trained nurse, Roslyn Emblin, to the post of Matron (now titled Chief Nurse). Miss Emblin had an outstanding record and curriculum vitae, with management experience to match. She was subsequently to demonstrate the wisdom of the appointment by going on to introduce changes to nursing practices throughout the Hospital, which were to prove of fundamental importance to its survival and progress in the brave new world of the modern NHS (see Part 2).

Primary-care strategy

It is difficult today to envisage a world without the concept of primary care, and yet before the 1980s it was not a term with which most of us, brought up in the old-style NHS as we had been, were really familiar. So used were we to the notion that Moorfields was a centre of excellence, with an over-riding commitment to tertiary care beyond all else, that when in the mid-1980s primary care began to assume fundamental importance in strategic planning, few of us stopped to think about this new buzz-word and what it meant. Indeed, it seemed to be a rather simplistic piece of jingoism. Notwithstanding the scepticism felt by many at the time, there is no doubt, looking back, that the vision of Atwill and the Board and their drive, foresight and determination, together with the commitment of Desmond Greaves, Noel Rice, John Wright, Arthur Steele, Bob Cooling and other members of the Medical Committee, transformed the Hospital's outlook. From then on, it changed from a comfortably elitist institution into a modern, forward-looking organization, able to reach out and provide ophthalmic services of the highest quality to the community as a whole. Furthermore, their commitment to a strategy devised and drafted by a group of the younger consultants whose future careers depended on it was truly enlightened.

It is difficult to put a finger on the precise circumstances in which the new philosophy of Moorfields as a centre of primary care, providing a 'bread and butter' service with highly specialized expertise in support, and of its inclusion in the strategic plan for the Hospital, came about. Nevertheless, it would seem that the broad concept was John Atwill's, long before it became a reality. Probably more fundamental to its inception, however, were the informal discussions that took place between Bob Cooling and David McLeod (both at that time consultant members of the Vitreoretinal Surgical Unit), following Atwill's demand in 1985–86 for a Clinical Strategy Document, to point the way forward for the medical services. Certainly Cooling is convinced that he drew inspiration for the idea from McLeod (who subsequently left Moorfields to take up the Professorial Chair in Manchester), before adopting it as the plank of Moorfields' clinical strategy. This was later shaped (in conjunction with John Lee and John Dart) by the Clinical Strategy Group, during the period between 1986 and 1990. (So far as the outreach concept is concerned, its precise origin is even more obscure than that of the primary-care service, John Atwill claiming that it was a chance remark by Peter Hamilton, an energetic and mercurial consultant surgeon, that 'Moorfields ought to stop contemplating its navel and look outside itself more', which sowed the seed.)

The plan for a primary-care, one-stop service, providing an economical facility for large numbers of patients from all parts of London, without the need for large numbers of beds and expensive resources, was much in tune with the government's new thinking. It provided the Hospital with the means of spreading its net widely and offering ophthalmic services in any part of London, instead of sitting and waiting for patients to come to the centre, as had always been the case in the past. By creating a first-class service with clinics to screen out serious conditions from the trivial, backed up by a full range of specialist out-patient clinics of the highest calibre, to which serious cases could be speedily referred, very large numbers of patients could be seen safely and efficiently. This revised structure lent itself well to the foundation of an outreach programme and was the basis on which Bernard Tomlinson in 1991 came to reconsider his opinion about the Hospital and its ability to continue as a free-standing, single-specialty unit. While other SHAs sank, almost without trace, unable to justify their existence as free-standing units because of their small size, narrow range of services and high running costs, Moorfields, working within tight budgetary restrictions and stringent financial controls, was able to sail on successfully towards independent NHS Trust status.

The new hospital takes shape

Redevelopment of the Hospital continued more or less smoothly throughout the 1980s, four new operating theatres being completed and opened at the City Road branch in 1986, and new outpatient clinics, on the ground floor, somewhat earlier. The most important development, however, and one that actually increased the working area of the Hospital, without extending beyond its existing confines, was the conversion of the basement area to clinical use. During the Second World War, this area had been reinforced with concrete to provide Anderson shelters for the protection of patients and staff in the event of bombing raids. The downside to this piece of foresight now became apparent. An estimate of the costs of demolishing the reinforced walls, in order to open up the space and provide clinical workareas, was prohibitively high and could not be achieved within the budgetary constraints of the redevelopment plan.

A chance meeting, one day over lunch, between crucial members of the Planning Committee, Lawrence Green (ex-marine commando), Reg Fryer (ex-beachmaster), Francis Cumberlege (ex-Royal Signals) and John Atwill (ex-RASC officer) (**Figure 11**), provided the solution. Blow it up!

John Atwill's somewhat unorthodox career had brought him, while serving in the army, into contact with an explosives expert, whose unusual hobby consisted of sculpting pieces of rock with controlled explosions, thereby demonstrating how elegantly, in expert hands, explosives could be

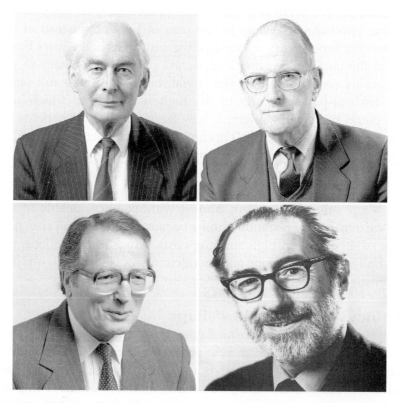

Figure 11   'Bomber Command' – Members of the Planning Team (all of whom had served in the Armed Services), who formed the idea of using explosives to 'open up' the reinforced basement of the Hospital for redevelopment: (*top left*) Francis Cumberlege (Chairman of the Board of Governors – Royal Signals); (*top right*) Lawrence Green (Chairman of the Finance and Planning Committees – Marine Commandos); (*bottom left*) John Atwill (House Governor – RASC); (*bottom right*) Reg Fryer (Board Member – D-Day landings beachmaster).

controlled. A firm of demolition experts was located, who, happening to be idle at this time between large contracts in the Far East and Africa, were prepared to undertake the (to them very small) task at Moorfields, for a sum one-third of that previously quoted by other companies.

Unfortunately, no insurance company was prepared to provide third party cover for such a potentially dangerous activity in an occupied building. On this occasion, however, the DHSS reacted with uncharacteristic insouciance, sanctioning the scheme, provided that the Board of Governors were prepared themselves to accept the risk. This, to their everlasting credit, the Board were, the only doubt in their minds being registered when it was noticed that the director of the demolition company was missing two fingers from his right hand! In the event, the demolition was carried out with only the faintest thump and vibration to alert the more sensitive doctors and patients to what was going on beneath their feet. Thus was the euphemistically named Lower Ground Floor (LGF) clinical area developed, creating much needed space, to accommodate numerous out-patient facilities.

It is no exaggeration to say that the refurbishment of the Hospital was a triumphant success (**Figures 12, 13 and 14**, Plates 5, 6 and 7). The new entrance hall and out-patient foyer were modern and attractive, the new clinics were patient-friendly and efficient, with colour coding and clear labelling to help the visually handicapped, and they were superbly well equipped. The lower ground floor in particular was an architectural feat, housing as it now did, not only a large and flexible open clinic space but also the brand new Retinal Diagnostic Department and the Department of Medical Illustration, a large laser suite, and the Orthoptic and Ultrasound Departments, as well as numerous non-clinical functions, such as the Central Sterile Supply Department, Medical Records Library and Laundry. Coupled with the extended operating theatre suite and improvements to other in-patient facilities on the upper floors, the Hospital was more than ready to face up to its new responsibilities.

Rebirth of medical management

As the 1980s entered its second half, the demands on the Planning Committee receded and the paramount objective became the development of a clear strategy for future clinical practice in the newly developed Hospital. For this, Atwill wisely looked to the younger members of the consultant staff, whose careers would thereby either flourish or wither. One of the youngest and most able of these, in both managerial terms and with respect to political nous, coupled with ruthless determination, was Bob Cooling.

Robert James Cooling was born in 1948 and received his medical training at Liverpool University, winning most of the available undergraduate prizes and awards for which he was eligible to compete, including the Leverhulme Travelling Scholarship and a First Class Honours degree. He arrived at Moorfields in 1975 and, after his time as a Resident and then a period as a clinical lecturer on the Professorial Unit (during which he initially thought to go into orbital surgery, but on John Wright's advice decided to specialize in vitreoretinal surgery), was appointed to the consultant staff in 1982. A fine surgeon, with a razor-like intelligence and single-minded focus, he soon attracted the attention of senior management, both medical and non-medical. Not long after his appointment to the consultant staff, he was asked to join the Planning Committee for the new, amalgamated Hospital, where he soon showed a keen interest in and capacity for, strategic development. As the need for supervision of the 'bricks and mortar' of the new Hospital diminished, the House Governor set up executive committees to oversee the implementation of strategy for both in-patient and out-patient services. Bob Cooling was appointed to chair the Out-Patient Executive Committee (OPEC) and Arthur Steele the In-Patient Executive Committee (IPEC). These two committees became fundamental to the progress of the Hospital, both physically and strategically. This was particularly true of OPEC, critical as it was to the evolution of primary care-based community eye services.

Cooling soon showed himself to have considerable foresight and political acumen, as well as total commitment to the task in hand. He learned avidly and rapidly from his more experienced colleagues on the Planning Committee and in its working parties, in particular John Wright and Noel Rice (Chairman of what had become the Joint Medical Committee of the two branches of the Hospital), and also absorbed some of the accumulated wisdom of the previous Medical Committee Chairman, Desmond Greaves. With the strong support of Atwill and Rice, he became responsible for preparing a Clinical Strategy Document, which contained, amongst many other proposals, the principles of developing primary-care services, restructuring the outpatient clinics and promoting wide provision of community eye services throughout the London Region.

To drive forward the concept of primary care and make it a major arm of the Hospital's clinical activities, a prototype primary-care clinic was established in 1986 on an experimental basis. Cooling himself was the clinical lead, but saw the need for a generalist of high calibre, with the knowledge, skills and leadership potential to direct this new service.

By great good fortune, such a person was already on the Hospital's payroll. Rhodri Daniel, a General Practitioner possessing the Diploma of Ophthalmology, was working as an out-patient officer at Moorfields. A man with commitment to the highest standards of practice and not inconsiderable ambition, he agreed to run the pilot clinic, and it was soon highly successful. In 1989 Rhodri Daniel took and passed the Fellowship examination of the Royal College of Ophthalmologists and was then appointed Fellow to the Moorfields Accident and Emergency and Primary Care Services. This was an experimental post and one that it was accepted could lead, in due course, to an appointment to the consultant staff. This it duly did and in 1992 he took over from Cooling as the first director of the Accident and Emergency and Primary-Care Service.

The 'internal market'

In January 1988, four years after the Griffiths management reforms were introduced, the Prime Minister announced a Ministerial Review of the NHS, and in July of that year the Department of Health was separated from the Department of Social Security, with Kenneth Clarke as Secretary of State for Health. After much debate between the Prime Minister, the new Secretary of State, the Chancellor (Nigel Lawson), the Chief Secretary of the Treasury (John Major) and senior civil servants, a fundamental change in the philosophy of the NHS was agreed, the main thrust of which was to establish a clear split between consumer and provider. In fact, Margaret Thatcher was keen to see a move away from funding from direct taxation, to a means-tested, insurance-backed scheme, along the lines of that already in place in some European countries and in the USA – one favoured by Kenneth Clarke's predecessor, John Moore – but Clarke opposed this. He was nevertheless determined to instigate a major change in the management structure of the NHS, building on the recommendations of the Griffiths Report, by introducing competitive bargaining, through a purchaser/provider divide (an idea first mooted in 1985 by an American economist, Alain Einthoven).

Even though in this so-called 'internal market' both purchaser and provider were ultimately being funded from the same source, Clarke thought that it would still provide the stimulus to make them compete for the most cost-effective outcomes. Throughout its entire life, the NHS had been a political football (perhaps more so under Barbara Castle's stewardship than any other), but now the government sought to distance itself from the agonising and often contradictory decisions relating to the provision of healthcare. What better way of doing this than to create a market for healthcare and let 'market forces' take control, the providers of healthcare being forced to fight amongst themselves to satisfy the insatiable demands of patients for free health services.

At the very least, Kenneth Clarke must be credited with steering Margaret Thatcher away from the concept of a privatized health service, and for succeeding in maintaining its status as a service, free at the point of delivery and fully funded from taxation. Ironically, however, as his successor, Virginia Bottomley, was later to remark, Clarke was castigated by the doctors for introducing measures that in effect preserved the fundamental concept of a free health service available to all – albeit by persuading the Prime Minister that, rather than remove the burden of it from general taxation by passing responsibility for it to the private sector, he could drive through unpopular managerial changes in the NHS that would deliver greatly increased efficiency and accountability.

The managerial stress that having to tender their services to purchasers (the so-called commissioning process) placed on hospitals was enormous. Furthermore, unlike a general hospital (especially a district general hospital, serving a clearly circumscribed population, often under the aegis of a single District Health Authority), Moorfields found itself contracting with multiple health authorities and, when GP fundholding was introduced between 1991 and 1994, with literally hundreds of different GP practices. It was extremely difficult to administer the contracts and even more difficult to collect the money. A small (in global terms) eye hospital did not rank high on the priority list of a cash-strapped HA or fund-holding GP practice, while, because of the failure of the government to provide adequate resources for improving and expanding healthcare and its blatant denial that there was any need to ration services, the purchasers were chronically starved of money. Although Clarke's strategy proved correct, in that the purchaser/provider divide promoted greatly increased competition within the NHS – providers struggling to achieve greater economic efficiency and purchasers looking for the best value – the cost to staff morale was enormous, while the ever-burgeoning size of the administrative infrastructure and its costs, unsupported by extra funding, militated against a successful outcome.

Amalgamation and diversification

In retrospect, 1988 proved to be a momentous year for Moorfields. In July, just as the new Health Secretary took over, the High Holborn branch finally closed and all the activities of the Hospital were concentrated on the redeveloped City Road site. This move went with surprising smoothness, thanks largely to the detailed prior planning and skil-ful liaison undertaken by Professor David Hill and his colleagues on the Transfer Liaison Committee. The actual transfer occurred on 19 July and, after a two-week theatre closure, normal activities resumed at City Road, without problems. On the 26 October the redeveloped Hospital was officially opened by its patron, Her Majesty the Queen (**Figure 15**, Plate 8).

It should not be assumed that the amalgamation of the two branches was achieved without some delay. When the present author was appointed to the consultant staff in December 1980, with duties almost exclusively at the High Holborn branch, he was assured that this would be for a period of two years at the most, before the proposed move to City Road. In fact, Hospital Reports indicate that as late as 1982 it was anticipated that the transfer would take place by the end of 1985. The planning and implementation of the amalgamation, with all that it signified in terms of the future viability of the Hospital, was neverthe-less a feat of very considerable magnitude, and one of which the Board of Governors, the House Governor and all members of staff could be justly proud. In the event, the Department of Health too did very well out of the deal, finally selling off the Holborn site to commercial interests for a sum in excess of £24m, while still insisting that Moorfields adhere to its original promise to save £360 000 in annual running costs.

The 1990s: a decade of upheaval

Lest it be thought that the main battles were now over, it soon became apparent that they were only just beginning. The 1990s were to see changes in the Health Service as never before, not only in the spheres of management and macroeconomics, but also in its very culture and means of healthcare delivery, as well as the organization and financing of teaching, training and research.

At Moorfields, in the clinical field, the 1990s heralded the creation of Clinical Directorates, leading up to the granting of independent Trust status. Nine Specialist Clinical Directorates were formed, each with a Director and a Training Director: the Adnexal (orbital and oculo-plastics), Anaesthetic, Cataract (comprising a number of consultant surgeons, all of whom were also members of one or other of the specialist services), Corneal and External Disease, Glaucoma, Medical Retina, Physicians, Strabismus and Paediatric, and Surgical Vitreo-retinal Services. In addition to these, Accident and Emergency (A&E) and Primary Care now formed a major service of their own. All the specialist services rapidly expanded during the 1990s, not only in response to the cry for more accountability and a consultant-based service but also to provide staffing levels and expertise to match the increased workload created by the outreach community services.

The Primary-Care Service developed rapidly, not only at City Road but also in the Outreach Community Eye Units as these were inaugurated, firstly in Bow in East London, and later more widely across London (**Figure 16**, Plate 9). In parallel with this development, the A&E service at City Road was compelled to alter its focus and the role of nursing staff in both departments took on a wider remit, involving triage, diagnosis and treatment. The age of the nurse-practitioner had arrived and the Casualty Training Course took on a new significance. Not only were nurses encouraged to see and treat the simpler cases, they also began to acquire special expertise in glaucoma, medical retina and other specialist areas.

The adnexal service found itself in especially great demand, partly as a result of the move towards greater accountability but also because of the changes wrought by the introduction of structured training, whereby consultants and more senior ophthalmologists were required to perform, or at least to supervise, even minor plastic or reconstructive operations. The range and sophistication of oculoplastic procedures also increased rapidly during this decade, while the reputation of Richard Collin and the success of his textbook attracted an increasing number of young ophthalmologists to Moorfields. With the retirement of John Wright and Peter Fells in 1995–96, a new consultant was appointed to take over the orbital and thyroid work, while a further consultant appointment was necessary to service the outreach programme.

Demands on the anaesthetic services during the last two decades of the century altered completely, as the changing face of cataract management led the way to an entirely different approach to patient care, and outreach units opened, capable of undertaking day-case surgery. General anaesthesia (GA) soon became a comparatively uncommon event, reserved as it was mainly for children, and adults undergoing prolonged and stressful operations. New preparations of drugs for intravenous use and ones that could be rapidly and completely reversed after surgery became readily available for cases requiring GA, while the methods of local anaesthesia multiplied with extraordinary speed. Not only did some surgeons choose to give their own anaesthetics, sometimes using only topical agents, but anaesthetists became adept at giving retrobulbar, peribulbar and sub-Tenon's injections, often more so than the surgeons themselves, and took to teaching these methods to others.

Developments in cataract surgery continued apace, not only because of the technological advances associated with phacoemulsification and small-incision surgery, but also because of the mounting pressure to undertake surgery on a day-case basis. With the increasing focus on costs and value for money, initiated by the Thatcher government and continued relentlessly under John Major and then by the New Labour administration, there was constant pressure during the 1990s to cut bed occupancy and increase patient throughput. The Tomlinson Report of 1991 had specifically targeted the London hospital services, with recommendations for bed closures throughout London, and the then Health Secretary, Virginia Bottomley, had implemented these mercilessly, even going so far as to threaten St Bartholomew's Hospital with closure. Small-incision cataract surgery, mostly carried out under local anaesthesia, was therefore not just a desirable advance, but an essential development in the drive to increase efficiency, and Moorfields seized on this opportunity with relish. Phacoemulsification, via tiny corneal incisions and the insertion through these of foldable or injectable lens implants, rapidly became the method of choice, as the decade progressed, for treating uncomplicated cataracts. Patients could be discharged the same day, with only a single postoperative check, so accurate were the pre-assessment ultrasound biometry scans and so thorough the preoperative examinations by doctors and nurses.

The vast majority of cataract operations were now performed under local anaesthesia, after pre-assessment in daily anaesthetic clinics set up for this purpose, and, even if a general anaesthetic was for some reason preferred, most could still be done as day cases. The operation had become so predictable and visually successful that the threshold of indications for surgery had fallen to a level where almost any symptoms of visual impairment were sufficient to warrant intervention. Furthermore, cataract surgery was now offered to the desperately ill and even those with terminal illnesses.

The New Labour administration, obsessed as it was with the length of waiting lists, saw cataract surgery as an ideal opportunity to demonstrate their commitment to bring these down. In 2003 they introduced the concept of Patient Choice and Diagnostic Treatment Centres (DTCs), whereby patients who had been waiting six months or longer for their cataract operations could phone up a Patient-Choice Centre, which would offer a choice of DTCs to which they could be directed for immediate surgery. Moorfields responded to this challenge by equipping and opening a DTC at St Ann's Hospital Tottenham and a further one in the newly refurbished unit at St George's Hospital Tooting.

In corneal and external diseases there were advances not only in the management of corneal grafts but also in the treatment of autoimmune diseases such as Stevens–Johnson disease and ocular pemphigoid and of a wide variety of devastating infections, with the introduction of an increasingly diverse range of second- and third-generation antibiotics and antimicrobials. Perhaps the most significant advances, however, were made in refractive surgery. From its early days in the early 1970s, when Fyodorov in the Soviet Union, by creating a series of radial scars, devised a method of altering the contour of the cornea, there was widespread interest in this treatment on the part of both patients and surgeons alike. The notion of doing away with the need for glasses and contact lenses was an appealing one.

At Moorfields, Arthur Steele was the first to attempt it, in the early 1980s, and taught it to his assistants, albeit without great enthusiasm. The method was crude and its outcome unpredictable, and treatment was difficult to justify unless the patient was unable or unwilling to wear either spectacles or contact lenses. In 1988, however, a dramatic advance was made, when new technology enabled corneal remodelling with the excimer laser, a technique that, combined with developments in wave-front technology and computerized sampling of corneal aberrations, transformed the procedure (see Part 2). A new consultant appointment was made, with Julian Stevens, a computer-literate technocrat, joining the staff to spearhead the advances in refractive surgery, which were quite clearly going to be a major addition to clinical practice. Later developments quickly advanced the technique further, with the introduction of laser intrastromal keratectomy (LASIK) making refractive surgery both safe and predictable, and Stevens and the other anterior segment surgeons at Moorfields soon adopted this method, not only for correcting conventional errors of refraction but also for remodelling the cornea scarred by trauma or disease (see Part 2).

In the glaucoma service, the development of new surgical methods was paralleled by the evolution of ever more sophisticated drug preparations, including topical preparations of alpha blockers, acetozolamide and prostaglandin agonists, while trabeculectomy surgery was enhanced by the use of antiproliferative agents. Peng Tee Khaw was appointed, with a 50/50 clinical/research contract, to take over the paediatric glaucoma work, on the retirement of Noel Rice, and to continue his pioneering work in wound healing, being, in the course of time, awarded a personal academic Chair. The Directorate quickly expanded, with the appointments of more consultants to manage the services in the outreach units, as well as at City Road, while the increasing need for more and better-quality research into the cause, pathology and outcomes of treatment in this devastating condition led to the appointment of young consultants on partly research-based contracts. Meanwhile, Roger Hitchings relinquished the directorship of the service to become the President of the International Glaucoma Association and was appointed to a Professorial Chair funded by that organization.

Advances in the medical retinal field were no less dramatic, not only in the field of genetics, under the auspices of Barrie and Marcelle Jay and Alan Bird, which grew steadily, but also in that of immunology and the treatment of uveitis, the special interest of Susan Lightman, who transformed the outlook in a condition in which previous attempts at treatment had been less than successful. Furthermore, the upsurge in the spread of the human immunodeficiency virus (HIV) and the acquired immune deficiency syndrome (AIDS) presented a whole new spectrum of retinal disease and treatment modalities with which to treat it, and Lightman was at the very forefront of the field. Indocyanine green fundus photography and photodynamic therapy, in the identification and treatment of age-related macular degeneration (ARMD), however, proved less effective than had been hoped.

The 1990s was the last decade in which a general physician was on the staff of the Hospital. David Galton, an endocrinologist at Barts, with special expertise in lipid metabolism and a keen interest in ophthalmology, retired in 2002 and was not replaced. This marked a change in emphasis that had previously been signalled by the appointment in 1994, for the first time, of a neuro-ophthalmologist. Prior to this, Moorfields had always been well served by the presence on the staff of consultant physicians, who, although usually neurologists, were expected to provide a wider service. The new appointee, Paul Riordan-Eva, was a fully trained ophthalmologist specializing in neuro-ophthalmology, with both clinical and research sessions at the National Hospital for Neurology and Neurosurgery, Queen Square and sessions at Moorfields, but with no surgical commitment. He was immediately inundated with work and within a short space of time fell seriously ill, precipitating his resignation. His replacement, James Acheson, similarly had sessions at Queen Square, but no research component, and he had operating sessions at the Hospital, joining the Strabismus and Paediatric Service. With Gordon Plant's full-time commitment to neurology at St Thomas', Queen Square and Moorfields, and Acheson's to neuro-ophthalmology at the latter two institutions, there was now an over-riding commitment to this particular sphere of expertise.

Changes to the pattern of management and treatment of squints centred on the decreasing incidence of amblyopia (lazy eye), a reduction in the number of children undergoing surgery for squint and a parallel increase in adult squint surgery. The increasing use of botulinum toxin and adjustable sutures, together with higher expectations and greater demand for adult squint correction, were overshadowed, however, during the latter half of the decade by the change in attitude to the management of children in all branches of medicine. The National Service Framework for children outlined in the NHS Plan (2000) and the appointment of a lead clinician to oversee it (Professor Aynsley Green at the Institute of Child Health), together with guidelines from the Royal College of Paediatrics, meant that child-friendly policies assumed overriding importance, and Moorfields struggled to keep pace with these developments. The concept of an International Children's Eye Centre, to separate paediatric care from the main hospital and further research, was a sensible and timely response to the introduction of this new doctrine (see Part 2).

In vitreoretinal (VR) surgery there were notable advances, in particular the successful treatment, with restoration of central vision, of retinal holes at the macula, a condition affecting large numbers of elderly women and previously considered inoperable. Subretinal surgery for ARMD, a condition accounting for the majority of blindness in the over-65s, was excitedly heralded as the new panacea, but proved to be less effective than was hoped. Meanwhile the fight to improve the results of surgery for complicated retinal detachments, by vitrectomy methods combined with the use of intraocular gases and silicone oil, continued, as did research into the causes of retinal scarring (proliferative vitreoretinopathy, or PVR) and its possible prevention. Collaboration between the VR surgeons and Peng Tee Khaw's wound-healing group led to the exciting discovery of a cocktail of drugs for the prevention of PVR, a multicentre clinical trial of which was extremely encouraging.

Development of community ophthalmic services

Allusion has already been made to the steps taken by Moorfields in 1986 to reinvent itself, with the initiation of a primary-care clinic, and the appointment of Rhodri Daniel to the post of Fellow to the Primary-Care Service. This was an inspirational move on the part of Bob Cooling and John Atwill, in their quest to transform the hospital from an esoteric centre of excellence (and provider of tertiary care) into the central hub of ophthalmic primary-care provision for London, but it had some unwelcome implications. The most immediate consequence was a radical and uncomfortable rationalization of the medical workforce (see Part 2). Out-patient officers and chief clinical assistants at Moorfields, some of very long standing, were asked to re-learn specialist skills or step down. Moreover, Fellows, many of them from abroad, who had come to Moorfields with the averred aim of picking and choosing the clinical experiences most suited to their esoteric interests and did not expect to do general work, were corralled, shamed and sometimes bribed into serving in the Primary-Care Service. Meanwhile, the need to expand and extend the Hospital's sphere of activities widely, throughout North London and beyond, in order to satisfy the new-found appetite for community services, was paramount. Overtures were made far and wide and, aided by the frequently impossible demands imposed on weaker units by the internal market, met more often than not with a variable and grudging, if not openly hostile, response. Moorfields tried hard to project a non-predatorial mien and to be seen, far from as seeking to take over other units, rather as a knight in shining armour come to rescue them from the dragon of financial and professional ruin. Needless to say, in many instances, this perception was rather different from the reality.

In some instances, the Hospital was able to take over the work of struggling units and offer their consultants places on the staff at Moorfields. In others, outreach clinics were set up under the Moorfields name and with Moorfields staff and equipment, sometimes alongside existing services provided by the local unit. Despite all best efforts to the contrary, a great deal of bitterness accrued in the ophthalmological community, both in London and in the country at large, sometimes the result of personal resentment and envy and in other instances arising from a sense of humiliation and helplessness felt by members of small eye units at the low priority that they were given by managers looking desperately for savings.

Whatever the rights and wrongs, one man stood alone and unmoved as the storm raged around him. While the vision of primary care and specialist services as the saviour of Moorfields may first have originated with John Atwill and the concept of outreach with Peter Hamilton, it was Bob Cooling who, in the final analysis, stood alone on the bridge in the teeth of the ensuing storm. Apparently impervious to much of the bile and invective engendered amongst its competitors by the new strategy, and totally convinced that the future of Moorfields depended on the success of this venture, Cooling sailed on relentlessly. In this endeavour he had the unconditional support of the House Governor and the Board of Governors – if not always that of all his consultant colleagues, some of whom were alarmed at the prospect of being censured by fellow members of the ophthalmic community.

By 1995, Moorfields offered community eye services at St Andrew's Hospital Bow, Northwick Park and St Mark's Hospital and Upney Lane Health Centre Barking, and two years later there were outreach units at St Ann's Hospital Tottenham, Potters Bar Community Hospital (see **Figure 16**, Plate 9) and Ealing Hospital. In 1994 the Hospital was asked to take over the management of vitreoretinal surgical services at St George's Hospital Tooting, while five years later retinal outpatient services were being supplied by Moorfields at Watford General Hospital, and both vitreoretinal and oculoplastic services at the Mayday University Hospital Croydon. In 2001 St George's asked Moorfields to take responsibility for the entire ophthalmic service there, and a year later Moorfields offered outreach facilities at Homerton Hospital in Hackney. In some of these outlying units outpatient facilities alone were set up, but in others such as the units at St Ann's Tottenham, in Barking and Ealing and at Northwick Park, facilities for cataract surgery were provided, and yet others were equipped for a wide range of ophthalmic surgery. In this latter respect, the widespread adoption of day-case and short-stay surgery, under both local and general anaesthesia, had facilitated the provision of surgical treatment in the outreach setting, where formerly this would have been difficult and costly.

Moorfields NHS Trust

In 1991, with the creation of the first wave of NHS Trusts and GP Fund-Holders, it became clear that Moorfields would need to achieve Trust status if it was to remain independent and self-governing, and it was now evident that the policy of expansion had been a far-sighted one. Indeed, while many had seriously questioned the tactics pursued by Moorfields in actively seeking out new sources of custom, some-times at the expense of weaker units, it seemed doubtful if those same critics would have come dashing to its rescue had it failed to look to its own salvation. Certainly, the present author is not alone in believing that John Atwill's vision and Bob Cooling's courage and commitment were crucial to the survival of the Hospital as an independent unit dur-ing this turbulent period of its history, nor was Atwill's successor as House Governor, Ian Balmer, slow to grasp the importance of the new strategy and nail his colours to the mast.

In simple terms, the introduction of the purchaser/provider split and of fund-holding by GPs meant that many of the patients who had previously been readily referred to Moorfields by their local Health Authorities and General Practitioners, from districts far and wide, were now expected to be seen and treated by their local service-providers. Those patients would be lost to Moorfields unless it could provide a competitive service in their locality. Cooling and Balmer therefore set about offering such a service, wherever they could see that 'business' would be lost if Moorfields could not provide it locally. To do this, they had to go out and seek contracts with the local purchasers, the GP fund-holders and health authorities, always being careful to ensure that they were invited to provide the service, but inevitably engendering the opprobrium of many of their professional colleagues, forced as they were into this competitive arena by the government's divisive policy. Moorfields owes much to Balmer and Cooling, their courage and their conviction, in establishing so many successful outreach departments. Nor should the dedication of the new clinical 'leads', such as John Wright at Northwick Park, in gaining the confidence and respect of the host Trusts be forgotten (although, in all fairness, it must also be admitted that some consultants who agreed to work in the outreach centres were shrewd enough to realize the opportunities for practice outside the NHS that working locally provided).

The central plank of Kenneth Clarke's scheme for the new NHS was the move to create self-governing hospitals and self-determining general practices, operating within the framework of the purchaser/provider split. His experience as a Minister of State for Health between 1982 and 1985 had convinced him of the wisdom of funding the Health Service fully from taxation and of the importance of the General Practitioner as a unique and central part of it. Sadly for him, although he was keen to see his reforms through, Margaret Thatcher for once lost her nerve and, realizing that Clarke was to the medical establishment like a red rag to the proverbial bull (*he had once famously remarked that they had, in the BMA, the most unscrupulous trade union with which he had ever had to deal (The Politics of NHS Reform 1988–1997,* Chris Ham, King's Fund, 2000, p.10)), decided in 1990 to reshuffle her cabinet, replacing Clarke as Health Secretary with William Waldegrave, a far more conciliatory character. Indeed, she is credited with saying to Waldegrave (of the doctors), on the occasion of his appointment: '*Kenneth has stirred them all up. Now you have to calm them down' (The Politics of NHS Reform 1988–1997,* Chris Ham, King's Fund, 2000, p.13). Nevertheless, Waldegrave was a keen supporter of both the purchaser/provider split and of self-governing hospitals, and the scheme went ahead as planned under his stewardship, continuing to do so after Margaret Thatcher was unceremoniously ejected from power, under John Major's administration.

So far as hospitals were concerned, this entailed conversion from a position of financial dependence to one of independent management, through the creation of self-governing Trusts. In Moorfields' case, as a single-specialty hospital, this meant that it had to demonstrate its ability to remain independently viable and solvent, and, due to the enormous restructuring that had gone before, it was in a good position to do so. Broadly speaking, the Hospital was required to purchase its own assets from the government and pay interest of 6% per annum to the Department of Health on the loan enabling it to do so. By virtue of its increased patient base throughout London, and greater capacity to meet the demand for its highly specialized services, it was in an eminently good position to seek, and subsequently gain, NHS Trust status. The Hospital was, however, first required to complete a period as a 'shadow' Trust, before applying for and finally becoming, in April 1994, Moorfields Eye Hospital NHS Trust.

The Tomlinson Report

Meanwhile, the government, alarmed by reports of widespread confusion and inefficiency among the hospitals in London, and the impact the reforms were having on the provision of services there, asked Sir Bernard Tomlinson, a distinguished and respected Professor of Pathology from Newcastle, to carry out an inquiry into the provision of health services in London. As with the Todd Report some 20 years earlier, Tomlinson recommended that all undergraduate medical schools and postgraduate research institutes should be part of multi-disciplinary teaching and research institutions. (Michael Peckham's Department of Research and Development had already identified four such schools in London: Imperial College in the West, Queen Mary Westfield in the East, University College in the North and Kings College in the South; with the disbandment of the British Postgraduate Medical Federation, in 1995, the Institute of Ophthalmology would be absorbed by University College.)

When Professor Tomlinson came to visit Moorfields, early in 1992, he was therefore in a mind to insist that a single-specialty postgraduate hospital should, logically, be merged with a large undergraduate teaching hospital, able to provide facilities for all branches of medicine. This notwithstanding, he was clearly impressed with the work that had been done to redirect the hospital, and listened carefully to the arguments put forward by the management team and the chairman of the Medical Committee, John Wright, in support of Moorfields remaining independent. So impressed was he, in fact, that, to the great relief of all concerned, there was nothing in his report to suggest that it should not remain so (*Report of the Inquiry into London's Health Service, Medical Education and Research*, HMSO, London, 1992).

It is alleged that, when the Medical Committee Chairman was asked what he thought should be done about ophthalmic services in London, John

Wright said he would put all the in-patient work into Moorfields and get Moorfields to manage all out-patient ophthalmic services, throughout London.

Academic revolution

It is worth recording here that the Institute had by this time already undergone major changes in its governance. In the early 1980s Whitehall began to demand greater accountability for their financial support of research activities and instigated periodic inspections by the Higher Education Funding Council for England of institutions receiving money for research, the so-called Research Assessment Exercises (RAEs). These were carried out at approximately five-yearly intervals, followed by the award of a grade to each research institute, from 1 (very poor) to 5 (good) and 5* (excellent). The Institute of Ophthalmology had been graded 1 at its first attempt and 3 at the second, leading to a warning from the Chairman of the University Grants Committee, Sir Colin Dollery, that if things did not improve then financial support could be withdrawn – in effect, it could be closed down.

Rolf Blach's appointment as Dean in 1985 had brought a considerable improvement in its rating, and the arrival of Adam Sillito in 1987 consolidated and improved this dramatically when he took over as head of Visual Science. Thereafter, the Institute's RAE grading improved steadily. Meanwhile, Peckham's antipathy to medical deans of research institutes led eventually to the replacement of the post of Dean by that of Director of Research, Professor Sillito becoming the first non-medical Director of the Institute in its history. A more detailed account of these events is given later (see Part 3), but suffice it to say here that, from 1990 onwards, the Institute of Ophthalmology consistently scored 5 or 5* in all RAE ratings, albeit at the cost of shedding from its staff most of the incumbent academics, and all but a very few of the clinical academics whom it shared with the Hospital.

Self-government

As far as the Hospital itself was concerned, the repeated reorganizations and reviews during the 1980s and early 1990s had left it relatively unscathed, albeit with a very different management structure and ethos to that prevailing in the years before. Application for and the subsequent achievement of Trust status had forced it to become a leaner, more efficient and accountable organization, albeit at the cost perhaps of some degree of professional and cultural harmony. It had also entailed the appointment of a Medical Director, and it was little surprise that this was Bob Cooling. As has already been noted, surviving in the 'internal market' placed considerable strain on resources, both clinical and managerial, while the extension of the outreach programme stretched them even further. The Medical Director, Chief Executive and their management team worked tirelessly to sustain Moorfields' continued prosperity throughout a period that was to prove one of the most difficult in the Hospital's history.

The changes at the top were rendered even more radical by the retirement in 1991 of Francis Cumberlege, who had been Chairman of the Board of Governors of Moorfields for 22 years and had had a profound influence on the development of the Hospital during a crucial period of its history, and in 1993 by that of John Atwill, also a pivotal figure. Nevertheless, contrary to what so often happens on the departure of powerful personalities central to development and progress, the Hospital battled on without pause – a fitting tribute, perhaps, to the strength of the organization that these two men had left behind and to the quality of the new management team. (Some indication of this can be gauged from the fact that, in the five-year period between 1995 and 2000 revenue increased by 33%.)

The new chairman of the Board of Governors (and two years later of the Board of Directors when the Special Health Authority became a NHS Trust) was Hugh Peppiatt, senior partner in a distinguished firm of lawyers (and a legal adviser to the Bank of England), while Atwill's place as House Governor was taken by Ian Balmer, who had been Planning Officer under him at Moorfields 10 years earlier (before going to St Thomas' Hospital). The new management team brought to the task a very different approach to that of their predecessors – and arguably one more suited to the prevailing socio-political climate. Hugh Peppiatt proved to be a subtle and calculating operator, a man of the world, with an iron fist in a velvet glove, well able to cope with the hard-edged demands of realpolitik. Furthermore, Ian Balmer brought to the post of House Governor and Chief Executive shrewd political judgement and an appreciation of the need for first-class presentation to complement underlying excellence, something that he had come to appreciate from spending some time in the independent health sector. Once again, Moorfields had acquired the 'right men for the job', at a crucial time in its history.

The retirement of Cumberlege and the appointment of Peppiatt heralded a new era, for although the Hospital remained a Special Health Authority for the time being, its progress along the path to self-governance and the change to a 'hub and spoke' structure were now inevitable, and the NHS and Community Care Act (1990) required a more streamlined management structure. The Board of Governors was accordingly reformed, with 12 members in addition to the Chairman: 6 executives [the House Governor, Chief Nursing Officer (and Deputy General Manager) and Director of Finance, and the Chairmen (all consultants) of the Medical Committee and Out-Patient and In-Patient Executive Committees], and 6 non-executives, including the Dean of the Institute (**Figure 17**).

The acquisition of Trust status two years later demanded further changes in management, there being a requirement that each Trust should have a Board of Directors consisting of a non-executive Chairman chosen by the Secretary of State, five executives and five other non-executives. The executive members were the Chief Executive (House Governor), the Medical Director, Chief Nursing Officer, Finance Director and the Director of Research and Teaching. The director of the Institute, Professor Sillito, joined the four independently selected members of the new Board as a non-executive director.

The running of the Hospital had been completely taken out of the hands of the consultant staff, with the Medical Committee, formerly a key influence in the management process, relegated to an advisory role, and renamed the Medical Advisory Committee (MAC). Executive decision-making was henceforward informed by the Clinical Management Board (CMB), chaired by the Medical Director and consisting, in addition to the House Governor and his most senior managers, of the directors of Research, Education, Contracting and Strategic Development, and Human Resources (Personnel), the chairman of the MAC, and the nine Specialist Service directors.

The loss of influence felt by the consultant staff was, however, for a number of reasons, not as great or as significant as might at first appear. For one thing, as recorded, with the change to Trust status the opportunity had been taken to abolish general out-patient clinics and form Clinical Directorates (Specialist Services) in each of the key areas of clinical interest, and each Service Director had a seat (and voice) on the CMB. For another, teaching and training were under the overall direction of the Director of Education, advised by a Training Director in each service, and similar arrangements were in place for research. Considerable power of decision-making was therefore at the disposal of the consultant body, if they cared to exercise it, and, in accordance with the recommendations of the Griffiths Report 10 years earlier, there was now, at last, clearly defined line management.

New government, new governance

The introduction of the internal market in 1991, and the huge admini-

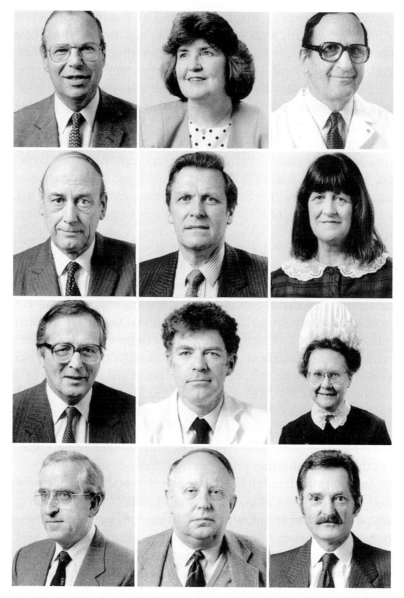

Figure 17 The new-style Board of Governors (resulting from the NHS and Community Care Act of 1990) consisted of six non-executive and six executive members, in addition to its Chairman, Mr Hugh Peppiatt. The non-executive members are: (*top row, left to right*) Mr J Bach, Mrs K Bennett, Mr R Blach; (*second row, left to right*) Mr J Brighouse, Professor A Elkington, Mrs J Smith. The executive members are: (*third row, left to right*) Mr J Atwill (House Governor), Mr R Cooling (Chairman OPEC), Miss R Emblin (Matron); (*bottom row, left to right*) Mr P Fells (Chairman of the Medical Committee), Mr D Rhys-Tyler (Treasurer), Mr A Steele (Chairman IPEC).

strative burden that this placed on Moorfields, contracting, as it had to do, with a multiplicity of purchasers, led to the appointment of a Director of Contracting and Strategic Planning, Brian Benson, who had previously served with a prestigious firm of chartered accountants and had a PhD degree. He became part of the Clinical Management Board and Management Executive, and with him came a whole new tier of managerial infrastructure. The weight of managerial responsibility, increasing regulation and demands for evidence of accountability was unrelenting.

In 1993 the Hospital received an official visit from the Minister of Health, Brian Mawhinney, a tireless critic of the medical profession and of the hospital service, who came to find fault and made this quite clear. Irritated by his attitude, the Chairman, Hugh Peppiatt, gave back as good as he got, pointing out to him that his criticisms made it plain that he knew very little about Moorfields. The Minister was affronted, terminated the meeting and strode from the Boardroom abruptly and in high dudgeon, with the clear intention of gaining the high ground by leaving so precipitately. Sadly for him, however, not only did he find, when he reached the front door, that it was raining, but his driver, not expecting him to emerge for some time, had retired to a local hostelry for some light refreshment. The official limousine was not to be seen, leaving the unfortunate Minister high and dry (literally), to wait alone in the front hall of the Hospital, his dramatic exit, much, no doubt, to Peppiatt's satisfaction, reduced to a humiliating charade.

Not only were the managers put under severe pressure as the 1990s began, but the medical staff were for the first time under official scrutiny, when medical audit, both general and specialist, was introduced as a statutory requirement. The entire staff were required to attend formal meetings, lasting two to three hours (the loss of clinical activity costing the Hospital thousands of pounds in lost income) every month, at which members of individual services were expected to present papers demonstrating the statistical data relating to their activities. Much further time was consumed in researching these figures, many of which were scarcely relevant to the day-to-day practice of the Hospital. They did nevertheless concentrate peoples' minds on what they were doing and hoping to achieve, initiating thereby a process of self-questioning and quality assurance that was to become the central theme of the decade ahead. The practice of holding plenary meetings, however, soon gave way to individual specialist audit within the emerging specialist services and to the formation of a Medical Audit Committee, whose task it was to review their findings.

In 1996 a Director of Operations, Christine Miles, was appointed, to oversee the day-to-day running of the Trust, or, as she confided to the present author, *'to do all the jobs Ian Balmer did not want to do'*. A pharmacist by training, with a Masters degree in Business Administration, who had learned and honed her NHS management skills in a Health Authority nearby, she displayed a ruthless determination to introduce accountability and efficiency, unmatched either before or since her four-year tenure. This caused considerable resentment and disquiet in some quarters, and indeed it has to be said that her approach was not always helpful. Nevertheless, by her single-minded commitment and boundless energy, she achieved some remarkable improvements in the running of the support services, including the merger of the contact lens department with optometry, and the maintenance of the fabric of the Hospital. More importantly, it was Christine Miles who was responsible for seeing that the new Outreach Units and the Mobile Medical Retina Unit became a reality, and, with Ian Balmer, she masterminded the concept of the new Manufacturing Pharmacy Unit.

Christine Miles was also responsible for organizing the official visit of Her Majesty the Queen in June 1999, on the occasion of the centenary of the opening of the Royal London Ophthalmic Hospital's new premises on City Road. This she undertook with military precision, and it all went like clockwork. One of her tasks was to ensure that the floors of the Hospital were polished, and she did this with characteristic zeal – so much so that when the police security men came to check the building for hidden explosives or other hazards, their sniffer dogs, unable to gain any purchase with their paws, on the mirror-like surface, took to the air like ice-skaters and kept tumbling over.

With the change of government in 1997, the philosophy and mechanics of health provision changed yet again, as contracts with Health Authorities gave way to Service Level Agreements (SLAs) and Fund-Holding General Practices were subsumed into Primary-Care Groups and thence into Primary-Care Trusts. Furthermore, New Labour was as concerned as the Conservatives had been, not only with patient choice and empowerment, but also with quality assurance. They lost no time in addressing the problems of the NHS, immediately producing a command paper 'The New NHS – Modern, Dependable' (1997), which was followed a year later by 'A First Class Service – Quality in the NHS.' Unable simply to steal their predecessors' clothes, they introduced a brand new concept – Clinical Governance, the responsibility, vested in Chief Executives and Medical Directors, for ensuring that there was '*a framework through which NHS organizations were accountable for continu-*

ously improving the quality of their services and safeguarding high standards of care, by creating an environment in which excellence of clinical care would flourish'. Moorfields promptly set up its own Clinical Governance Committee, chaired by a member of the Board, with the Medical Director, Director of Education, Director of Research, Chief Nursing Officer and Chairman of the Medical Advisory Committee as members. Nor was it long before the need for explicit quality assurance became paramount, following the arraignment and subsequent conviction of the Chief Executive, Medical Director and a Consultant Paediatric Cardiothoracic Surgeon at a Trust in the West of England, on charges of incompetence and dereliction of duty. What is more, the NHS was to see many more such assaults on its integrity, as it approached and then entered the 21st Century. At Moorfields itself there were to be suspensions and enquiries (albeit of surgeons who had joined the staff of Moorfields as a result of mergers with other hospitals) where standards were found to be unsatisfactory – something which would have been unheard of 10 years before. The Hospital responded boldly, going a step further and appointing a consultant in Public Health Medicine, Dr Parul Desai, to oversee the Trust's Governance procedures and risk management strategy.

Teaching and training in the new NHS

Further change, of the most elemental kind, had also begun to influence the conduct of teaching and training. In 1992, in response to political pressure from the European Parliament, the Chief Medical Officer (CMO), Kenneth Calman, was asked to carry out a wide-ranging review of specialist medical training in the UK. Following acceptance within the European Union of a Certificate of Specialist Training for each specialty, acceptable to all member states, it soon became apparent that, to comply with European Law, the UK would have to carry out modifications to its educational procedures and qualifications. Accreditation by the Medical Royal Colleges for entry to independent practice, on the basis of criteria laid down by them, was no longer acceptable in European Law. The UK was obliged to have its own Certificate of Competence, to be issued by an over-arching Competent Authority, answerable directly to Brussels in accordance with European practice, and to accept the certificates awarded by other member states when appointing the consultants of the future.

Kenneth Calman was a man of very considerable vision, allied with political acumen, and saw this as an opportunity to undertake a radical reform of teaching and training in the UK. The Report of the CMO's Working Group to advise on Specialist Training in the UK (1993) recommended sweeping changes throughout the NHS. Most notable among these were a shorter period of Higher Specialist Training, with precisely defined criteria for entry and exit, in each specialty (a total of some 39 specialties were defined), a single Higher Specialist Training Grade (the Specialist Registrar), to replace the Registrar and Senior Registrar Grades, and continuous monitoring of progress within the grade by means of annual assessments, the so-called RITA process (Record of In-Training Assessment). The whole process was to be centred on structured training programmes, usually involving rotation around several different trainers in different institutions, and controlled and implemented by the Regional Postgraduate Deans.

This was a profound change to the established order, wherein, from time immemorial, apprenticeship had been the quintessential feature of the British model of training. No longer were consultant 'chiefs' to be indulged with entourages of compliant students and enslaved juniors. Credit for teaching and training was henceforth to be granted to those with demonstrable teaching and training skills, trainers must observe and be able to fulfil the curricula prescribed by the relevant Medical Royal Colleges, and junior staff must rotate to other units, as and when the curriculum demanded it. This meant that patronage was (almost) abolished overnight, while trainees could cheerfully rely on the knowledge that, however they behaved towards their seniors, provided that they could satisfy the requirements of the RITA process, they would move seamlessly through the continuum of higher specialist training. Furthermore, the successful acquisition of a Certificate of Completion of Specialist Training (CCST) at the end of this period would entitle them to apply for a consultant post here or anywhere else in the European Union.

The Postgraduate Medical Deans, who had been nominally in charge of teaching and training for a long time, were now for the first time given ultimate responsibility for implementing the training curricula specified by the Medical Royal Colleges, and the power to go with it. Already employees of the Universities, they now became civil servants, answerable to the CMO, via him, to the Secretary of State for Health. The Medical Royal Colleges set the standards for postgraduate medical training by designing strict syllabi defining every aspect of its content, while the Deans were required to implement the curricula of training. In addition, by virtue of paying half of the trainees' basic salaries, they had the power to exercise control over the quality of training opportunities provided in the hospitals. (The Deans could, if necessary, withdraw their contribution to trainees' salaries if training was unsatisfactory, effectively closing down the posts, a measure that guarded against exploitation of trainees by the Trusts, who might otherwise have been tempted to demand their services alone, to the neglect of training.)

The effects of this change on the Moorfields training programme were at first only marginal, because the Hospital was still at this stage a Special Health Authority and therefore not subject to Regional authority. The Postgraduate Dean could not therefore appoint a Clinical Tutor, pay trainees' salaries or exert any direct influence over its activities. Later on, however, when it became a Trust (1994), and thereby under Regional control, the effects were wide-ranging: first because the Royal College of Ophthalmologists required all higher trainees to undertake structured training in rotating programmes around their Region (in this case, North Thames), the Moorfields Residents were no longer the Moorfields trainees of old, but rather North Thames trainees, spending a period of their training at Moorfields (with allegiance now to their Deanery, rather than to the Trust); and secondly because, as a consequence, the period of time that each trainee could spend at Moorfields (and therefore the amount of teaching and training available to them there) was necessarily much reduced. Furthermore, because the Trust had amongst its consultants by far the greatest proportion of specialist expertise in North Thames, all trainees were required, and in most cases wished to spend, as much of their available time as possible training at Moorfields.

The introduction of the Calman reforms, subsequently nicknamed 'calmanization', was indeed a defining event in the changing culture of the NHS and one that deserves fuller exploration and consideration (see Part 3). Suffice it to say here that from the trainers there came almost universal condemnation of the demise of the apprenticeship system so beloved by consultants of the past, while from the point of view of the trainees, there were, as in most things, gains to be made on the swings that balanced the losses on the roundabouts. Furthermore, although their effects were also blamed on Calman, it was the reduction in hours of work resulting from the Department of Health's 'New Deal' for junior doctors and the European Union's 'Directive on Working Hours' that further reduced 'hands-on' training opportunities, and amplified the problems associated with the shortened training period.

Research funding

In research, too, there was great turbulence, largely stemming from the government's growing preoccupation with cost-effectiveness and 'value for money'. During the late 1980s and early 1990s, due to the obsession with uncompromising scientific exclusivity, support for hospital-based research became more precarious, and laboratory-based research at the Institute, which attracted the highest grades (and thereby funding), became increasingly divorced from clinical application. In 1994 Professor Anthony Culyer was deputed to enquire into and report to the government on funding for clinical research throughout the NHS. His findings were disturbing. Much of the money provided was either being redirected by hospitals with shortfalls in their budgets to shore up patient services, or being used to support research of indifferent quality, with little evidence of benefit to healthcare, either present or future.

It was therefore decreed that in the future government funding for clinical research would be carefully monitored and that each hospital would receive an agreed annual sum, at first based on previous funding and thereafter on the basis of accurate information provided by the Director of Clinical Research in each institution. This allocation became known as 'Culyer' and the government expected that the sum of money granted annually in the Culyer exercise would be matched by research grants of 'soft' monies, awarded to research workers in each unit. When New Labour came to power in 1997, they proved to be just as concerned with getting value for money as their predecessors, if not more so. They recognized however, that support for clinical research required wider and less rigidly defined resources of material and manpower than that provided by full-time academics working in the laboratory, and renamed the funding 'Support for Science, Priorities and Needs'.

In 1996 the Trust decided to appoint its own Director of Research, to coordinate and direct clinical research throughout the hospital. Sadly, however, the first appointee to this post failed to live up to the part and, after a period of ill health, resigned. His place was eventually taken by Roger Hitchings, consultant surgeon and director of the Glaucoma Service, who had previously stood in as acting Director of Research prior to the department's formal recognition in 1998, and who subsequently performed with distinction in this complex and demanding position.

The cultural gap that developed between the Hospital and the Institute during this period was in large part a direct result of the government's research and development strategy, whereby funding of research was made conditional on a grading based on high-quality laboratory-based work, irrespective of its relevance to improvements in healthcare. As a result, there was now only a small handful of university-funded clinical academics at Moorfields, most clinical research being undertaken by Fellows and junior doctors, on 'soft' monies. In response to this unsatisfactory state of affairs, the Trust took the initiative by doing two things. The first of these was to appoint an increasing number of consultants to posts with several research sessions per week built into their contracts, fully funded by the Hospital, a measure enabled by 'pump-priming' monies from the Special Trustees. The second was for the Special Trustees, at the request of the Board of Directors, to provide £2m towards the building of Phase VIa of the new Institute, to provide shared space in which clinicians could undertake laboratory work. These measures attracted candidates with proven track records of commitment to top-quality research, to fill the new-style consultant posts, and it was confidently expected that constructive dialogue and mutual trust between the Hospital and the Institute would, as a result, be re-established.

Ever-increasing accountability

Perhaps the most striking change in the culture of the NHS, during the period after the election of New Labour in 1997, was the drive towards total accountability. While there was clear evidence of a move in this direction under the Conservative administration of John Major, with the publication in 1991 of the 'Patients' Charter', performance review and analysis during the latter half of the decade escalated beyond anything the medical profession could have imagined. As has been noted, less than a year after their election, the new government produced two papers, 'The New NHS – Modern, Dependable' and 'A First Class Service – Quality in the NHS', setting out their vision for the future. These included the creation of National Service Frameworks, Primary Care Groups, Health Action Zones and Health Improvement Programmes, the introduction of Clinical Governance, and a pro-gramme of lifelong learning for staff – all aimed at improving the quality of patient care and the degree of accountability in the NHS.

It was not long, however, before Frank Dobson, the first New Labour Secretary of State for Health, a populist, back-slapping 'man of the people', was replaced by Alan Milburn, altogether a different political animal, hard-headed and hard-hitting, with a confrontational style and only thinly veiled antipathy towards doctors. Furthermore, so alarmed was he by stories in the popular press of dirty hospitals, bed-shortages forcing patients to wait for hours or days on trolleys in A&E departments, and low morale amongst staff, that the Prime Minister himself intervened. Tony Blair announced his intention to bring annual spending on healthcare in the UK up to the same proportion of GDP as that spent by other EU states. Another White Paper soon followed, 'The NHS Plan – A Plan for Investment, A Plan for Reform', backed by a huge injection of much needed cash (£28bn over three years), which set out detailed plans for modernization that were to justify this investment. As the government's critics were quick to point out, however, the NHS had been so seriously under-funded (to the tune of some £267bn) over the course of the previous 20 years, that no amount of cash now could hope to solve its problems at a stroke.

A multitude of professional bodies designed to monitor and control the behaviour of the medical profession sprang up in the wake of disturbing reports in the popular press concerning poor performance and incompetence. Among these were the Commission for Health Improvement (CHI), the National Clinical Assessment Authority, the National Audit Commission, the NHS Modernisation Agency and the Clinical Negligence Scheme for Trusts, while, in an attempt to control costs (particularly of drugs), a watchdog – the National Institute for Clinical Excellence (NICE) – was created. Never had there been such a high level of political interference and control, and there was no sign that the tide of micromanagement would recede. In 2002 the NHS Reform and Health Care Professions Act expanded the remit of CHI, which was radically restructured (and retitled) to give it more sweeping powers, with a high-profile lawyer and ethicist, Sir Ian Kennedy, at its head, and the avowed intention of re-examining the roles and performance of NHS staff at all levels. No longer was it simply a watchdog – now called the Commission for Health-Care Audit and Inspection (CHAI), its aims were to rein in the medical profession and enforce strict guidelines in all aspects of clinical practice.

Because of its relatively small size and tradition of 'hands-on' management, Moorfields was peculiarly well placed to respond positively to such measures. The Turnberg Report on modernizing London's health services in 1998 had gone some way to boosting the morale of hospitals in London and was the trigger for Moorfields to launch its 'Moorfields Direct' helpline (see Part 2) and later the Patient Advice and Liaison Service (PALS). An inspection by CHI in 2002 was followed by a satisfactory report (they were particularly impressed by Clinical Governance and Risk Management procedures in the Trust, ably presented to them by the consultant in Public Health, Parul Desai). Performance indicators suggested that targets continued to be met satisfactorily and the Trust was well placed in the so-called 'league tables', with the award by the Department of Health in the summer of 2002 and again in 2003 of its highest (3★) rating.

Nevertheless, the constant scrutiny, with the thinly veiled threats that accompanied it, was not always productive, or good for morale. The effects of high-profile cases such as the Bristol heart surgery debacle and the highly publicised trial of the serial murderer Dr Harold

Shipman were felt keenly throughout the profession, and Moorfields was acutely aware of the dangers of complacency in its own affairs. Clinical governance and risk management were the watchwords of the day, and many hours were spent each week ensuring that they were rigorously applied throughout the Trust and its outreach satellites.

A more gracious interlude

In the midst of it all came the start of a new millennium, an event that the whole wide world, let alone Moorfields, felt moved to celebrate. Not only that, but the Hospital was taken up with a concatenation of events: the founding of the Royal London Ophthalmic Hospital's new building on City Road in 1898, its opening a year later, the millennial celebrations, and the bicentenary of the Hospital's foundation shortly thereafter. It was decided to mark the centenary of the opening of the Royal London Ophthalmic Hospital on City Road with a grand Open Day and to invite Moorfields' patron, Her Majesty the Queen, to visit and perform the ceremony. This she graciously did, on a miserably wet day in June 1999, attired in strawberry pink, bringing to the event a glorious air of radiance and colour that raised spirits all round. Speaking to the assembled company, she reminded them that her great grandfather and grandfather had respectively laid the foundation stone and opened the new premises on City Road. She could also have mentioned that she and her father and mother had all visited the Hospital at significant moments in its history and that royal patronage had made a long and important contribution to its pre-eminent position (see Volume II of this *History:* pp. 27, 235 and 236). A clock, fashioned in the shape of an eye, was commissioned and dedicated by Her Majesty to adorn the Hospital's façade (**Figure 18**, Plate 10), a commemorative plaque unveiled, and a beautifully illustrated com-memorative book was produced to mark the occasion. The entry into the 21st Century itself six months later was, as far as the Hospital was concerned, a more muted affair, national and international celebrations taking pride of place in everyone's affections.

The proposal to promote the best-performing Trusts to Foundation Hospitals, with increased freedom to manage their own affairs, first mooted in late 2002, was seized upon eagerly by Moorfields, its specialist nature and the high scores it had achieved in national tests of quality fitting it well for such special status. The Health and Social Care Bill, abolishing government control of NHS Trusts by turning them into competing independent corporations (Foundation Trusts), came before Parliament in the summer of 2003. Moorfields' application to become one of the first Foundation Hospitals was accepted in April

2004, although the furore that broke out amongst politicians of all complexions at the decision to create elitist institutions that might prosper at the expense of weaker ones threatened to derail the process. It certainly seemed likely that the freedom of action so readily promised initially for Foundation Hospitals would be so watered down in the final event that, while their obvious drawbacks remained, most of their apparent advantages would be lost. Nevertheless, the huge advantages of legally binding and enforceable contracts with commissioners of its services, together with the opportunity of greater freedom to borrow money (for instance, to underwrite the ICEC), still made the prospect of being awarded Foundation Hospital status particularly attractive to Moorfields.

There was little sign, however, that the national sense of insecurity and dissatisfaction would abate. Doubts about the medical profession's ability to regulate itself effectively were magnified and distorted by politicians and the media alike, with a view to 'bringing the doctors down a peg' or as a result of the commercial possibilities inherent in a good newspaper story or television scandal. It was an age when instant information, often wrongly or thinly researched and presented, was projected as the given truth and the medical profession was ill-prepared to cope with such distractions. Slogans from the very top of the political tree, such as Milburn's 'the NHS is a 1940s system operating in a 21st Century world', were not only untrue but deeply hurtful and insulting to NHS staff who had been struggling for years, with restricted resources, to keep British medicine at the forefront of scientific and cultural advance. Even the General Medical Council came under attack, and an over-arching public body, the Council for the Regulation of Healthcare Professionals, answerable only to the government, was established to control and manipulate the medical profession still further. Significantly perhaps, while CHAI was to be headed by a lawyer, a senior policeman was appointed to lead this new body – it seemed that the medical profession was heading for both arrest and prosecution.

Not content with attempts to cut waiting times by setting up the London Patient Choice Project (LPCP) with Diagnostic Treatment Centres (DTCs) to utilize spare capacity within the NHS, the Government decided to woo the electorate by sending patients abroad for treatment when this was not readily available in the UK. Furthermore, they set about employing surgeons from outside the UK, including some from the USA, to carry out waiting-list initiatives and undertake cataract surgery in the UK. Moorfields saw the need to remain ever vigilant and to maintain the high standards of care that it had set and achieved so far. The Trust worked with the LPCP to open DTCs at St Ann's Hospital Tottenham and St George's Hospital Tooting. This was a necessary step to protect the Hospital against the threat delivered to other eye units by independent DTCs that were being set up in other parts of the country. Likewise, the appointment of architects and preparation of plans for the proposed International Children's Eye Centre, in 2003, was an important step towards strengthening the Trust's paediatric base, in the face of increasing pressure to isolate paediatric care from that of adults. In other areas too, the Hospital sought to tighten its grip, including the appointment of a consultant in medical retina to supervise screening for diabetic eye disease, in line with the criteria demanded by the National Service Framework.

With the appointments of both a new Medical Director and a new Director of Nursing in 2002, Moorfields saw the need to espouse the National Eye-Care Plan, especially in the direction of patient-focused initiatives, by modifying patient-care pathways to reduce waiting times and delays inherent in some of the established procedures at the Hospital. To this end, the newly appointed Medical Director, Bill Aylward, and Director of Nursing and Development, Sarah Fisher, produced a joint plan to move the clinical services away from procedures centred on the function of professional groups, towards those that were of direct benefit to patients. They also saw the need to participate actively in the London Strategy for Eye-care, although the Trust's vision of this was not always widely shared by other units in London. Nevertheless, a new generation of movers and shakers had taken the helm and, as had happened so often before, saw the need for the Hospital to set a different course if it was to pursue its destiny with success.

A view from the past

It may be helpful at this point to step back and take a look at Moorfields in 2004, to see how it compares with what an aspiring young ophthalmologist found in 1967, the year in which the present author first entered its hallowed portals. As can be seen from photographs of the time, the exterior appearance of the City Road branch has not greatly changed, because its façade has been preserved and there is little room on its City Road aspect for expansion. The island site as a whole has, however, undergone radical redevelopment, with the building of the new operating theatres, out-patient facilities, Professorial Unit and School of Nursing, the relocation of the Institute of Ophthalmology and the conversion of Peabody Buildings to Fryer House (now soon to be the International Children's Eye Centre). It is within the hospital building that the real changes are to be found, however – not only structurally, but in every aspect of its activity. Nor should we forget that the Hospital at City Road is now the hub of an institution providing eye-care London-wide.

When the author first walked into the City Road branch of the Hospital in the autumn of 1967, there was a large front hall and waiting area, in which stood a desk with a signing-in book for visiting medical staff below the rank of consultant. Much of this space has since been eroded for use as office space, but the fabric has been nicely refurbished and it is generally brighter and more comfortable. In 1967 two ladies, Maureen (Hamilton-Smith) and Mona (Farrell), worked in a small back office and 'were' Medical Staffing, while Wendy Meade struggled with the administrative burden of the Medical Committee, under mountains of paperwork in equally cramped conditions. The out-patient clinics were divided between the old and the new, the former being open-plan and the latter with cubicles. Each consultant had two outpatient clinics weekly: Monday and Thursday, Tuesday and Friday or Wednesday and Saturday. Special clinics were a novelty, and apart from Fison's Retinal Clinic at City Road and Hudson's at High Holborn, and Miller's Glaucoma Clinic there, were exclusively the province of Barrie Jones' Professorial Unit. The operating theatres were still on the second floor, at the front of the Hospital, and were an antiquated relic of the past, but the new suite was in the process of construction.

The High Holborn branch of the Hospital, although housed in a more modern building than the Hospital at City Road (see **Figure 1**, Plate 1), functioned in a similar fashion. The building itself comprised eight floors above ground, as well as a basement below it, but its overall area was severely restricted by its location between adjacent buildings. A friendly atmosphere prevailed. There were six consultants, six Residents, brand new operating theatres were under construction on the eighth floor and it was a flourishing institution of its own. An argon laser was installed in 1970, and Tim Ffytche started a fluorescein fundus angiography service. In 1973 Professor Hill's Retinal Unit moved there from the Royal Eye Hospital. Miss Mostyn kept the medical staff in order and worked from an altogether more prepossessing and spacious office than that granted to the ladies in Medical Staffing at City Road. The hospital closed in July 1988 and the original building was pulled down to make way for a more modern one, so that now there is nothing in High Holborn to show that it ever existed.

In 1967 cataract surgery had only recently changed from extra-capsular to intracapsular, silk sutures were used to close the wound and iris prolapse was a not uncommon complication, necessitating further surgery. The postoperative in-patient stay was commonly 10 days or longer. Cataract extraction was usually delayed until the visual acuity in the better eye fell to 6/18. Postoperatively, patients were issued with temporary spectacles and, about two months later, were refracted and given their definitive prescription. This was usually high (+10.00 or +12.00 dioptres) and the lenses were thick, making the glasses heavy, unsightly and uncomfortable. Cystoid macular oedema, resulting from disturbance of the vitreous dynamics, occurred postoperatively in as many as a third of cases, often precluding recovery of good visual acuity.

There were more than 300 beds at the two branches, and no day-surgery unit or hostel at either. Wards and accommodation for nursing staff occupied most of the available space on the upper floors. The ground floor at City Road was almost entirely given over to out-patient clinics and a huge open waiting area. There was no information desk, shop or cafeteria. There were high ceilings and no fire doors. Secretaries shared a large space known as the 'goldfish bowl' and there were no computers (or even electric typewriters). Most of the clinics were open-plan in design, with tall desks at which doctors and patients (two of each to a desk) stood for consultation (**Figure 19**). There was no privacy. Dark rooms housing slit-lamps ran along the back of the

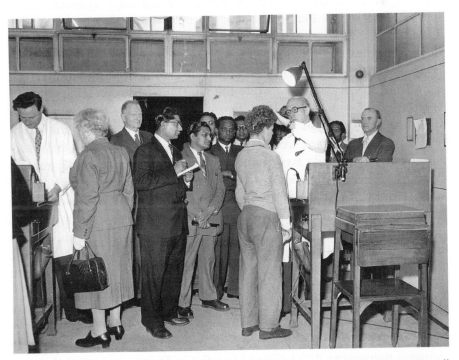

Figure 19 In the old style of out-patient clinic, doctors and patients alike stood at tall desks during consultations. There was little privacy or opportunity for personal discussion.

clinics. Many of the slit-lamps were antiquated (the Haag-Streit 900 was only just coming in). Refraction was frequently done on the spot, by out-patient officers, in the refraction 'boxes'. The basement housed the old air-raid shelters, stores and some other non-clinical services. You could park your bicycle there.

There was no such thing as a Primary Care Clinic, nor was there a Retinal Diagnostic, Electrodiagnostic or Ultrasound Department. Lasers, phacoemulsification, small-incision surgery, adjustable sutures, botulinum toxin, vitrectomy and refractive surgery, in common with much else, had not been heard of. Implant surgery had been tried and abandoned. Silicone oil was used only by John Scott, in Cambridge. Treatment of chronic simple glaucoma (now termed primary open angle glaucoma) consisted of pilocarpine, Eppy (adrenaline) and eserine drops and oral Diamox. Idoxuridine (IDU) ointment for herpetic keratitis was new. Oculoplastics was as yet an unrecognized specialty. Trabeculectomy was the talk of the town. Xenon-arc photo-coagulation and cryotherapy were new and exciting innovations. HIV infection did not exist (or if it did, no-one knew about it). Almost all operations were done under general anaesthetic. Retrobulbar injection was the only effective means of administering local anaesthesia for intraocular surgery. Halothane was the new wonder agent for general anaesthesia. Giant jars containing leeches still lined shelves on the walls of the pharmacy.

The nursing staff of 1967 wore smart green uniforms with crisply starched aprons and caps, while the Matron, Miss MacKellar, was a towering and much respected figure, held in awe, both within the Hospital and throughout the ophthalmic nursing community. The majority of the nurses worked on the wards, which were of the old-fashioned Nightingale type, with masked windows to reduce ambient light. Their roles were very different from those of today and their appearance reflected this (**Figure 20**, Plate 10). They performed basic nursing duties and minor ophthalmic ones, such as instilling drops, irrigating the conjunctival sac and syringing lacrimal canaliculi, but few of the sophisticated procedures carried out by nurses today. There were no nurse-practitioners. The notion of calling Matron by her first name would have called for mental certification.

One need only look at the staff numbers, bed occupancy and activity statistics to see how much things have changed during the past 35 years. In 1967, taking both branches together with the Highgate Annexe, there were 310 beds at Moorfields. In the year 2000 the total was 80. In 1967 there were 7400 discharges, while in the year 2000 a total of 18 500 operations was undertaken – two and a half times the number of procedures from a quarter of the beds, or 10 times the surgical activity per bed. The Hospital, its outreach units and staff are all today geared to rapid patient turnover.

Surprisingly, overall nursing numbers have only risen by about 30% during this period – an indication of the increased intensity of work and multifarious nature of the tasks undertaken by today's nurses. Their skills have shifted away from those of the bedside nurse towards more technical activities, including pre-assessment of cataract patients and the many tasks that modern ophthalmology demands, such as biometry, tonometry and detailed clinical assessment, while operating theatre duties may even involve them in minor surgical procedures. Each specialist Clinical Service at Moorfields now has a senior nursing sister as part of the clinical team, with specialized knowledge and skills in its particular field. Their pay and conditions are better and the work is more interesting, but it is more intensive, with higher levels of responsibility and stress.

Appointment to the Resident (formally titled Resident Surgical Officer) training programme in 1967 was a more personal affair than it is today – one's 'face had to fit' to be successful, and personal knowledge of and by the consultants was important.

The present author had no powerful connections (and a not very attractive face!) so he had to apply five times (twice at High Holborn) before he was finally successful in getting on to 'the House' at City Road.

At the High Holborn branch, the criteria for selection were different from those at City Road. It was generally reckoned to be more 'civilized' at Holborn and purely scientific prowess was not deemed sufficient, so that it tended to attract candidates with wider interests than those at City Road. Once 'on the House', residents at City Road felt obliged to compete with others appointed at the same time, while at High Holborn, appointments were made singly, so that competition between contemporaries was impossible and the atmosphere was in consequence less highly charged. Once 'on the House' at one or other branch, Residents stayed at that branch alone, there being little or no intermingling or overlap between the two; indeed there was always some degree of rivalry between them.

As a result of the Clinical Professor's origins, there was throughout the 1970s a disproportionately large number of New Zealanders on the training programme at both branches. Together with others who came as Fellows, the present author was blessed throughout his career with knowing more

ophthalmologists, pro rata, from that country than any other, some of them,
like Philip Boulton, remaining firm friends for a lifetime.

In 1967 there was no Director of Education, no Training Prospectus,
no Clinical Tutorial Complex, and no Skills Laboratory. The residency
programme was for a fixed period of three years. Unlike today, when
Specialist Registrars (SpRs) spend five years in the North Thames
training programme, of which only two are spent at Moorfields, the
entire three years was spent at the Hospital. After two years in the
registrar grade, Residents were automatically upgraded to Senior
Registrar, without any formal test or interview, provided that (as was
almost invariably the case) the consultants supported this promotion.
At the end of the three-year period of training, Moorfields trainees were
judged to be competent to enter independent practice, and it was not
uncommon for a trainee to leave 'the House' and obtain a consultant
post at another hospital, without undergoing further training.
Paradoxically, this bears some striking similarities with the situation
today, following 'Calmanization': today's higher specialist trainees,
once appointed to SpR posts, have no need to compete for more senior
positions and are judged competent to become consultants, provided
that they pass through all their RITA assessments satisfactorily, a
process which relies heavily on the opinions of their consultant trainers.

Clinical research at Moorfields in 1967 was still in its formative years.
There was no Department of Research and Development and there
were no 50/50 clinical/research consultant posts. Barrie Jones had been
in the Chair of Clinical Ophthalmology for only four years, and his
department on the second floor at City Road was small and cramped.
He had nevertheless already attracted a number of clever and ambitious
young men to his department, as lecturers and senior lecturers, to work
jointly in the laboratory and the special clinics that were developing in
several fields as a result of his pioneering work. At the Institute in Judd
Street they and other aspiring academics and clinicians were also busy,
but it would be several years before the development of the new,
expanded Clinical Department at City Road (1973) and many more
years before the opening of the Department of Preventive
Ophthalmology (1981) and finally (1991) the transfer of the entire
Institute of Ophthalmology to its present building on the island site.

Governmental control in 1967 was light, and Moorfields and its
consultants were largely autonomous, while patients were, for the most
part, compliant and accepting. (Ironically, in spite of all the medical
advances and the greater degree of respect for their wishes and feelings,
they seemed to be happier with their lot and to complain less than is the

case today.) The enormous cultural change that has taken place amongst hospital staff is well illustrated by the change in dining arrangements. In 1967 there were three separate dining-rooms: one for the Consultants, one for the Residents and one for 'the rest'; now there is just one dining room for staff and anyone else who chooses to eat there. For the medical staff, there were no watchdog bodies other than the General Medical Council and the Medical Royal Colleges. Standards were one's own. Professional pride and respect were strongly felt and were sacrosanct. European influences were negligible, Postgraduate Medical Deans of little consequence, and most clinical research was ad hoc.

There were 18 consultants at Moorfields in the early 1960s. The Hospital is now staffed by specialists and there are more than 60 members of the consultant staff, many of them, unlike 40 years ago, female (**Figure 21**). There are 65 SpRs on the North Thames training programme, compared with 18 Residents, almost all of whom were male.

Indeed, the only female Resident ever to be appointed to the High Holborn branch of Moorfields, Marion Handscombe, explained to the present author that she was only appointed as a result of a complaint made by one

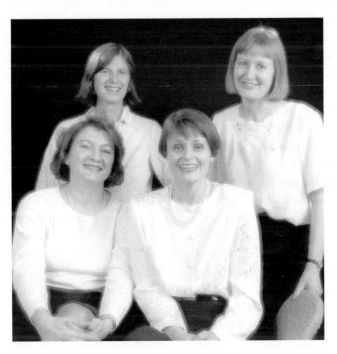

Figure 21   The 1980s saw the first of an increasing number of women appointed to the consultant surgical staff of the Hospital. Pictured here are the first four such appointees: *Clockwise from top left:* Miss Linda Ficker, Miss Wendy Franks, Miss Gillian Adams and Miss Michele Beaconsfield.

of her female colleagues about the openly chauvinist nature of the
advertisement for Resident posts at the High Holborn branch of Moorfields.

In the space of 40 years ophthalmology has grown into a highly
sophisticated specialty and in the developed world the truly general
ophthalmologist rarely exists. Increasing specialization is the price paid
for constant advances in knowledge, technology and expertise, and
changes in standards and expectations. The short comparative
description given here goes some way to show how great have been the
changes during the past 40 years. Moorfields and the Institute of
Ophthalmology have managed to keep pace with them, and must
continue to do so if they are to survive as independent institutions.

Moorfields in the future

As one looks North across City Road in the New Year of 2004, to the
new building housing the pharmacy manufacturing unit (see Part 4),
South to the site of the International Children's Eye Centre (see Part 3
and **Figure 50**, Plate 26) and more widely across London to the
Community Outreach Units, it is clear that the future of Moorfields is
going to be no less exciting and challenging during the next 40 years,
than it has been during the past 40. In spite of all attempts by the forces
of bureaucracy to stifle innovation and initiative in the name of safety
and quality control, today's Board of Directors, with their management
and staff, continue with vision and enterprise to plot the best course
onward. Some things on the horizon seem clear, while others remain
difficult to define. The steady increase in skills-base and autonomy, and
of nurse-practitioners working to strict protocols, combined with the
unremitting progress of high-technology medicine, seem set to continue. Increasing empowerment of patients is unstoppable (in spite of
the government's decision, after 30 years, to scrap the patients' watch-
dogs, the Community Health Councils). So is the trend towards more
community-based eye-care. The future of Foundation Hospitals is less
certain.

As long as Moorfields remains true to its ideals and, together with
the Institute, remains at the centre of clinical innovation, teaching and
research, the outlook appears bright. Wider involvement in the running
of the Hospital by a Board that is broadly representative of the local
community, in tune with the philosophy of Foundation Trusts, could
restrict the Hospital's freedom of choice and muddy the waters, rather
than smooth its passage. This and other issues surrounding the future
of the NHS are foremost in the path of the Trust as this history goes to
press, while the controversy surrounding the recent rejection (2003) of

the consultant contract and the reluctance of the Secretary of State (now John Reid instead of Alan Milburn) to renegotiate it, has fuelled mistrust between the Department of Health and the consultants. Just as in 1975, when the then Health Secretary, Barbara Castle, almost capsized the vessel and drowned its crew, Moorfields righted itself to battle through the waves and sail on regardless, so it must now be prepared to do so again, for the wind of change is unlikely to abate and the storm of progress is even less likely to die away.

PART 2

The Clinical, Nursing and Clinical Support Services

CHAPTER 2

Clinical Services

Background

Profound and far-reaching changes in clinical practice have taken place during the last four decades in every branch of medicine. In ophthalmology not only are these manifest in the way in which doctors, nurses, other healthcare professionals and their patients think and behave, but also in an explosion of technology that has raised everyone's hopes and expectations. Improvements in the management of eye disorders, both medical and surgical, have led in most instances to greater numbers of patients receiving treatment, while the speed of recovery from surgery and the increasingly sophisticated nature of interventions have reduced the need to stay in hospital. It follows that surgeons have had to become highly skilled superspecialists, and nurses to become specialist nurse-practitioners, based not on wards but in primary-care and pre-assessment clinics, while a host of expert paramedical technicians has emerged to provide technical back-up. All this has had to be achieved within much the same budgetary restrictions that have prevailed throughout the NHS since soon after its inception. For, while its most ardent protagonist, Aneurin Bevan, at first believed that a free health service would mean better health for all with a commensurate fall in demand, it soon became obvious that demand was insatiable and that, without strict budgetary controls, costs would spiral upwards.

One consequence of this new world has been the relentless erosion of medical traditions, such as the spotless, highly polished floors, neatly ordered rows of perfectly made beds, and the starched caps, cuffs and aprons of the nursing staff, so beloved of those with cherished and romantic memories of the past, and their replacement with the high-tech (but expensive) tools of modern medicine. It is a strange anomaly that changes in practice brought about by the enormous improvements in diagnostic and therapeutic methods during the last 40 years are often seen, by patients and staff alike, only as part of the sad demise of the 'good old days'.

The change in culture at Moorfields was spearheaded in the 1960s and 1970s by Professor Barrie Jones, who established the concept of subspecialization, thereby setting a new pattern for the entire hospital. Nor was this revolution confined to the Professor's own chief interests, in external eye disease and disorders of the adnexal tissues. Not only did he, with Lorimer Fison's support, encourage new developments in the treatment of diseases of the posterior segment, but he also introduced the Hospital to intraocular microsurgery.

Fluorescein angiography and laser photocoagulation, introduced in the late 1960s, led to the development of the Retinal Diagnostic Department, started by Alan Bird in 1970 at the City Road branch. This burgeoning new clinical service, at first housed in a corridor of the Professorial Unit, with one slit-lamp, two fundus cameras and three stools, soon found a home on the second floor, previously occupied by the operating theatres, but grew so rapidly, such was the demand for its services, that it was forced to move after a few years to a larger area that became vacant on the closure of one of the wards. Similarly, the electrodiagnostic service expanded rapidly and required more space, as did new diagnostic methods such as ultrasound – a pattern that was to become a familiar one from then onwards, as in-patient services contracted, technology advanced and out-patient facilities expanded, and in the 1990s as the provision of day-care facilities mushroomed.

Because of the limited opportunities for expansion beyond the Hospital's existing boundaries, to accommodate the constantly changing pattern of ophthalmic practice, there was, throughout the 1970s and 1980s, prior to and alongside the redevelopment of the City Road branch, a gradual, amoeba-like shift of new facilities into spaces that became vacant through the redundancy of others. At High Holborn these changes were less dramatic, first because there was less incentive, as it was a smaller unit with fewer consultants, and secondly because its projected closure precluded on practical, economic grounds expensive reorganisation. Nevertheless, the provision there of new operating theatres, with operating microscopes, soon brought in microsurgical practices, while Tim Ffytche established a retinal diagnostic facility in 1970, and, with the transfer of Professor David Hill's department from the Royal Eye Hospital in 1973 and the installation of an argon laser, this aspect of the service was considerably strengthened.

Provision of modern out-patient clinics, operating theatres and other facilities was always a priority of the Board of Governors, new theatres of the very latest modular design being built at both branches in 1968, courtesy of the Hayward Foundation and the Department of Health, with four more at City Road, together with new out-patient clinics,

Plate 1

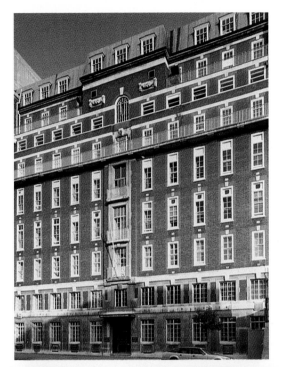

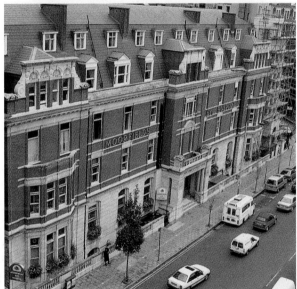

Figure 1 *Top*: The Royal Westminster Eye Hospital building in High Holborn, opened in 1916, and amalgamated with the Royal London Ophthalmic and Central London Ophthalmic Hospitals, in 1946, as a branch of the 'Moorfields, Westminster and Central Eye Hospital'. (The building was closed in 1988, when the Hospital merged on the City Road site, and was subsequently demolished for commercial redevelopment.) *Bottom*: The Royal London Ophthalmic Hospital building in City Road, opened by the Duke of York (later King George V) in 1899, now Moorfields Eye Hospital NHS Trust.

Plate 2

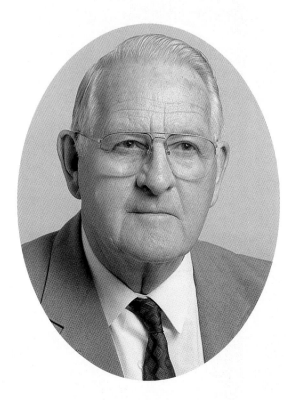

Figure 3 Professor Barrie Russell Jones CBE, first Professor of Clinical Ophthalmology (1963) and Director of the Department of Clinical Ophthalmology, Institute of Ophthalmology, University of London. In 1981 Barrie Jones founded the International Centre for Eye Health, Department of Preventive Ophthalmology, at the Institute of Ophthalmology, and was its Head until his retirement in 1986.

Born and trained in medicine in New Zealand, he came to England in 1951 and remained here until 2002, when he finally returned home. This volume of the Moorfields History is dedicated to him, recognising that he was the principal architect of the Hospital's conversion to modern methods of ophthalmology, and thereby of its continued prosperity.

Plate 3

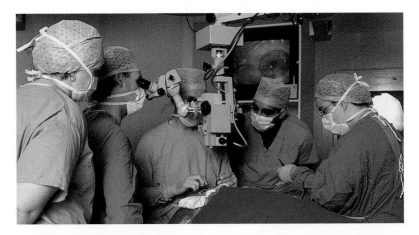

Figure 4 The introduction of the operating microscope was fundamental to progress in the surgery of cataract and most other forms of eye surgery.

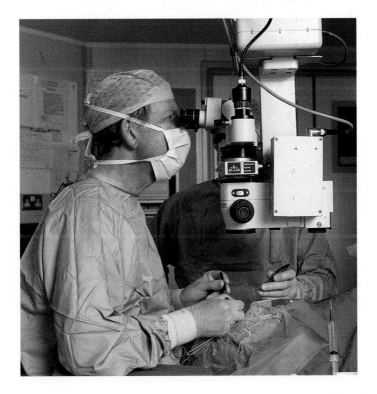

Figure 5 Closed intraocular microsurgery for the treatment of complicated surgical conditions of the posterior segment of the eye was enabled by the introduction of vitrectomy instrumentation at Moorfields in 1974.

Plate 4

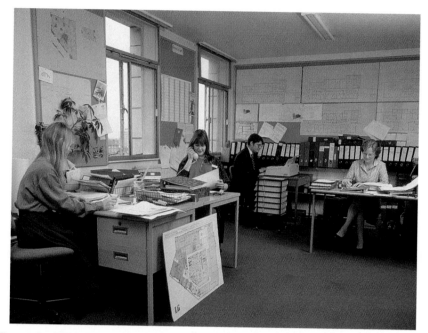

Figure 9 The team in the planning office was indispensable to the redevelopment project. (See p. 24.)

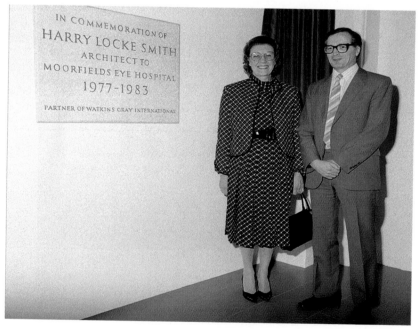

Figure 10 Mrs Locke-Smith pictured with Mr John Atwill at the unveiling of the plaque commemorating her late husband's contribution to the Hospital's redevelopment. (See p. 24.)

Plate 5

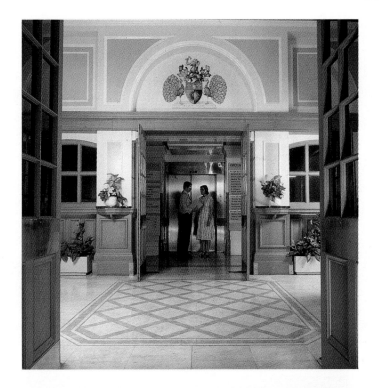

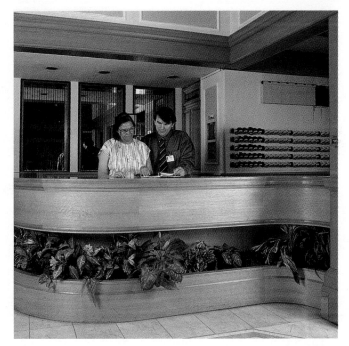

Figure 12   The Front Entrance (*top*) and Front Desk of the Hospital (*bottom*), as they appeared after refurbishment.

Plate 6

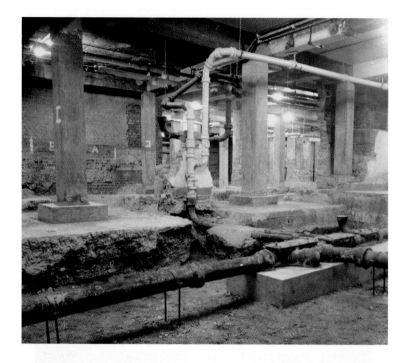

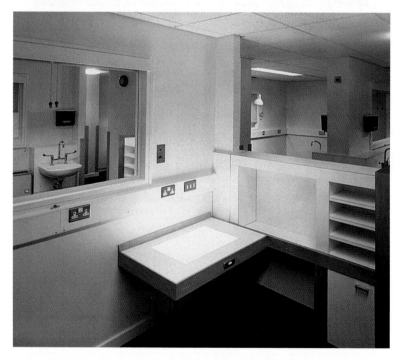

Figure 13 The basement of the Hospital at City Road, as it was during redevelopment (*top*). One of the new clinics on the lower ground floor, following its refurbishment as a clinical area (*bottom*).

Plate 7

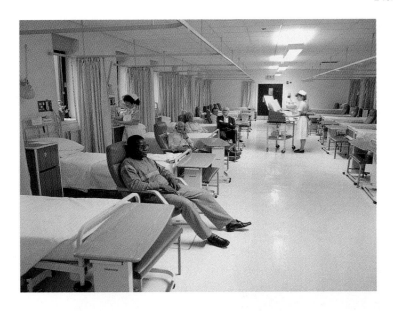

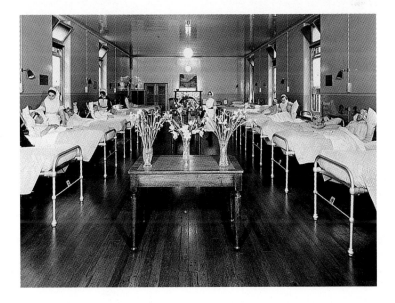

Figure 14 The appearance of a ward following the redevelopment of the Hospital during the 1980s (*top*). An old-fashioned ward (*bottom*).

Plate 8

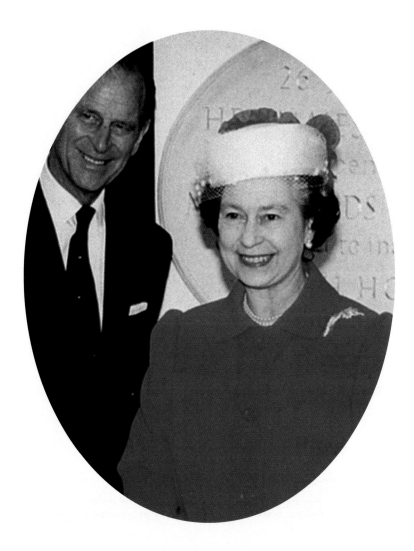

Figure 15   Her Majesty Queen Elizabeth II and HRH The Duke of Edinburgh visited the Hospital on the occasion of the formal opening of the newly developed building, on 26 October 1988. They are seen here after Her Majesty had unveiled a commemorative plaque.

Plate 9

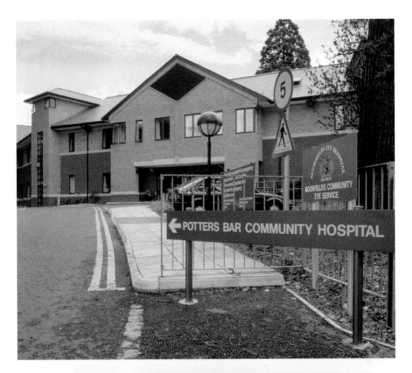

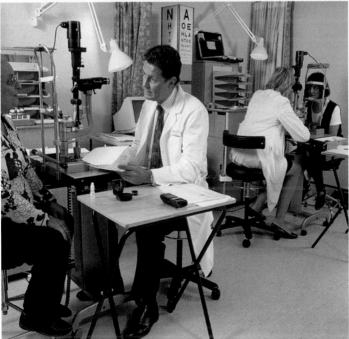

Figure 16 Outreach Community Eye Units were opened throughout the 1990s. Pictured here is the unit at Potters Bar. The Director of Primary-Care Services at Moorfields, Rhodri Daniel, is seen in the foreground.

Plate 10

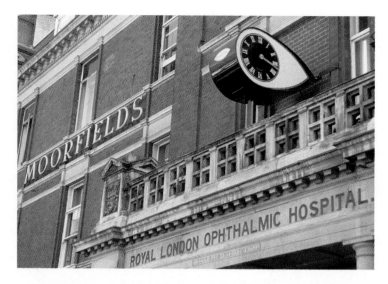

Figure 18   The Moorfields clock, erected to mark the centenary of the Hospital on the City Road site, and dedicated by Her Majesty the Queen at a ceremony on 23 June 1999.

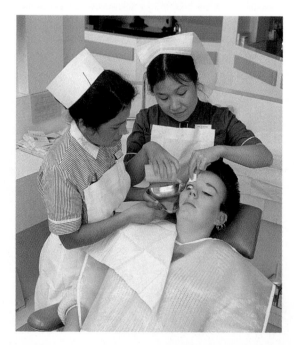

Figure 20   Nursing has seen huge changes. The Sister and nurse pictured here undertaking an irrigation procedure are dressed in traditional, old-style uniforms. Moorfields nurses now wear blue and white tunics, commonly with matching blue trousers. They acquire a wider knowledge of ophthalmology and are trained to perform many procedures previously considered to be the prerogative of doctors. (See p. 66.)

Plate 11

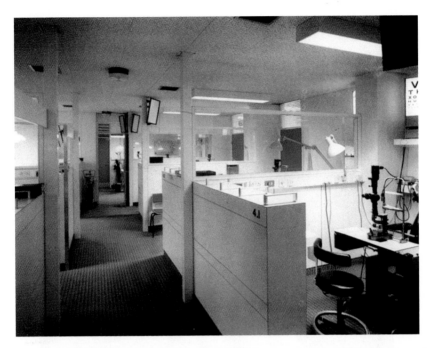

Figure 22   The prototype clinic (the Red Clinic) was set up in 1978 to explore the possibilities for modernizing the clinics throughout the Hospital. This clinic incorporated many new ideas, including half-glass partitions dividing the clinical space into cubicles. Equipment was provided, on a trial basis, by a number of optical instrument suppliers. The scheme was a resounding success and laid the foundations for the future redevelopment of all the out-patient clinics.

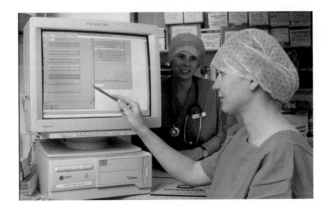

Figure 23   Introduction of a computerized administrative system in the operating theatres, seen here in use, transformed the organization of operating schedules throughout the Trust and facilitated the tracking and identification of instruments used in a given case. (See p. 79.)

Plate 12

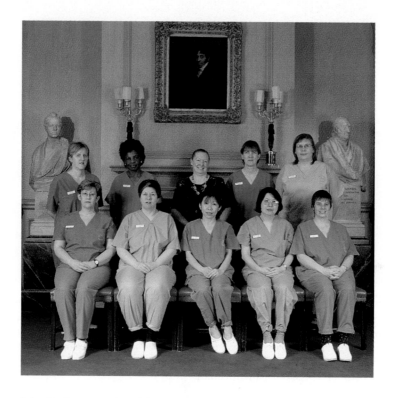

Figure 24 Senior operating theatre nursing staff at the start of the new millennium (2000). Seated, left to right: Miss Debbie Green, Miss Natalija Mihalovic, Mrs Joyce Morrin (Nursing Superintendent), Miss Poh Heoh Theam and Mrs Siobhan Taylor. Standing, left to right: Miss Carmel King, Mrs Rhoda Ubani, Mrs Linda Mepham (formerly Nursing Superintendent), Miss Lyn Marsh and Miss Jane Knowles.

Plate 13

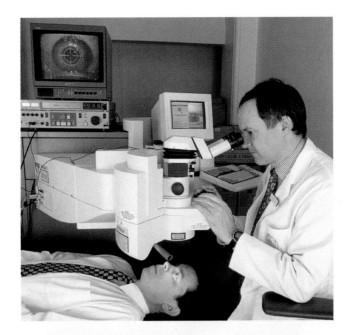

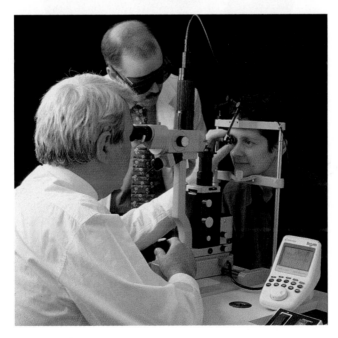

Figure 25 *Top*: Photorefractive surgery was introduced at Moorfields in the late 1980s. LASIK (laser intrastromal keratectomy) using an excimer laser, as pictured here, did not come in until the latter half of the 1990s. *Bottom*: The argon laser came into use at Moorfields in the late 1960s, and was from then on employed with increasing frequency for the treatment of disorders affecting the retinal vasculature and some types of tapetoretinal degenerative disease.

Plate 14

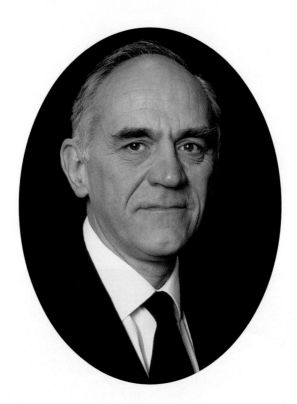

Figure 27 Professor Alan C Bird, first Director of the Retinal Diagnostic Department (RDD) and recognized as one of the foremost world authorities on medical retinal disorders and genetically determined eye disease. He trained at the High Holborn branch of Moorfields before undertaking a Visiting Fellowship at the Bascom Palmer Eye Institute in Miami.

Plate 15

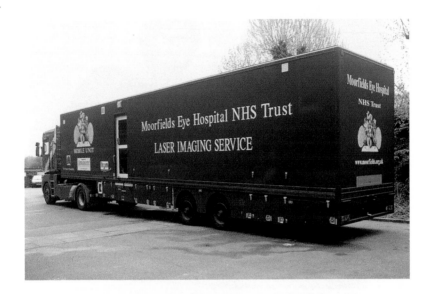

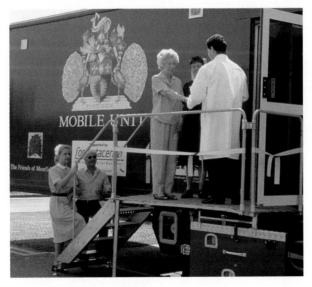

Figure 28   The Mobile Unit was an enterprising innovation, but proved to be less useful than was at first envisaged. Its large size and limited manoeuvrability, together with a capacity for the disruption of sensitive medical equipment, limited its usefulness. (See p. 134.)

Plate 16

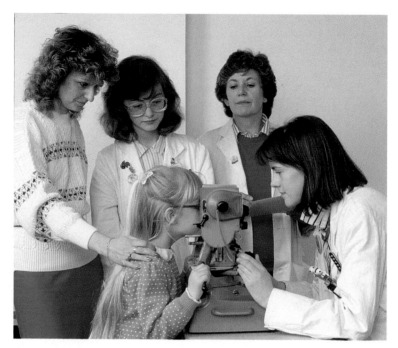

Figure 29 Mrs Ann McIntyre (*standing, right*), Head of the Orthoptic Department, pictured teaching student orthoptists in the department at City Road.

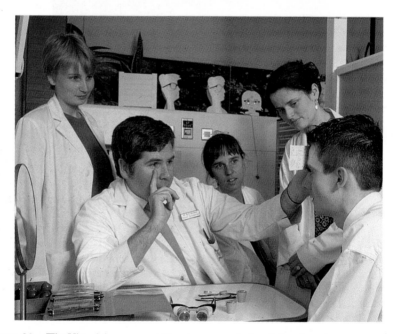

Figure 30 The Visual Assessment Service expanded and developed enormously during the 1980s and 1990s, playing a vital part in supporting the Hospital's clinical activities.

during its refurbishment, prior to amalgamation. The old style of out-patient clinic, with tall desks at which doctors and patients stood during consultations, was finally abandoned at City Road, in favour of cubicles with half-glass screens. This followed an ingenious and novel trial period in 1978–79, during which a prototype clinic (the Red Clinic) was established and equipped (cost-free to Moorfields) by a number of different instrument manufacturers, to test out the best format (**Figure 22**, Plate 11). At High Holborn, the out-patient clinics had, in any case, been designed on a more modern plan and did not require such extensive modification.

Similar updating of the fabric at City Road took place on the first and second floors, with new consulting rooms for Residents and the gradual replacement of wards throughout the 1970s and 1980s, to accommodate expanding out-patient clinical services, notably the Retinal Diagnostic and Electrodiagnostic Departments, and the expansion of the Professorial Unit. Meanwhile, the lower ground floor was re-modelled as part of Phase I of the redevelopment, and opened in 1986, to accommodate, amongst many other things, modern out-patient facilities, including the definitive home for the Retinal Diagnostic Department with its concomitant Department of Medical Illustration, both of which had already outgrown their previous accommodation.

Operating theatres

It says much for the excellence of their design and the quality of their construction that the operating theatres at City Road had, up to the time of writing, undergone only relatively minor changes since their construction. The original theatres at both branches were replaced in 1968 by the latest modular design, two at High Holborn and four at City Road, and inaugurated by Her Majesty Queen Elizabeth the Queen Mother (see Volume II of this *History*, p.235). In 1986 a further four theatres, very similar in design, were added to the existing suite at City Road, in anticipation of the amalgamation. The two theatres at Holborn were situated on the top (eighth) floor, offering surgeons the pleasant reward of commanding views over London while scrubbing up. Both were equipped with ceiling-mounted operating microscopes, which were transferred to the theatres at City Road when the hospital closed.

In the City Road suite there was a large recovery bay, nursing administration office and small anaesthetic office, together with men's and women's changing rooms and a small laboratory for the Pocklington corneal transplant unit. Part of the recovery area was originally divided off for use as a light coagulation room, housing the 'jumbo' xenon arc light coagulator. Later, when that instrument became obsolete, this became an office and then a storeroom. The theatre suite also housed the Eye-Bank and, from 1981, the Pocklington Research Laboratory after its transfer from the Institute to City Road.

Even though operating microscopes were available, either ceiling- or floor-mounted, for use in all the theatres, some surgeons were slow to take advantage of this new technology and loupes were at first still in common use. Nevertheless, in due course of time microsurgery took over, as younger surgeons were appointed who had been brought up to use the operating microscope. Likewise, needles threaded with silk were replaced by monofilament nylon and disposables became the norm, so that the late evening nursing staff were no longer required to sit washing instruments and threading needles into the small hours of the night. More and more machinery appeared, and scrub nurses handpicked by the surgeon for their manual dexterity and skill at reflecting the corneal flap were no longer in such great demand. Even so, it was not until the early 1980s that the last Graefe section was performed and still, up until the late 1980s, general anaesthesia was used for almost every surgical case.

At the High Holborn branch, until the early 1980s, Charlie Smith ruled the theatres (most of the Hospital, in fact) and taught generations of porters and young surgeons the tricks of their trade, including Graham Nunn, who subsequently went on to become the vitreoretinal technician at City Road, and Frank Zinsa, who became an operating department assistant there. At City Road, Charlie Whipp, who joined in 1939, played a similar role, although his influence did not extend so far outside the theatres, while Sister Watkins ruled the roost there (see **Figure 45**, p. 212), followed over the years by Linda Mepham, Susan Humphreys and Joyce Morrin. Talking to the present author, Joyce Morrin recalled that when she first arrived, in 1982, things were very different from today. Much of the sterilization was done in the theatres, each one having its own 'little sister' sterilizer, the instruments being washed by hand, sterilized then and there, and re-used for each subsequent case. When the additional theatres were opened in 1986, a Theatre Sterile Supply Unit (TSSU) was opened at the far end of the suite. In 1992, however, a fire broke out in this unit during the course of one weekend, causing serious damage and rendering it unusable for several months, with the happy result that many instruments were replaced with more modern ones, at the Department of Health's expense.

The resurgence of Creutzfeld–Jacob Disease (CJD) in the 1990s, caused an enormous change in practice. Department of Health regulations forbade the re-use of many instruments and devices that could not be guaranteed free of all contamination by normal methods of sterilisation, so disposables were increasingly used. Furthermore, in order to be able to track down any possible source of infection should this occur, the clinical path of any device used more than once was required to be clearly traceable. This was at first achieved using stickers, but was never easy, especially as only half the equipment could be accommodated in the TSSU, the other half having to be sterilized in the Central Sterile Supply Unit (CSSU) in the basement. In 2002 an inspection by the NHS Estates Department threatened closure of the theatres if this deficiency was not corrected within one week, thereby precipitating a rapid purchase of extra equipment and the refurbishment of the CSSU, so that all sterilization could be accommodated there. Necessity being the mother of invention, this near miracle was somehow achieved by the deadline and the operating schedule was unaffected. The subsequent introduction of the Galaxy (Sanderson Ltd) software system into the theatre complex in 1997 greatly improved the capability of tracing instruments, as they were from then on tagged electronically (**Figure 23**, Plate 11). Operated by Gary Coplen, this computerized management system was soon extended to the operating theatres at the outreach units, enormously simplifying coordination of operating lists throughout the Trust.

Increasingly intense operating schedules (14 000 operations a year compared with 7000 twenty years before), speed of surgery and the increase in private work at Moorfields all had marked effects. In 1982 there was a complement of 38 nurses, 10 of them at the Holborn branch. In 2003 there were 101 nurses in the theatres at City Road. Formerly, when almost all patients arrived in the theatres on trolleys, cohorts of 'outside' and 'inside' porters were required, to bring them from the wards, take them into the theatres and put them on the operating tables, and then to take them to the recovery bay and later back to the wards. With day-case surgery under local anaesthesia, this all changed, many patients walking into theatre in their ordinary clothes and walking out again after the operation. Porters were no longer needed to fetch the majority of patients, and the system of 'inside' and 'outside' porters became redundant. So, while the complement of nurses increased, the numbers of porters decreased. Furthermore, the numbers of patients recovering from operations at any one time, and the speed at which they did so, bespoke a much larger recovery area, with more staff. Some portering staff saw these changes as an opportunity and went on to train and take examinations to become anaesthetic assistants (operating department assistants, ODAs) Similarly, some nurses who saw openings trained to became become operating department practitioners.

The opening of the Diagnostic Treatment Centre at St Ann's Hospital Tottenham and the new theatres at St George's Hospital Tooting threw additional strain on the operating department at Moorfields, while the increase in private work at City Road itself, especially from five o'clock to ten o'clock in the evening, was an extra commitment, in effect signalling the arrival of a three-session working day. In spite of all this, Sister Morrin and her nurses appeared to cope well with the increase in work intensity (**Figure 24**, Plate 12). Notable amongst the latter were Sisters Poh Heoh Theam and Natalija Mihailovic, and Senior Nurses Denis Weekes, Malitat Phanthumkumol and Rhoda Ubani, ably supported by the ODAs, porters and managers. This ability to handle the powerful and often unexpected undercurrents that have been a feature of the NHS during the past 20 years has been a hallmark of Moorfields, and its capacity to 'raise its game' when necessary has been central to its survival.

The new culture

The call to convert from a self-contained establishment to the hub of a community-orientated organization had been recognized at an early stage (see Part 1). In the 1990s the new Moorfields Community Eye Services, at Bow, Northwick Park, Barking, Potters Bar, Tottenham and Ealing, were all equipped and staffed to the highest standard from their outset, as was the Mobile Diagnostic Unit, built and introduced in 1998 (see page 134). Likewise, the importance of modernizing teaching and training to comply with the increasing attention paid to self-regulation by the Faculty of Ophthalmologists and the Royal College of Surgeons (and later of the Royal College of Ophthalmologists), not to mention the Royal College of Nursing and other professional bodies, was quickly recognized.

As practices and culture changed, so did the Hospital and its staff adapt – first to the technological revolution during the late 1960s and early 1970s, when the introduction of microsurgery, fluorescein angiography and lasers transformed the face of ophthalmology, thereby shifting the priorities for allocation of space and resources, and later, in the 1980s and 1990s, to the demands for community care, greater accountability, patient empowerment, self-regulation and evidence-based medicine. All this was in the face of an ever-increasing demand for clinical services. In 1967 there were 7400 discharges from 345 beds. This compared with 14 300 from 80 beds at City Road in the year 2000, and a further 4200 operations done in the Outreach Units – a tenfold increase in productivity. The average in-patient stay, in the mid-1960s was 12 days, falling to 7 days in the early 1970s and to less than

2 days at the turn of the century, the pressures on all members of staff increasing commensurately, only partially mitigated by the considerable increase in their numbers and attempts to reduce their working hours.

Until the publication of the government White Paper 'Working for Patients' in 1989, when it became apparent that the Special Health Authorities were to lose their special status and would henceforth have to compete openly in the 'marketplace', there was little incentive to develop specialist services beyond the point of general 'firms', headed by a consultant with a specialist interest. Most of those appointed to the consultant staff at Moorfields, from the 1960s onwards, had acquired a more or less well-developed special interest, but none was appointed specifically to take charge of a particular subspecialty, to the exclusion of all else. Thus, Desmond Greaves, Redmond Smith and Patrick Trevor-Roper, all appointed in 1961, were content to be general ophthalmologists, and Greaves and Trevor-Roper remained so until they retired, maintaining an interest in and undertaking surgery for all manner of eye problems. Even Redmond Smith and Stephen Miller, although they were the recognized glaucoma experts at the two branches, ran general clinics and operated over a wide spectrum. Likewise, the other surgeons at both branches, although they each had an overriding special expertise, maintained their general interests (and were expected to do so). As recently as the 1970s and 1980s, although surgeons were appointed to provide special expertise in areas of practice that the Hospital needed most, they were all required to hold general out-patient clinics and undertake surgery for most conditions, provided a case was not too complex. The creation of the Primary Care Clinic in 1986 was a bold and imaginative move, laying as it did the foundation for genuine specialization at Moorfields, when this became necessary.

The consultants were ably and loyally supported in their clinics by a large contingent of clinical assistants, many of whom, like Michael Hollis, Muriel Rolfe, Hugh Fagan, Jean Vasey, SV Elbogen, Geoffrey Collyer and Helen Casey, were extremely experienced and widely knowledgeable. They served the Hospital with great distinction and were the willing mentors of a large number of aspiring ophthalmologists like the present author, who valued both their wisdom and their friendship. However, like their bosses, few of them specialized in one aspect of ophthalmology to the exclusion of all else. For those who had reached or were nearing retirement age, the change in philosophy was not of particularly serious import, but for others it meant a drastic revision of their entire professional lives, sometimes with serious consequences for their own health and well-being. Some, such as Mala Viswalingam, Lalitha Moodaley, Kamal Sharma, Joe Preziosi and Banoo Shariff, readily adapted to the modern trend and took steps to develop a special interest in depth. Their careers prospered and their standing was enhanced, most of them becoming Associate Specialists in their chosen fields. Similarly, in the new Outreach Units, where demand for their services was seemingly unending, Marwan Zeidan, Margaret Leigh, Zia Swe and others were the mainstays of the clinical services, and the Trust relied on them heavily. It was a difficult and sometimes stormy period, however, and the transition from the old way to the new saw its fair share of casualties, the out-patient medical workforce, at its end, being greatly reduced in numbers as well as a great deal more sceptical in outlook.

Nevertheless, in 1990, when the NHS and Community Care Act came into force, Moorfields was as a result of all this upheaval in an excellent position to 'enter the marketplace', since the preparatory groundwork had already been done. Six core specialties were identified: Adnexal, Corneal and External Disease, Glaucoma, Medical Retina, Strabismus and Paediatrics, and Surgical Vitreoretinal, while several other disciplines of a broader nature also formed service directorates, namely Anaesthetics, Physicians, Primary Care and the over-arching Cataract Service (drawn from members of several specialist services). The formation of these directorates and their increasing accountability, as a result of the demands made by the government and its electorate for consultant-based services, led to the appointment of many more consultants during the 1990s, chosen specifically for their specialist expertise. While there was no absolute regulation forbidding a member of a specialist service to operate outside his or her special interest (and the medical Royal Colleges had taken no steps to licence their members to practise only in a specific sphere – or spheres – of interest), it was recognized that anyone straying outside their area of expertise could not easily be supported by the Hospital if things went wrong, and few would have been prepared to take the risk of doing so, even were they so tempted.

With the formal recognition of specialist services, there was clearly a need to integrate this with multidisciplinary working practices, especially nursing, and in 1995 specialist nursing sisters were appointed to each new service (see Chapter 3). This concept was an immediate success, although it took longer in some services than others for these nurses to integrate fully with their activities. Each of the service nurses was free to develop her role as she saw fit, influenced by both the way in which the service functioned and by her own personality and inclinations. Thus some were predominantly clinical, some administrative and some academic in their activities, a good example being the nursing sister appointed to the adnexal service.

In common with the other core specialist clinical services, a Service Nursing Sister was appointed in 1996 to play a key role in establishing multidisciplinary working practices in the adnexal service. Sophie Lewis, who was the first to fill this role, did so with charm and distinction, carving out a distinctive place of her own, by dint of energetic attention to the administration of the service and her unique ability to drill her sometimes wayward medical colleagues into order. It was not long before she had made herself an indispensable part of the service, not only contributing to the general administration and running of out-patient clinics and operating lists, but also sitting on appointment panels for junior medical staff and taking part in policy decisions with Richard Collin and his consultant colleagues, who were more than happy to accept her generous help and advice.

When Moorfields achieved Trust status in 1994, the administrative structure had to be changed, not only to accommodate the conversion to subspecialization and the increasing size of the consultant body, but also to reflect the shift in responsibility for the delivery of clinical services, which now rested with the directors of the 10 services, in their turn responsible to the Medical Director. The administrative instrument by which coordination and communication was established, the Clinical Management Board (CMB), was chaired by the Medical Director, and comprised the directors of all the clinical directorates, as well as senior members of management and the directors of Research and Education. This forum for debate and direction of policy met monthly and enabled the greatly enlarged consultant workforce to participate in the strategy and direction of the Trust (though this was not a view shared by all the consultants, however, some of them feeling that far from increasing their opportunities to participate in the decision-making process, it had eliminated their capacity to do so). The Medical Committee, previously the mouthpiece of the consultant body, now assumed an advisory role only, with no executive power, and as such was renamed the Medical Advisory Committee (MAC). In this way, for better or worse, was subspecialization finally established at Moorfields on an official basis, bringing it into line with the principles laid down for NHS Trusts and giving it a viable structure for the future.

From the foregoing, it will be appreciated that although the following account describes the primary care and specialist clinical services as individual units, at the time of writing, specialist clinical services had only existed as free-standing directorates for a little over 10 years.

Accident and Emergency Service and Primary Care Clinic

How the Hospital had, by the late 1980s, already adapted itself to the different way in which the NHS would function in the brave new world, has already been described. It has also been noted how, stemming from the planning process begun in the late 1970s, a 'think tank' of forward-looking consultants comprising Noel Rice, John Wright, Arthur Steele, Bob Cooling and David McLeod devised a scheme for primary-care and specialist services to supplant the existing model of consultant-led general clinical services. Prior to this, each consultant ran his own general clinics, patients attending for the first time and then being referred, if necessary, for investigations and/or specialist advice, to other departments and clinics, before returning to the general clinic or coming into hospital for treatment, under the care of the original consultant. Under the new system, a patient referred by his or her GP, without specifying a particular consultant, would be seen in the Primary Care Clinic (PCC), a diagnosis made, and the patient either discharged or referred to the appropriate specialist service. (Strictly speaking, the PCC was a secondary-care clinic, patients attending with a letter, albeit undesignated, from their doctor.)

The scheme demanded a skilled general ophthalmologist to run a pilot clinic and put theory into practice. By a happy coincidence, just such a person was already working at Moorfields in 1986, as a Clinical Assistant in Rice's and Steele's out-patient clinics. Rhodri Daniel, a GP with a declared interest in ophthalmology, had already taken and passed both the Diploma of Ophthalmology and the first part of the examination for Fellowship of the Royal College of Surgeons. He agreed to pilot the prototype PCC, housed in a small room adjacent to the Accident and Emergency Department, working with Sue Mulligan, a visiting Fellow from Australia. The scheme was an instant success, and in 1989 Daniel gave up general practice, passed the Final Fellowship examination and became a full-time Fellow under the aegis of the Department of Clinical Ophthalmology, with Honorary Registrar status. Thus was the PCC at Moorfields founded. It quickly went from strength to strength, paving the way for the momentous changes that were to take place in the 1990s and, in particular, demonstrating to Sir Bernard Tomlinson's 1991 enquiry into London's hospital services Moorfields' ability to survive as a single-specialty hospital in the new 'market' environment, by providing primary care on a large scale that, allied with top quality specialist facilities at the centre, could meet the needs of the wider community.

In 1991 the Clinical Strategy Implementation Board, chaired by Bob Cooling, formally approved the adoption of this new concept throughout the Hospital, while accepting that it would take some time to implement, particularly in specialties such as glaucoma and medical retina where patients were often required to continue attending for long periods and could not simply be discharged or transferred abruptly from a general clinic to a specialist one. Nevertheless, within a short space of time, up to 50% of patients referred to the Hospital with suspected glaucoma were being screened out by the PCC, thereby relieving the pressure on the glaucoma service, and more than half the total of referrals were being seen there in the first instance.

Hand in hand with the strategy for developing primary-care services at City Road went that of offering high-quality ophthalmic care to the community at large. The development of outreach facilities, first at St Andrew's Bow in 1993, followed by Northwick Park (1994), Barking and Potters Bar (1995), St Ann's Tottenham (1995–96), and Ealing (1996–97) (see Part 1), demanded a huge expansion in primary care, each unit being led by a consultant with a supporting staff of non-consultant career-grade Clinical Assistants, a body of experienced and skilled ophthalmologists, most of whom had transferred from posts in general out-patient clinics as these metamorphosed into specialist clinics. They, in their turn, were backed by well-trained and experienced nurse-specialists and nurse-practitioners, without whom the new strategy would have been impossible to implement. Further developments took place in 1998 when the outreach unit at Bow was transferred to Mile End, and in 2001 when an outreach service was started at the Homerton Hospital in Hackney, culminating in the inauguration in 2002 of the Duke-Elder Eye Clinic at St George's Hospital Tooting.

Successful development of the Primary Care Service could not have been achieved without changes in the provision of Accident and Emergency services, the two necessarily running hand in hand with one another and their roles frequently overlapping. Broadly speaking, patients who walked in off the street were seen in A&E, while those with a doctor's letter were given an appointment for the appropriate PCC (clinics were weighted towards a particular diagnosis, e.g. glaucoma, and staffed accordingly). In practice, however, if appointment slots in the PCC were free, or a casualty clearly had an urgent problem more appropriately seen in the PCC than A&E, then cross-referral took place on an ad hoc basis. As soon as the strategy for developing the new type of service was decided, the Chief Nurse, Roslyn Emblin, under the aegis of Bob Cooling, the consultant lead for A&E and Primary Care services, together with Lyn Heywood, Director of Out-Patient Nursing Services, began to initiate the training of nurses capable of undertaking the duties involved in its implementation. The Casualty Course for nurses, which already included training in the use of the slit-lamp, was upgraded to include a greater awareness of diagnostic criteria and the skills required to carry out triage, as well as the ability to carry out applanation tonometry, and even recognition of abnormal optic disc appearances. A new breed of nurse-practitioners soon emerged, including three who were to become the senior nursing sisters in the combined A&E and Primary Care department: Linda Langton, Eleish Quinn and Jan Scudder. Their job descriptions and working conditions, not to mention their uniforms, were altogether very different to those in the days of Sister Pugsley's reign, 35 years before.

The PCC was at first conducted in a separate clinic (the Green Clinic), but as soon as it was clear that primary care was here to stay, the A&E and primary care departments were merged into one area, at the expense of the Brown Clinic's demise. This provided adjacent A&E and PCC facilities, which, although actually less capacious than the previous arrangement, ensured better coordination of their activities. Strict protocols were drawn up so that nurses and doctors alike knew precisely the limits of their respective remits. Gone were the days when all cases – however trivial – were seen by the Casualty Officers, a practice which sometimes led to impatience and frustration on the part of the doctors and to comments written in patients' notes which today would be considered unacceptable.

It is alleged that Mr Arthur Lister, sensitive and conscientious as always, noticed a reference recorded by the Casualty Officer, in the notes of a patient who had been seen many times in the A&E department with trivial complaints, which simply stated 'CRUD'. Summoning the doctor concerned to his presence, he demanded to know the meaning of this comment, fully expecting a contrite and embarrassed response. Not so, however: 'Chronic, Recurrent, Unexplained Disease, Sir' was the prompt reply.

In the PCC all patients were seen by a doctor, in the final analysis, but in A&E there gradually emerged a triage policy enabling senior nurses to assess, diagnose and treat some cases, including the supply of medications, without direct medical supervision. True nurse-practitioners had finally arrived at Moorfields.

Modules in the training courses for nurses could be easily modified to include new knowledge and skills (see Chapter 3), while the development of the skills laboratory as a teaching facility, proved invaluable. Nurse-practitioners' performance was monitored and audited as time went on and the standards of professional practice were shown to be high. The numbers of patients attending both A&E and PCC rose steadily, possibly as a result of the higher level of patient expectations, kick-started by the introduction of the Patients' Charter, combined with decreasing accessibility of their GPs. Pressure on the service eventually led to changes in its operation, nurses being divided into Red and Green teams, the former seeing patients with urgent problems such as acute glaucoma, or complicated and serious disorders such as retinal detachments or uveitis, and the Green Team the less urgent ones. In 2002 the Trust received a grant of £35 000 from the King's Fund to refurbish the A&E waiting area, to which the Special Trustees generously contributed a further £45 000, enabling extensive modifications to make it more user-friendly. At the Outreach Units, while PCCs were run on much the same lines as those at City Road, no Moorfields A&E service was provided, except for urgent cover for their general Casualty Departments, at units such as that at Ealing, where such existed.

Adnexal services

Prior to the advent of sub-specialization, one man towered over ophthalmic surgery in the UK. Hyla Bristow ('Henry') Stallard, consultant ophthalmic surgeon to St Bartholomew's Hospital and Moorfields, had dedicated his career to the advancement of eye surgery, developing new techniques and teaching and writing extensively. His textbook *Eye Surgery* was the standard text and he was the foremost exponent of surgical technique, especially in surgery of the lids, orbit and lacrimal drainage system. Although at this time all ophthalmic surgeons practised lid and other adnexal surgery to the best of their abilities (frequently with the help of Stallard's book), his retirement in 1966 created a yawning gap. Barrie Jones, himself a gifted surgeon, had already established a reputation as far as lid surgery was concerned, this sphere of activity having particular bearing on his special interest in trachoma, a condition that frequently caused lid scarring. He had already set up a lid clinic, and, with his interest in sophisticated techniques of lacrimal surgery, had also established a lacrimal clinic. In other areas of adnexal disease, however, the lines of engagement were less obviously drawn.

In the late 1960s a number of bright and ambitious young men who had recently finished their resident training at Moorfields could see the direction in which the wind was beginning to blow. Peter Fells, although he had already displayed a special interest in disorders of ocular motility, was also interested in thyroid eye disease and trauma of the orbital tissues, while John Wright had, during his residency, done some original research with Glyn Lloyd, consultant radiologist to the Hospital, into radiological methods of demonstrating orbital tumours, and had visited Milan to study methods of orbital venography. When Fells returned after a year in the USA as a Harkness Fellow, both he and Wright joined the Professorial Unit as lecturers. Wright had meanwhile secured a grant of £100 000 from the Medical Research Council and, by the early 1970s, encouraged by Barrie Jones, they had both established their positions in their chosen spheres of expertise. It was not long before Dick Welham too was encouraged to join the Professorial Unit, to do lacrimal surgery, and he too became an acknowledged expert, all three eventually becoming consultants at Moorfields. Thus did Barrie Jones ensure that, after Stallard's death from cancer in October 1973, his mantle was not discarded, and that the progress that he had begun in surgery of the adnexal tissues would continue.

Orbital disease

Barrie Jones, realizing that he had in his department two men with a special interest in orbital surgery, asked them to set up an orbital clinic and, in April 1968, this they did. In 1970, together with Fells, Wright and Lloyd, he presented a series of orbital cases at the meeting of the Ophthalmological Society of the UK, summarizing their experience. It soon became clear that Fells' special interests lay in thyroid disease and in fractures of the orbital walls, while Wright had developed, with Lloyd, sophisticated methods for diagnosing and demonstrating orbital tumours. With the retirement of Alex Cross in 1973, John Wright was appointed to replace him, while Fells, who was already on the consultant staff, took his place as Director of the Orthoptic Department, Barrie Jones thereby securing the simultaneous appointment of both a world-class orbital surgeon and a squint surgeon (albeit the latter with an additional interest in thyroid eye disease and orbital trauma). The subsequent break-up and divergence of the original orbital partnership was inevitable, Peter Fells setting up his own thyroid clinic with Nick Lawton, and John Wright establishing the Orbital Clinic with Glyn Lloyd and members of the Pathology Department. The latter was the first of its kind worldwide and was soon attracting large numbers of patients. Postgraduate students were attracted to the clinic from all over the world, Wright going on to modify and improve the surgical approach to the orbital contents, and in so doing establishing himself as one of the world's foremost orbital surgeons.

John Wright's advances in the surgery of orbital tumours deserve special attention, Moorfields rapidly becoming, and thereafter remaining for a period of 25 years, the foremost centre for this type of surgery. Wright was a man of steely determination and single-minded ambition, with the ability to focus on a problem to the exclusion of all else going on around him. When he started his residency at City Road he had already obtained his MD and, as noted above had, whilst on the training programme, teamed up with Glyn Lloyd to explore ways of elucidating the nature of orbital disease, long before the introduction of computed tomography (CT). On his appointment to the consultant staff, they continued to work together, becoming adept at recognizing patterns of abnormality in the orbit typical of neoplastic disease, and thereby developing unique expertise in the field.

In his own words: *'At this time orbital disease was poorly understood and its treatment haphazard, mainly because orbital tumours were uncommon and investigative techniques relatively crude. With the influx of these patients to the Orbital Clinic it became apparent that a team effort was needed to deal with their problems. A weekly, open clinical meeting was started, in 1974, and was held for an hour before the start of the Orbital Clinic. Every new patient was discussed, together with the surgical and histological findings from those who had been admitted for treatment. The expert opinions of Dr Lloyd, members of the Pathology Department and the clinicians always resulted in a lively and productive discussion of each case. These meetings kept everyone up to date and cemented the feeling that the management of these patients was a joint effort.'* Not only did they interact with one another and with the Pathology Department, but also with Ian McDonald, the consultant neurologist, whose clinic followed the meeting and ran in parallel with the orbital clinic, thereby enabling ready consultation about cases involving the optic nerve and foramen. *'Within a few years, the combination of a relatively large number of patients and the increasing clinical experience of the group resulted in the publication of a number of landmark papers on previously unrecognized patterns of orbital disease.'*

The first patients with orbital tumours ever to have CT scans were sent to Dr Ambrose at the Atkinson Morley Hospital, where Dr Hounsfield and the prototype scanner were installed. As each machine with the capacity for higher resolution was developed, it was tested on patients from the Moorfields Orbital Clinic, part of the early history of CT scanning.

Lacrimal surgery

In addition to his special interest in orbital and adnexal disease, Barrie Jones had early on developed an interest in surgery of the lacrimal drainage apparatus. This included using plastic tubing to maintain patency postoperatively and, his own microsurgical tour-de-force, the canaliculodacryocystorhinostomy (CDCR), when obstruction of the lacrimal duct was complicated by obstruction of the canaliculi.

The root cause of his special interest in this field was to be found far back in his medical career when, as a registrar in Dunedin, a woman attended the hospital with intractable watering of her eyes. On investigation, she was demonstrated to have obstruction, not only of the lacrimal sac, but also of the canaliculi. Neither young Jones, nor his boss knew what best to do for her. The standard operation, dacryocystorhinostomy (DCR) would be sure to fail in the face of blocked canaliculi. Her surgery was therefore deferred, until such time as they could think of something better.

In the meantime, as a result of her poor vision on looking down, occasioned by the accumulation of tears in the inferior fornices, she one day missed her footing and fell down a flight of stairs, shortly thereafter succumbing to her injuries. Although this unhappy event relieved the surgeons of their immediate problem, her death so upset Barrie Jones that he was inspired to invent a new operation, the CDCR, to ensure that such a thing should never happen again; so a patient's otherwise untimely death was, in the end, not devoid of a positive outcome.

His capacity for delicate and time-consuming surgery and the patience required to achieve success in these cases were legendary, but it soon became clear to the Professor that a younger surgeon was needed, with the time and energy to concentrate wholly on their management. So it was that Richard ('Dick') Welham, who had demonstrated his interest before being appointed to a consultant post elsewhere (and had carried the burden of lacrimal surgery at Moorfields in an honorary capacity long after that), was finally appointed in 1975 as lacrimal specialist at Moorfields. He brought to the post great technical skill, a lively (some might say ribald) sense of humour, and exceptional teaching ability, an attribute that enabled him to pass on the knowledge bequeathed to him by Barrie Jones, to generations of Moorfields Residents and Fellows until, in the early 1990s, the increasingly unreasonable demands for personal commitment and accountability finally forced his resignation.

A joint Fellowship Programme was started, in 1974, in orbital and lacrimal disease. Surgeons in training were keen to spend either 6 or 12 months studying the new investigational methods and being trained in the innovative surgical techniques developed by both John Wright and Richard Welham. Over the succeeding 22 years, some 26 such individuals from a wide variety of countries underwent this training, many of them starting up similar departments of their own after returning home.

Developments in orbital and lacrimal surgery
Welham's replacement on the consultant staff, not only as lacrimal surgeon but also to understudy John Wright's orbital role, was Geoffrey

Rose, formerly a Fellow on the Adnexal Service, and an exceptionally able surgeon with a forceful personality and an enquiring and innovative approach. He soon challenged the accepted views concerning healing of rhinostomies by primary or secondary intention, and with meticulous surgery defined the most favourable approach to lacrimal surgery, the Moorfields lacrimal service as a consequence achieving outcomes from healing by primary intention, unmatched elsewhere. Rose shared a period of six years alongside John Wright, acquiring the knowledge and skills developed by him in surgery of the orbit, before the latter's retirement, and along the way developed his own special expertise and understanding of thyroid eye disease. Before 1990, just as patients with disfiguring scarring and mutilation of the orbit had accepted their disfigurement, so had those with thyroid exophthalmos, surgical relief generally being confined to the correction of corneal exposure by lid-lowering surgery. (*One patient, treated in this way, is alleged to have remarked that the surgery had simply changed his appearance from that of a goldfish to a 'Garfield' – a popular cartoon character of a cat with bulging eyes and drooping eyelids.*) Rose set about changing this attitude, adapting the methods developed by John Wright for decompressing the orbital tissues, by an approach through the conjunctiva, via a small angular incision combined with a relieving incision in the upper lid, to reach the walls of the orbit with the minimum of cosmetic disturbance. So successful and popular was this method to become that, by 2002, two to three patients per week were seeking treatment at Moorfields. (*One such patient was referred not by her doctor, but by another patient who, spotting her while sitting opposite travelling on the Underground, recognized her condition and recommended that she seek Rose's help without delay.*)

Such was the increase in demand for adnexal surgery during the 1990s that two further appointments were made: Michelle Beaconsfield to take on lid surgery and establish an outreach service at Northwick Park and Tony Tyers, especially to help with teaching. Tyers was already an established consultant in Salisbury, a geographical obstacle that in the long term proved to be too demanding and that regretfully soon led to his resignation from the Moorfields post.

In 2002, in recognition of the huge workload in orbital surgery (twice that of any other unit worldwide, including between 500 and 600 new tumour cases per annum), a fourth consultant was appointed, Jimmy Uddin, with special expertise in the treatment of thyroid eye disease, who was also expected to take his share of lid, lacrimal and orbital surgery, and was charged with providing an outreach service at St George's Hospital.

Ear, nose and throat surgery

The physical proximity of the paranasal sinuses to the adnexal tissues of the eye has always engendered some degree of cross-boundary overlap and even, sometimes, of rivalry between ENT and ophthalmic surgeons. For this reason it was natural that there should be an oto-laryngological expert on the consultant staff at Moorfields, and this had indeed been the case since the 1920s. In 1962, on the retirement of Gilbert Howells, Brian Pickard was appointed to this position. Already on the consultant staff of St George's Hospital and the Atkinson Morley, and previously a senior registrar at the Royal Throat Nose and Ear Hospital (RTN&EH) in Gray's Inn Road, he was fast, decisive and a highly experienced and accomplished surgeon. He was also lively, energetic, boyishly engaging and slightly vain, with a penchant for flying his own aeroplane, fast cars and wearing brightly coloured bow-ties. His tenure at Moorfields, from 1962 to 1987, was happy and fulfilling from both his own and the Hospital's point of view.

In the early days of Barrie Jones's foray into the surgery of orbital tumours, abscesses and mucocoeles, Pickard was happy to be associated with cases involving the sinuses. When cases were beyond the scope of ophthalmological intervention, they were transferred to St George's Hospital Hyde Park Corner and on the latter's closure and transfer to Tooting, to the RTN&EH.

Perhaps unsurprisingly, given their uniquely antipathetic person-alities, Pickard and John Wright were not the easiest of bedfellows. This did not present serious problems, however, as Wright was quite happy and confident in transgressing outside the confines of the orbit, when necessary, without asking for assistance (he was appointed consultant ophthalmic surgeon to the RTN&EH in 1973). Peter Fells' interest in thyroid eye disease and orbital floor fractures was, however, a different matter. Fells was more inclined to seek advice and play second fiddle to others with special expertise, sharing his thyroid clinic with a consultant physician and happy to operate in tandem with Pickard, in the trans-sinusoidal approach to decompression of the orbit and in operations involving repair of orbital fractures, where there was extensive involvement of adjacent structures. It was a happy and fruit-ful collaboration.

On his retirement, Pickard's place on the consultant staff at Moorfields was taken by the Clinical Professor at the RTN&EH, Donald (later Sir Donald) Harrison, who regularly attended the weekly orbital meetings. He worked equally comfortably alongside Fells until the latter's retirement, and when he too retired, he was succeeded at Moorfields by Valerie Lund, who had been appointed to the Clinical

Chair at Gray's Inn Road. She was an equally able surgeon and continued to collaborate easily with Rose in his out-patient clinics, and to undertake surgery where there was extensive disease involving the sinuses.

Oculoplastics

In the latter half of the 1970s, as Barrie Jones' other interests widened, he foresaw the need for an oculoplastic surgeon to fill his shoes, especially in the field of lid surgery. In 1972 Richard Collin, a Resident at the High Holborn branch of the Hospital, had begun to take an interest in alternatives to conjunctival grafts and, while doing some experimental work at the Institute of Ophthalmology, had received encouragement and advice from Henry Stallard. Barrie Jay, then already on the consultant staff at High Holborn, had been deputed to undertake Stallard's conjunctival melanoma and ptosis work, so Collin was able to explore these interests during his residency. At the end of this period, he decided to pursue oculoplastic surgery further, going first for six months' general plastic surgical training with Robin Beare in East Grinstead, and then spending time in Scotland, as an observer with Jack Mustardé, as well as attending the American Society of Oculoplastics and Reconstructive Surgery, where he learnt the importance of a thorough understanding of the anatomy of the eyelids and adnexae (Collin was subsequently to write the chapter on eyelid malposition from the ophthalmologist's point of view, in the 3rd edition of Mustardé's book).

Encouraged by Barrie Jones, Collin afterwards went to San Francisco to work with Crowell Beard for a year, before returning to London in 1977 to work in the Lid Clinic at City Road, first as an out-patient officer, then lecturer and finally, in 1980, as senior lecturer with consultant status, taking over the direction of the Lid Clinic. In 1982 he was appointed to a substantive consultant post, assuming responsibility for Barrie Jay's patients, on the latter's appointment as Dean, and becoming the first formally recognized oculoplastic surgeon in the Hospital's history.

Throughout the 1980s, oculoplastics remained chiefly concerned with lid surgery and the correction of ptosis. Other defects, such as empty sockets after enucleation or injury, had traditionally been considered of relatively minor importance, patients being encouraged to put up with or ignore their disfigurement. The clinical burden of lid disease, especially from trachoma, and the increasing use and success of corneal grafting, which demanded prior correction of entropion and trichiasis, was sufficient to occupy most of Collin's time. Gradually, however, due to both clinical and cultural factors, this situation changed.

It had previously been the dictum that the eye socket should be left empty following enucleation for malignant melanoma, to facilitate palpation of the socket and detection of any tumour recurrence. The result was a cosmetically unsatisfactory, volume-deficient and sunken appearance of the socket. A retrospective study by Collin showed, however, that of 500 patients who had undergone enucleation for malignant melanoma, only six had developed local recurrence in the socket, while of those six, five already had distant metastases by the time of its discovery and the remaining one developed fatal metastases within 18 months of it. There was therefore no good reason to refrain from using implants in these patients, any more than in those with other indications for enucleation, and their use therefore rapidly increased. Moreover, the increased deployment of implants led to improvements in their design and the materials of which they were made, not only greatly to the immediate benefit of the patients, but also leading to greatly increased levels of expectation, so that before long, unsightly sockets were considered unacceptable.

Other events also modified the oculoplastic case-mix during the 1980s and 1990s, in particular changes to the law governing the wearing of seat-belts and improvements in windscreen manufacture, whereby serious ocular damage from motor accidents was practically eliminated. This was coupled with huge changes in patients' attitudes to their physical appearance. Thus, in parallel with the diminishing demand for lid surgery, consequent upon successful treatment of trachoma, its employment in other conditions increased. Patients with thyroid exophthalmos were no longer content to live with their disfigurement, nor were those with ptosis, while the parents of children with microphthalmos or anophthalmos became aware that, with the introduction of hydrophilic materials, most such children could have their sockets expanded sufficiently to accommodate an artificial eye.

While many of the advances in the field of oculoplastics took place elsewhere, the first use of hydrophilic material for babies with microphthalmos or anophthalmos was initiated in the Contact Lens Department at Moorfields, and further advances were made to this concept by a Visiting Fellow from Germany. The Hospital led the world in this field, not only in respect of surgery and implant technology, wherein Collin accumulated the largest series of such patients worldwide, but also as a result of collaboration with Dr Barry Jones, the Hospital's consultant paediatrician, and Professor Barry Jay, in genetic and supportive counselling. Furthermore, the oculoplastic service at

Moorfields is credited with the first use of Mersilene mesh to support the upper lid and the first use, in the UK, of Moh's technique for excising tumours. In the late 1990s, Collin collaborated with John Dart from the Corneal and External Disease Service and the maxillofacial surgeons in treating end-stage cases of dry eyes, with lid grafts and sub-mandibular gland transplantation. His election to the inaugural Presidency of the British Oculoplastic Surgery Society, founded in 2001, seemed a fitting recognition of both Collin's and of Moorfields' contribution in the field.

While the mainstay of practice throughout the period remained surgery to the lids, in blepharitis, trichiasis, entropion, ectropion and ptosis, the increase in surgery for exophthalmos and unsightly conditions such as empty sockets radically altered the case-mix during the 1990s. Furthermore, advances such as the introduction of botulinum toxin in the treatment of essential blepharospasm, which could be administered by a nurse-specialist, intravenous sedation for oculoplastic surgery and adjustable sutures for lid surgery brought about fundamental changes in practice. Other technological innovations, such as lasers and more sophisticated cryotherapy machines for treating trichiasis and tumours, and the introduction of better endoscopes and electrocautery instruments, also played their part in the process of modernization. These advances, together with the development of the outreach programme and Richard Welham's resignation in 1993, were to combine in reshaping the adnexal service as it moved towards the new millennium and thereafter.

Anaesthetic services

In some respects, Moorfields represents a microcosm of the NHS as a whole, but unlike larger institutions, it is able to react and adapt quickly to the changes going on around it. In no field has there been a greater degree of change than that of ophthalmic anaesthesia. In the 1950s and 1960s there was a small core of anaesthetists at Moorfields providing general anaesthesia for those operations requiring it. Such operations were, for the most part, short and relatively uncomplicated. For children, ether was still commonly used, as a safe and well-tried agent in experienced hands, although its volatility, despite being one of its advantages, could also be a hazard.

On one occasion it caused an explosion, when the waste vapour made its way along the gas scavenging pipe, thereby delivering it to a workman using a blow-torch on the roof of the operating theatre. The ether bottle on the anaesthetic machine shattered and there was great alarm amongst the theatre staff, but fortunately no serious harm to the patient.

There was no special requirement for those giving anaesthetics to children to have any special training or experience in paediatric anaesthesia. Adults commonly received trichlorethylene, later replaced by halothane, an excellent agent for inducing and maintaining tranquil anaesthesia and for permitting recovery without the risk of coughing, but a potentially dangerous agent (especially when administered over a prolonged period and/or repeatedly, as was not infrequently the case in patients with retinal detachments). Most patients needing surgery were required to be quite physically fit if they were to be considered for operation under general anaesthesia.

The advent of sophisticated retinal surgery and of microsurgery triggered a whole gamut of changes. It became possible to operate successfully on many patients previously considered beyond treatment, and these operations frequently took a long time and were often done in near darkness – conditions that rendered the environment unfavourable, as the anaesthetist had little means of observing the appearance of his patient, and the warm, dark atmosphere was not conducive to a high state of alert.

> *This state of affairs may have given rise to the tale (no doubt apocryphal) of an exasperated surgeon once saying to the anaesthetist 'If the patient can stay awake, why can't you?'*

Anaesthetists were sometimes required to administer general anaesthetics to patients undergoing minor procedures, or investigations, in the Out-Patient Department, using ether, without assistance and frequently in less than optimal conditions. One instance of the latter, in particular, was the early practice when carrying out ultrasound investigations of using a water-bath surrounding the eye, improvised by sticking a waterproof surgical drape to the patient's face, secured in a retort stand, thereby introducing the additional risk of drowning.

Dr Barry Smith was an officer in the Territorial Army and had innate abilities of leadership and organization. He was therefore an obvious choice as head of department, a role he fulfilled well for many years. His appointment as consultant anaesthetist in 1968 coincided with the provision of new operating theatres at both branches. Nevertheless, he found that there was no proper recovery room at either branch, only one technician at each (albeit as skilled and stalwart as were the two Charlies: Whipp at City Road and Smith at High Holborn), no secretarial support, office or library space at either, and a small complement of part-time anaesthetists, one of whom would only do private cases. Barry Smith's arrival heralded a new approach to anaesthesia at Moorfields, and gradually, over a period of several years, a whole range of modern equipment and methods was introduced.

This was not without some opposition from the surgeons; Barry Smith asserts that when he arrived at Moorfields, he was told that he was at liberty to attend the meetings of the Medical Committee, but should not expect to say anything.

Neither sophisticated anaesthetic and monitoring equipment nor consultant anaesthetists come cheaply, but Barry Smith nevertheless managed to build up the department, acquire office space and secretarial support, and modernize both equipment and practices in line with the latest developments. This he was able to do by dint of strong leadership and by fearlessly warning of the dire consequences that would ensue if patients were to suffer as a result of deficiencies in staff or equipment. Not only was the complement of medical staff increased, but anaesthetic nurses and operating department assistants were employed, until the Anaesthetic Service became one of the best of its type, Barry Smith's textbook *Ophthalmic Anaesthesia* soon becoming required reading for would-be ophthalmic anaesthetists.

In step with advances in surgical technique, anaesthetic practice rapidly became more sophisticated. The old methods of anaesthesia were no longer considered safe and, in any case, the introduction of new anaesthetic agents, together with sophisticated monitoring equipment, soon made them obsolete. Not only did the monitoring equipment, notably the pulse oximeter, sound an alarm if anything untoward occurred, but also the introduction of closed-circuit television rendered the operation intelligible and interesting to doctors and nurses alike. It soon became possible to give a general anaesthetic safely to any patient, however frail, elderly or sick, so skilled was the modern breed of anaesthetists and so safe the anaesthetic agents and equipment at their command.

The increasing popularity of intra-ocular lens implantation and the change from intracapsular to extracapsular cataract extraction during the late 1970s and early 1980s heralded a new direction, not only for cataract surgery but also for ophthalmic anaesthesia. As the design of lens implants improved and their use became routine, the role of general anaesthesia in this type of surgery was called into question. The need for patients to stay in hospital for cataract extraction was much reduced, while the introduction of phacoemulsification during the latter half of the 1980s further hastened the demise of general anaesthesia for cataract surgery. During the 1990s, small-incision surgery and foldable implants, with no need for sutures and with recovery of vision so good and so swift as to be little short of miraculous, finally opened the door to day-case cataract surgery, so that the prevalence of day-case surgery under local anaesthesia during the last decade of the 20th Century rose from 10% at the outset to 90% or more at its close.

This trend, especially in the Community Outreach Units, coupled with new joint guidelines from the Colleges of Ophthalmologists and Anaesthetists, encouraged ophthalmic anaesthetists during the next 15 years to take on the administration of local anaesthetics more and more, thereby making day-case surgery safer, faster and so agreeable to patients that it soon became the method of choice. In situations where no anaesthetist was actually present in the operating theatre (although, as dictated by joint College guidelines, one was always available at immediate notice, if required), as was the case in some of the Outreach Units, patients were now able to walk into the theatre, be given their local anaesthetic injection by the surgeon, have their surgery, walk out of the theatre, have a cup of tea and go home, all within the space of a few hours. Furthermore, specially trained nurses were able to undertake their pre- and postoperative assessments, reducing the need for them to wait to see a surgeon, either before or afterwards. This was a fundamental change, especially when considered in the context of Moorfields' ambitious outreach programme. Furthermore, the new breed of anaesthetists showed themselves to be not only much quicker and safer giving locals than many of their surgical colleagues, and excellent at teaching the juniors how to give them, but also able and willing to help in the smooth running of operating lists, by carrying out delicate adjustments to the microscope, phacoemulsification and laser equipment.

Not only did the use of local anaesthesia increase, so also did the variety of methods for its administration. Retrobulbar injection, formerly the only recognized method of achieving adequate anaesthesia and akinesia for cataract surgery, was, during the late 1980s and early 1990s, largely replaced by peribulbar injection. This change in method, although it minimized the risk of retrobulbar haemorrhage, increased the hazard of ocular perforation. Progressively atraumatic methods of surgery, however, in particular the use of small incisions, led some surgeons and anaesthetists to adopt a modified sub-Tenon's capsule injection, a method that became very popular amongst both patients and surgeons at Moorfields, or even to use topical application of local anaesthetic alone.

Where general anaesthesia was still required, new agents for total intravenous anaesthesia, such as ketamine for children, were introduced, and for more extensive procedures in adults drugs such as propofol (previously used only as an induction agent), combined with the fast-acting opioids derived from fentanyl, became in the 1990s popular for speedy induction and recovery, without the need for volatile, potentially toxic, gases such as halothane. These agents were almost free of side-effects, patients awaking clear-headed, rational and feeling well, so permitting their early mobilization and discharge. They had the additional advantage that they could be used safely in retinal cases where intraocular expanding gases were employed, as they reduced the need for nitrous oxide, a highly soluble gas that diffuses freely into the eye from the bloodstream, thereby causing the intraocular gas bubble to expand rapidly, with a coincident rise in intraocular pressure.

As a consequence of Peng Tee Khaw's pioneering work on paediatric glaucoma, which entailed long periods under general anaesthesia, and the large volume of paediatric strabismus cases, nearly 15% of the anaesthetic workload in 2001–02 was in children, while the advent of the International Children's Eye Centre seemed likely to increase this figure. Guidelines from the Colleges of Anaesthetists and Paediatrics during the 1990s dictated that only paediatric anaesthetists were allowed to anaesthetize children, increasing the pressure on the department at Moorfields. In the mid 1990s Jonathan Lord, who had trained at Moorfields as a registrar, and who had a special interest in paediatric anaesthesia, was appointed to the consultant staff. The trend towards subspecialization was in anaesthesia, as in ophthalmology, ever growing.

The huge increase in surgical work, from less than 7500 cases per year in the 1960s to more than 18 500 at the beginning of the new millennium, combined with the involvement of anaesthetists in the administration of local as well as general anaesthetics, led to a steady increase in the number of consultant staff in the Anaesthetic Service. In 1993, in the run up to Trust status, Pam Stracey took over as director of the service, soon followed by Suzanne Powrie. The latter had joined the staff in 1977, at the High Holborn branch, and was a popular choice, with wide experience not only in ophthalmic but also in cardiothoracic anaesthesia. She continued to head the service for four years, before Caroline Carr, who had been on the staff at Moorfields since 1986, and was also on the staff at the Eastman Dental Hospital, took over. In 2001, however, with the introduction of the tridivisional management structure, Carr was appointed to the post of Divisional Clinical Director and Jonathan Lord became Director of the Anaesthetic Service. Where, in the 1960s, there had been a total of 8 part-time consultant anaesthetists covering both branches, by the year 2000 there were 12 consultants, most of them all but full-time, as well as a complement of 4 registrars. The service was obliged to supply not only staff to cope with the increasing load at City Road but also staff for the Community Outreach Units at Mile End and St Ann's Hospital Tottenham, where skilled ophthalmic anaesthetic cover was not otherwise available. As this, together with increasing patient expectations, the drive towards greater and greater efficiency, and the demands imposed by clinical governance, all became more demanding, anaesthesia for ophthalmic surgery, far from becoming less important, appeared to have become more so.

Cataract surgery

Since the latter half of the 1970s, cataract extraction had gone through a momentous period of change. In the first half of that decade the intracapsular method, using capsule forceps or cryoprobe, to remove the lens in one piece, via a limbal corneal incision, under a limbus-based conjunctival flap, was still in all but a few cases the method of choice in adults. The introduction of intra-ocular lens implants in the mid-1970s changed this entirely, extracapsular extraction soon becoming universal, along with 10/0 nylon sutures instead of 9/0 silk, and corneal incisions under fornix-based conjunctival flaps. These innovations notwithstanding, Moorfields was slow to embrace modern trends, due to a number of historical factors, the most influential of which was Harold Ridley's adventurous and pioneering foray into the use of lens implants two decades earlier.

Just after the Second World War, Ridley, by then a senior member of the consultant staff at both Moorfields and St Thomas's Hospital, devised a uniquely daring and innovative approach to the treatment of cataract, involving the implantation of a Perspex lens. Neither a discussion of the technical details nor of the ethical or scientific arguments relating to this pioneering work would be appropriate here, but its sociopolitical fallout bears heavily on the subsequent course of events at Moorfields. To understand the situation fully, it is necessary to bear in mind that Sir Stewart Duke-Elder was, both during and after the Second World War, the unchallenged leader of British ophthalmology. By all accounts, he and Ridley were at odds, while relations between the latter and his colleagues at Moorfields, in particular Henry Stallard, the most brilliant and innovative surgeon of the day, were never easy. The implants devised and used by Ridley, in spite of opposition from his colleagues at Moorfields, were untested and untried and gave rise to many complications, his continued use of them in consequence arousing the ire and opposition not only of Duke-Elder but also of most of the British ophthalmological establishment.

To put matters in slightly more balanced perspective and to be fair to Ridley, it is said that even when he offered to demonstrate the results of his work in this field by presenting a series of cases, and invited Duke-Elder to come and see for himself, the latter refused to do so.

Although he pursued his work mainly at St Thomas',* many of the complications were fielded by the consultants at Moorfields, who as a result, reacted strongly against implant surgery – a reaction that was to endure long after Ridley's retirement and the reintroduction of lens implants in the 1970s by Binkhorst in Sweden and others here and abroad. Furthermore, Peter Choyce, a disciple of Ridley's, continued to design and use his own anterior chamber implants, with questionable judgement and even more questionable results, throughout the 1960s and 1970s, causing further disquiet amongst the Moorfields surgeons, who were not infrequently called upon to deal with the resulting complications.

In the late 1960s and early 1970s a new generation of cataract surgeons emerged who took Ridley's revolutionary concept and allied it to modern science and thinking. Preservation of the posterior lens capsule to support the vitreous face and thereby protect the retina was considered important even in the early era of iris-clip and anterior chamber lenses, while the conversion to posterior chamber lens implants made it mandatory. The introduction of viscoelastic agents, to maintain the anterior chamber and protect the corneal endothelium, and sophisticated suction/infusion cannulae were notable advances, and the operation became steadily more sophisticated and safe. Advances in technique and instrumentation during the 1980s were enormous, and it was not long before phacoemulsification and capsulorhexis were introduced, flexible implants became the accepted norm, and small-incision surgery arrived. (Phacoemulsification of the lens had been tried, much earlier, in the USA by Kelman and in the UK by Arnott, but did not gain

---

* *The story goes that HR (as Harold Ridley was known) attempted to conceal his surgical activities from his Moorfields colleagues, by undertaking implant surgery at St Thomas', where they were less likely to be aware of it. On the consultant staff at the High Holborn branch of the Hospital, however, was Frederick Ridley, who, apart from sharing the same surname, had little else in common with HR and, indeed, was also at loggerheads with him. A patient who had undergone an intra-ocular lens implant operation by Harold mistakenly booked his postoperative follow-up appointment with Frederick, thereby in no uncertain terms letting the cat out of the (capsular) bag!*

popularity until the introduction of other techniques, in particular capsulorhexis, which made its use practical and safe.)

Moorfields, while it had been astute and forward-looking in so many aspects of the transition from the old to the new style of medicine, was slow to grasp the nettle where modern methods of cataract surgery were concerned. This reluctance was due to two things: first, there was a natural disinclination amongst the older consultants to alter their surgical practice in such a radical way and to re-train in the new techniques involved, when the old well-tried methods appeared to work well, and secondly, as already noted, there existed an entrenched antipathy to lens implantation, born of Harold Ridley's earlier experiments. As a consequence, in the latter half of the 1970s Moorfields lagged seriously behind other centres of excellence around the world. Although John Wright in particular bucked the trend and was proactive in the cause of implant surgery, it was nevertheless an instance, in which the Hospital for a time failed to lead the specialty, in an area crucial to the practice of modern ophthalmology, an omission that exposed it to adverse criticism.

Modern cataract surgery at Moorfields

This shortcoming, like so many others, was seized upon by Barrie Jones, who encouraged Arthur Steele to pursue efforts to rectify the situation, setting up a multicentre clinical trial of lens implantation, with Peter Hamilton at the Middlesex Hospital and Dermot Pierse in Croydon. Although the trial itself was soon abandoned as too unwieldy and cumbersome (the definitive trial was done by Hung Cheng in Oxford), this soon led to the method's general acceptance at Moorfields. The appointment of Steele to the consultant staff in 1976, on the early retirement of Derek Ainslie, was a defining moment in the development of cataract surgery at Moorfields. Steele proved to be not only an outstanding surgeon and technical innovator but also an excellent mentor, going on to teach and inspire generations of young ophthalmologists in the art of anterior segment microsurgery. Not only did he introduce the latest developments in instrumentation and technique, including phaco-emulsification and foldable and injectable lenses, but he also supplied the leadership that the Hospital needed in this field, soon making up for the period in which it had lagged behind. While the introduction of new high-vacuum and laser phacoemulsifiers, non-steroidal anti-inflammatory drugs (NSAIDs) and refinements in surgical technique have continued to make the surgery of cataract quicker, safer and more patient-friendly since Steele's retirement in 1996, his place in the pantheon of fame at Moorfields remains assured. Meanwhile, the development of new antibiotics such as ciprofloxacin and topical preparations of NSAIDs, combined with the increasing use of disposable equipment (driven by the fear of CJD), rendered cataract surgery safer than ever before.

The inauguration of the Moorfields outreach programme coincided with the government's drive for greater efficiency and the trend towards day-case surgery, especially for cataract, engendered by it. The Outreach Units with facilities for undertaking surgery (at Mile End, Ealing, St Ann's Tottenham and Northwick Park) were in an ideal position to promote day-case surgery under local anaesthesia. Away from the centre there was less resistance to changes in practice, while the viability of these units depended on providing facilities attractive to GPs and their patients. At Northwick Park, in particular, where John Wright promoted high-volume cataract surgery, in the mid 1990s an anaesthetist was the exception rather than the rule, and pre- and post-operative assessments by nursing staff enabled the surgeons to operate on large numbers of cases, with speed and safety. In 1999, when the government produced its 'Action on Cataracts' directive, surgeons were able to increase the number from five to seven patients per list, without detriment to patients' comfort or safety, an increase of four cases per day, or 40%. Nevertheless, a trial comparing outcomes of cataract surgery done by specially trained nurses that was proposed by Professor David McLeod in Manchester met with huge resistance from the Royal College of Ophthalmologists, of which he was a Vice-President, eventually leading to his resignation from that position. It was clear that the forces for change had their limitations.

With Moorfields' attainment of Trust status in 1994, it was obvious that cataract surgery warranted its own directorate, and the Cataract Service was created, establishing a management framework within which direction and policy could be formulated and by means of which the highest standards of practice could be assured. The service comprised surgeons from several of the existing specialist service groups, as well as those involved primarily in cataract surgery alone – in all a total of 11 consultants and 2 Fellows. By the time the millennium was reached, the service was responsible for doing more than 4000 operations a year in the Outreach Units, as well as 5000 at City Road, its first director Miss Carol Cunningham doing 98% of her cases as day-cases and 75% of these without an anaesthetist. Moreover, her preferred method of anaesthesia, like that of many of her colleagues in the service, entailed the use of topical amethocaine only (sometimes topped up with a sub-Tenon's capsule injection).

The idea of cataract surgery constituting a specialist service took a long time to sink in, while the notion of a Moorfields consultant specializing in the surgery of cataracts alone took even longer.

Nevertheless, with the emergence of the specialist service directorates, it soon became apparent that the Trust needed to embrace this concept, and Carol Cunningham was duly appointed as the first cataract surgeon (together with primary care), and soon afterwards asked to head the Cataract Service. Nor was it long into the 21st Century before it became obvious that there was a need for further such appointments, Vincenzo Maurino concentrating on cataracts alone and others on primary care coupled with cataract surgery, to confront the challenge thrown down by the government, demanding shorter and shorter waiting times. Two such appointments were made, one to serve the City Road site, Miss Seema Verma, and one to be at St George's, Alex Ionides. At the end of 2001, to support the cataract service further now that it comprised some 12 surgeons, Michael Miller, who had previously headed the Glaucoma Service and been the clinical lead at Northwick Park, switched to the Cataract Service and took over from Cunningham as its director.

More than in other services, there was a clear need for all members of the Cataract Service to follow the same protocols, while the introduction by the NHS Modernization Agency in 2002 of Diagnostic Treatment Centres (DTCs), aimed at providing patients who had been waiting for six months or longer for their operations with the choice of immediate surgery in a unit specially equipped, staffed and geared for this, was an opportunity not to be missed. The Moorfields Outreach Units at St George's Hospital Tooting and St Ann's Hospital Tottenham were felt by the Trust to be the most suitable to be DTCs and were equipped and staffed accordingly. Both Carol Cunningham and Michael Miller had contributed immensely during the previous two years to the groundwork necessary to establish and get them up and running so quickly. They began to take patients in September 2002 and were officially opened for business in March and June of 2003 respectively, by which time the centre at St Ann's had already done more than 1300 extra cataract operations. The vast majority of patients undergoing modern cataract surgery were delighted with the results and were more than happy to be operated on under topical anaesthesia, if necessary, although in practice an anaesthetist was usually present to give a sub-Tenon's block.

Only a few found the outcome disturbing, such as the lady who, when asked by Michael Miller if she was pleased with the result of her operation, replied: 'Oh yes, Mr Miller, but there is just one thing that I find distressing.' ' Oh dear, what is that?', he asked. 'Well', she answered, 'my cat no longer appears to be a tabby!'

Corneal and external disease

Background

Barrie Jones developed his lifelong interest in ocular infection as a result of the inspirational teaching he received while training as a junior doctor in New Zealand. After studying chemistry and physics in Wellington and obtaining a science degree, he went to medical school at Otago University, Dunedin, where he came under the influence of Rowland Wilson, a Scottish ophthalmologist who had been the Director of the Giza Ophthalmic Memorial Laboratory in Cairo, prior to becoming the first Professor of Ophthalmology in New Zealand. Wilson was an inspirational figure, an excellent surgeon with a superb understanding of external eye disease and extensive knowledge of microbiology (he later bequeathed to Barrie Jones his extensive and unrivalled collection of *Chlamydia* pathological material). After qualifying, Jones returned to Wellington, where the ophthalmology training posts were combined with otolaryngology, and then went back to Dunedin as a registrar, in both the ophthalmology and neurosurgical units, thereby acquiring extensive experience in neurosurgery and ENT, as well as ophthalmology. This was to stand him in good stead later, when his attention turned to the surgery of the orbit and lacrimal drainage system.

It was obvious to him, very early in his career, that the treatment of trachoma, the greatest cause of blindness worldwide (and the principal reason for which Moorfields had originally been founded), was still wholly inadequate and its cause poorly understood. When he came to London, he soon became aware that his old chief in New Zealand knew far more about trachoma than anyone at Moorfields and had all but proved its aetiology. Moreover, other infections, particularly those of fungal and viral origin, were often diagnosed at too late a stage, or not at all, and were resistant to treatment. For this reason, the first specialist clinic he established when he became Professor (with the laboratory at the Institute of Ophthalmology to back it up), was called the Virus Clinic, this title covering conditions caused by a multitude of different microorganisms. Enormous advances in the understanding and hence treatment of viral, chlamydial, fungal and amoebic infections, many of them caused by agents such as *Acanthamoeba* and mycobacteria, which had previously been thought to be commensals, soon followed. As a result, a generation of young ophthalmologists, the present author among them, grew up to recognize the signs and symptoms of a whole host of previously obscure but disabling conditions affecting the external ocular tissues.

Of special importance was the identification of *Chlamydia* as the causative agent in trachoma and its implication, at least in the developed world, as a major cause of venereal disease leading to low-grade pelvic infection and sterility. Barrie Jones noticed that individuals suffering from inclusion conjunctivitis in London in the 'swinging sixties' were typically young, sexually active people and that the female partners suffered from chronic infection of the genital tract, with cervicitis, while their offspring developed ophthalmia typical of infection with *Chlamydia*. Sexual promiscuity, like ocular promiscuity, encouraged the spread of infection, which gave rise to two very different diseases in different social and climatic environments. To prove the connection between the cervical pathology and that of the conjunctiva, Barrie Jones personally examined the cervical epithelium (upending both the patients and the portable Zeiss operating microscope at Moorfields to do so), as well as the conjunctiva, thereby demonstrating identical pathology in the cervical epithelium to that in the conjunctiva and labelling the ocular condition TRIC (trachoma inclusion conjunctivitis) and its cause TRIC agent. He cooperated closely with the venereologist at the London Hospital, Dr Eric Dunlop (see below), and set up special clinics to handle the problem. Nor did he stop there. He conducted epidemiological studies in the Middle East, in particular what was then Persia (now Iran), where trachoma was rife and demographical information exceptionally good, and demonstrated that it responded well to tetracyclines. This work encouraged the introduction of treatment programmes worldwide.

Initially, he established a close relationship with a member of the consultant 'old guard' at Moorfields, Arthur George Leigh, and together they set up a corneal clinic. Leigh was not only clinically excellent and a fine surgeon, but he had an especially good relationship with Duke-Elder and knew instinctively how 'the Duke' would view things. As a result of this relationship, the latter was well disposed to the idea of developing microbiology at the Institute and supported Barrie Jones in his endeavours. Duke-Elder helped him to set up his own laboratory ('the Duke' had not used generous funding from British Petroleum, made available for overseas projects, and was keen to be seen to use this for a worthy cause), ensuring thereby its independence from Ashton's laboratory (the microbiology laboratory was later funded by the Medical Research Council).

Nor should Frederick Ridley's influence go unmentioned. After Ida Mann set up the first contact lens clinic in the 1930s, in this as in several of her other brilliant initiatives, she appears to have soon lost interest. It fell to Ridley to promote the use of therapeutic contact lenses at the High Holborn branch of Moorfields, where he (with the aid and support of the then CMO, Sir George Godber) set up the first Contact Lens Clinic. This proved to be a catalyst for the development of many an interest in surface disease, Peter Wright, Roger Buckley, John Dart and Steve Tuft all serving their apprenticeships in the Contact Lens Department, run later by Monty Ruben, Ridley's successor, and in turn by Roger Buckley. Whilst Ridley had promoted the use of hard lenses for therapeutic purposes only, however, Ruben and Buckley were to carry this on into the modern world with soft lenses. Hard corneal and scleral lenses nevertheless still had their place, a Moorfields optometrist, Ken Pullum, going on to be one of the foremost international experts in scleral contact lenses.

The Corneal and External Disease Service

After Leigh's tragically early death in 1968, his replacement on the consultant staff followed the prevailing tradition of the time, taking no account of any particular deficiency in the Hospital's clinical armamentarium. Rolf Blach, as already noted, had already established an overwhelming claim to the vacancy, albeit with a reputation in disorders of the retina. By this time, however, the Virus Clinic and laboratory were well established and there were others to fill the vacuum, in particular Noel Rice, then a senior lecturer on the Professorial Unit, who had already made his mark as an outstanding anterior segment surgeon and who was appointed to the consultant staff the following year. Continuity was thus assured, Rice's appointment being the first among many to match the specific requirements of the Hospital in meeting its commitment to provide specialist excellence in all aspects of eye disease. Peter Wright, who had done his residency at High Holborn and had already been a consultant at King's College Hospital since 1965, was appointed four years later, on John Ayoub's retirement, continuing thereby to contribute to the service his unique knowledge and understanding of tear physiology and the pathology of lacrimal secretory disorders.

There was, in any case, another corneal surgeon on the staff during this period – Derek Ainslie, who had developed special expertise with the earliest attempts at refractive surgery, a technique he had learned from José Barraquer in South America. Sadly, however, Ainslie was forced to retire in the mid-1970s as a result of ill health, thereby creating a further vacancy in the field of external disease and surgery of the anterior segment. This led to the appointment of Arthur Steele.

Steele's appointment was a matter of expediency, and to some extent a volte-face for, as he related to the present author, although he had initially set out on the path of anterior segment microsurgery (under the tutelage and inspiration of Dermot Pierse at the Mayday Hospital, Croydon), he had subsequently been persuaded by Barrie Jones, who perceived the Hospital's weakness in this field, towards a career in oculoplastic surgery. On Ainslie's retirement, all this suddenly changed. Roger Hitchings took over in the interim, as locum consultant, and the professor asked Steele if he was prepared to switch from plastics to his previous choice of specialty. This he was only too happy to do, going off to Bogota to learn refractive surgery at the feet of Barraquer, before returning in 1976 to secure his promotion to the consultant staff. This was a change of direction that served the Hospital well, as Steele went on to promote new developments in microsurgical technique and left the path clear for Richard Collin to pursue his interest in oculoplastic surgery.

Arthur Steele's career followed a somewhat unusual pattern. An Australian by birth and upbringing, he did his medical training in Melbourne, but after qualifying as a doctor and undergoing training in a number of different surgical specialties, he felt dissatisfied and undecided about his future. He had always nursed a dream to become an actor. With a strong thespian streak, a fine baritone voice and a not inconsiderable measure of chutzpah, he felt the urge to try his luck on the stage. Working in general practice in Melbourne until he had sufficient money, he then set sail for England. A brief job as an 'extra' for the BBC brought him his Equity (the actors' trade union) card and he was soon 'on the boards' in provincial repertory. It was an experience that, after a year, convinced him he was not the next Sir John Gielgud, and having purged himself of the desire for a thespian career he returned to the study and practice of medicine.

He went back to medicine partly by examining people at Australia House, which was good quick money, and also by GP relief work, which could be done at night, whilst studying. In his own words, 'I was so pleased to be back...I remember tapping on my first chest and the patient saying "I have never been examined like this Doctor" ...and I thought "I enjoy this" and I never went back. When I had enough money I did my Primary. I knew I wanted to be a surgeon, but probably a plastic surgeon, and it was while I was doing the Primary that I met someone who said "instead of a plastic surgeon you should be an ophthalmologist".

'So I bought Trevor-Roper's little book Lecture Notes in Ophthalmology *and thought well yes there is a great deal more to this than I had thought and I decided to pursue it. I ran my finger down the page and it said Institute of Ophthalmology. I rang them up and said "who is in charge?" and they said "the Dean, of course", so I went along to see him. He (Alex Cross) was very kind and gracious, and I explained that I wished to take up ophthalmology and that he must tell me what to do to*

become a first-class ophthalmologist. He said: "Steele, you need a good first job, as a Senior House Officer, and you will need to do your training at Moorfields. Now you don't have a job at the moment. Would you like to just join the DO course, which is starting the week after next?" I said "Yes, I'll do that", so I joined the DO course and started hunting for a job.

'Two jobs came up, one at a prestigious London teaching hospital and one at the Mayday Hospital, a district general hospital in Croydon. I made an appointment to see the consultant at the teaching hospital and went along at the appointed hour to his out-patient clinic. After half an hour he hadn't appeared and I asked the clinic clerk where he was. She said "He's gone to his consulting rooms in Harley Street." I said "Has he!" and I went round to his Rooms too. I banged on the door and said "I had an appointment in your out-patient clinic and you did not see me and here I am." "What did you want to know?" he asked, and I explained my predicament. "Oh you don't stand much of a chance: (a) you are too old and (b) you have done no ophthalmology." So the job went to someone else and I ended up at the Mayday under Dermot Pierse; and the rest is history."

(In fact, a few years later, the consultant who had turned him down so abruptly was to become a close colleague on the consultant staff at Moorfields, but remained blissfully unaware, for ever afterwards, of their previous acquaintance.)

Together with Dermot Pierse, the team at Moorfields, comprising Barrie Jones, Noel Rice and Arthur Steele, conducted regular micro-surgical workshops, encouraging the innovation and spread of modern surgical practice throughout the country. Meanwhile, other senior members of the Professorial Unit were developing their own ground-breaking activities, amongst them Peter Wright in tear physiology and infections and Peter Watson in scleritis, both of whom became giants in their respective fields. As the 1970s progressed, it was obvious, even to the Professor, that his academic and clinical workload and spread of interests were impossible to sustain in the long term, and he persuaded a charming and able ophthalmologist who was due to retire from service in the Royal Navy, Surgeon Commander Crawford Barras, to join the staff at Moorfields and the Institute, with an administrative and teaching role. This imaginative and pragmatic solution worked well, until Barras developed a pituitary tumour that forced his early retirement.

During the late 1970s and throughout the 1980s, the trend towards increasing subspecialization, championed by the Academic Department, continued relentlessly, driven by a combination of worldwide technological advances and the prescient attitude of the hospital leadership. Thus, although there was no move, as yet, to abandon the principle of a general ophthalmological commitment from all the consultants, clinics were established in all areas of special interest, to which patients with complicated problems could be referred. The Corneal Clinic had, as noted above, been one of the first of these, and served to maintain continuity and cohesion between the consultants, lecturers and other staff specializing in corneal and external disease.

Up to the end of the 1980s, senior members of the Academic Unit, although full-time university employees, were still granted consultant status and employed by the Hospital largely to undertake clinical work, the quality and quantity of their research output being considered of relatively minor importance. In the 1990s, in tune with the new direction taken by the Institute, what had in truth become a somewhat laissez-faire attitude towards research, on the Professorial Unit, was no longer acceptable. Senior members of the clinical academic staff therefore moved on, some going on to academic appointments while others became NHS consultants; their academic posts in the Professorial Unit were not reinstated. When the time came for the Hospital to seek Trust status, therefore, corneal and external disease was already established as a free-standing entity, no longer tied to the Academic Department. There was little difficulty in forming a directorate incorporating the consultants who had trained under Barrie Jones, Noel Rice and Peter Wright in the 1960s, Arthur Steele in the 1970s, and Linda Ficker and John Dart (who had joined in the 1980s), together with a broad group of other clinicians, including the director of the Contact Lens Service, Roger Buckley, the role of service director being assumed by Miss Ficker.

Their special interests within the subspecialty were diverse. Furthermore, Rice had long since taken over the management of paediatric glaucoma, on Arthur Lister's retirement, so he also had a foot in the Glaucoma Service. Steele's mentor, Dermot Pierse, had famously asserted: *'The surgeon who goes on doing what he was taught in the first place, and does not, with experience, change his practice and search for new approaches, is a menace to both himself and to his patients,'* and he took it upon himself to bring in the latest microsurgical techniques, from intra-ocular lens implants to refractive surgery, and established an outstanding surgical reputation, while Peter Wright continued in his role as Moorfields' doyen of tear physiology and external eye diseases.

When Barrie Jones left to set up the Department of Preventive Ophthalmology in 1980, there had been no obvious successor to take forward the advances he had made in infectious disease, and although Douglas Coster held the fort until he went back to Australia, progress in this field languished for a time. This gap was later filled by John Dart, who, after finishing his residency, went to the USA and Australia to spend Fellowships with Dan Jones and Coster, before returning to the UK and to Moorfields in 1984. Initially funded by Fisons, the pharmaceutical manufacturers, to undertake research into allergic eye disease, he went to work with Roger Buckley in the Contact Lens Department, as a clinical lecturer, gaining enormous experience in ocular surface disease and completing his MD. When the resignation of David McLeod in 1988 created an opening, he was formally appointed to the consultant staff, to continue the pioneering work on infections begun by Barrie Jones long before. By providing a service, at all hours of the day and night, for patients with devastating infections, he rapidly gained unparalleled experience and established a world-class reputation for himself in the field, publishing widely, especially on microbial keratitis, *Acanthamoeba* keratitis and ocular cicatricial pemphigoid. Meanwhile, he worked closely with Peter Wright, seeing patients with autoimmune conditions, in the course of which he acquired an outstanding knowledge of Stevens–Johnson disease and ocular pemphigoid, so that, on Wright's retirement in 1996, he was able to take over the care of these patients.

As with most of the other specialist directorates, the development of the outreach programme and increasing demand for a consultant-based service brought ever greater numbers of patients, the Corneal and External Disease Service being uniquely exposed, because of its close alliance with the Cataract Service, whose day-case surgery programme dominated the outreach services. With the split into primary-care and specialist services, not only was the number of referrals with surface disease greatly increased, but most of the consultants were also actively involved in undertaking an increasing amount of cataract surgery. Furthermore, the greater sophistication, speed and lower threshold of acceptability for the latter did nothing to lighten the burden. With the retirement in turn of Noel Rice (1994), Arthur Steele (1995) and Peter Wright (1996), it therefore became necessary to strengthen the consultant team in Corneal and External Disease, as well as to appoint consultants to the Cataract Service alone.

Steve Tuft, who had worked with Roger Buckley in the Contact Lens Department and done major research into the effects of the excimer laser, was appointed in 1995, followed by David Gartry and Julian Stevens, also experts in excimer laser technology. Frank Larkin, specializing in corneal transplantation, and Bruce Allan in biocompatible materials research, both of whom had sessions from the Trust dedicated specifically to research, were appointed soon afterwards, not only to widen the areas of expertise in the service but also to provide it with a broad research base. By the end of the decade, therefore, the complement of consultants had increased from four to seven, the loss of the clinical academic posts in the old academic unit being more than counter-balanced by the '50/50' research members, while in 2002 the total number of senior staff included seven Visiting Fellows.

Because of the size and patient throughput of the Contact Lens Department at Moorfields, together with the special interests and academic skills of John Dart, Steve Tuft and Frank Larkin, the Hospital re-established its reputation for quality in the 1990s in the field of surface infection, deploying new antimicrobial agents and, in the case of *Acanthamoeba*, pioneering the use of a biguanide disinfectant anti-microbial, Bacquacil, formerly used as a swimming-bath cleaner. The latter was in contrast with the situation in the 1970s, when although Barrie Jones was the first person to describe a case of *Acanthamoeba*, it was a comparatively uncommon and untreatable condition, the herpes simplex virus being then a major scourge and fungal keratitis among his special interests.

Frank Larkin had spent a year training in corneal transplantation research with Douglas Coster in Adelaide. His special knowledge and understanding of graft rejection was of fundamental importance to progress in corneal transplantation at Moorfields, more than 350 corneal grafts being undertaken there each year. Nevertheless, storage of corneal graft material, introduced at Moorfields by Trevor-Roper in 1967, although it changed radically in the early part of the new century, was still considered to be unsatisfactory. Although the Eye-Bank facilities were refurbished and modernized by the Trust, at a cost of £80 000, in the prevailing climate of alarm and despondency engendered by high-profile cases of latent infection, they still failed to meet the demands of the Department of Health's inspection agency. The cost of the modifications to the preparation and storage areas and of the other changes demanded would have been colossal, and annual running costs similarly prohibitive. Despite the closest attention paid to the screening of donors for any history of unexplained neurological disease or infection with hepatitis B, syphilis and HIV, and the most stringent attention to hygiene in the department, the Eye-Bank was unable to satisfy the inspectors fully. Sybil Ritten, who had served as Eye-Bank Officer under Arthur Steele since the mid-1980s and then under Frank Larkin, found it an increasingly uphill task to provide a satisfactory service in the face of demands that were at best unreasonable and at worst ran counter to patients' best interests.

It is worth recalling here that the Pocklington Eye Transplantation Research Unit, originally founded by Sir Benjamin Rycroft, was trans-ferred to the Professorial Unit in the early 1970s, and became closely associated with the Eye-Bank when the latter moved over to City Road. This collaboration greatly enhanced the handling of donor corneas for transplantation, under the aegis of the Research Unit's scientist Emil Sherrard, whose interest in endothelial cell function led him to undertake pioneering work in specular microscopy.

Refractive surgery

As recorded, the first attempts at surgical correction of refractive error were carried out at Moorfields by Derek Ainslie in the 1960s, after he went to visit José Barraquer in Bogota, who was undertaking what was then called keratomileusis (flattening the cornea) and keratophakia (increasing its curvature). This was done by remodelling a lamella of tissue, cut from the cornea and frozen, using a micro-lathe, a difficult and relatively untried procedure requiring considerable manual dexterity. Sadly, no records of the cases done by Ainslie survive, so little is known about his results. In fact, the idea of reshaping the cornea to alter its refractive power was nothing new, it having been mooted at the beginning of the 20th Century, but it failed to gain acceptance at that time, owing to technical difficulties and the crude nature of the instrumentation. The concept was subsequently revived by Sato in Japan, using radial incisions from within the anterior chamber, but this method, not surprisingly, caused corneal endothelial damage, with subsequent decompensation. In the 1970s Fyodorov, working in the Soviet Union, free from the limitations imposed by ethical considerations or peer pressure, devised a method using partial-thickness radial incisions to cause flattening of the corneal curvature, which was successful in cases of high myopia and astigmatism. Thus was radial keratotomy born, an incisional procedure with unpredictable outcome and considerable risks, which nonetheless presaged the dawn of a new era of technological advance.

At Moorfields, Arthur Steele made a tentative effort to embrace the new technique, always mindful of its obvious shortcomings even in his hands, and taught it to his Fellows from the early 1980s onwards. Others throughout the UK and further afield, possibly recognizing its commercial possibilities, were less cautious. In 1988, however, a breakthrough was made that was to change the course of refractive surgery radically. As long as five years before, Troquel and Srinivasan in the USA had experimented with a new type of laser for sculpting tissues. The excimer laser produced light with a wavelength of 193 nanometres, capable of penetrating corneal tissue without being absorbed by it (thereby having the capacity to cut without carrying the danger of teratogenicity), but it at first proved difficult to control the depth of penetration. Finally, at Louisiana State University, New Orleans, in 1988 Marguerite McDonald undertook the first successful photo-refractive keratotomy (PRK) in a human eye, using the excimer laser.

In London, Steve Tuft and John Marshall (then Sembal Professor) at the Institute of Ophthalmology carried out extensive work on the effects of the laser on rabbit corneas. Marshall, who was already a world expert on laser technology, did more than anyone else to develop the excimer laser for clinical use, and in 1989 an excimer laser was installed at Moorfields and first used by Arthur Steele. In 1991 Marshall left the Institute and went to St Thomas' Hospital. The excimer venture at Moorfields was not at first entirely successful, the results being far from 100% satisfactory and the complication rate higher than was acceptable. The first laser was therefore returned to its manufacturers, and it was not until 1992 that a VISX excimer laser was installed at the Hospital, which proved to be reliable, relatively safe and highly effective (although even then the outcome of treatment was not entirely predictable) (**Figure 25**, Plate 13, top).

At this time, the Steele's Fellow was Julian Stevens, a technophile with an abiding interest in all things electronic and mathematical, who soon realized the huge potential, both clinical and commercial, of the new technology, and set about learning everything there was to know about PRK. In 1992 Steele and Stevens undertook 228 PRK procedures, doing one eye at a time and waiting six months before treating the second eye, in itself an indication of their uncertainty about its long-term outcome. During the next two years, 1800 eyes were treated at Moorfields and a total of 12 000 nationwide. With the retirement of Arthur Steele in 1996, Julian Stevens was appointed to the consultant staff, with the express purpose of promoting best practice in PRK and undertaking research at Moorfields. He was soon asked to chair a symposium at the Annual Meeting of the Royal College of Ophthalmologists, and to set guidelines for its practice nationally (including those for the Civil Aviation Authority). In the clinical arena he was ably assisted by David Gartry, who was appointed to the staff in 1997, and who became the President of the British Refractive Surgery Society in 2001, and by his other colleagues on the Corneal and External Disease Service, the number of cases treated at Moorfields rising by the turn of the century to 5000 per year. Of these, as many as 400 were NHS patients whose refractive errors could not be corrected with spectacles or contact lenses, and these were paid for by the NHS. With a facility fee charged by Moorfields in most cases, however, PRK represented a considerable commercial benefit to the Hospital, as well as a boon to the patients.

Between 1992 and 1995, a further development of great significance took place. Surgeons in Crete and Italy returned to the early concept of keratomileusis and keratophakia, this time using a manual micro-keratome to cut a lamellar flap within the anterior cornea, and marrying this with precision sculpting by the excimer laser – so-called laser intrastromal keratotomy (LASIK). Nevertheless, they still had great difficulty producing acceptably reliable and predictable results using manual techniques. The introduction of the automated micro-keratome, however, made a significant improvement, and the technique was first used at Moorfields in 1998. Automated instruments obviated the need for surgeons to be perfectly ambidextrous in sculpting lamellar flaps for right and left eyes, while further advances, mostly in wave-front technology, soon enabled precise corneal contour-mapping, the information being fed to the microkeratome electronically. LASIK became the method of choice in the majority of cases, being painless, quick and almost instantly effective, while corneal surgeons took to it seamlessly, finding the technique easy to acquire and extremely patient-friendly. Not only was it used in otherwise-healthy eyes, but cases of corneal dystrophy and scarring could also be treated by laser kerat-ectomy, with excellent optical results.

The spectacular advances in refractive surgery now seemed likely to lead to other exciting developments. Improvements in wave-front measurement (defects in the corneal contour being mapped at 200 separate points within the pupillary area), coupled with the introduction of femtosecond lasers, heralded the advent of intrastromal corneal remodelling without the need for lamellar keratectomy. This could enable the measurement and potential correction of complex spherical aberrations causing amblyopia in small children, as well as the treatment of corneal dystrophies and scarring. There seemed little doubt that the use of photorefractive surgery was set to escalate still further in the future, an opinion obviously shared by the equipment manufacturers, who were happy to provide Moorfields with the laser free of charge, for an initial period of five years, as well as an annual fee of $50 000, in respect of consultant time. Equally, Moorfields appeared to recognize its potential, when, in a short space of time, they purchased a second laser.

Glaucoma services

Background

Of all the subspecialties, none has seen more development and expansion than glaucoma, where advances in assessment and treat-ment, especially during the past 20 years, have transformed its management. Formerly within the ambit of all consultants, until the late 1960s chronic simple glaucoma (now termed primary open angle glaucoma, POAG) was a relentlessly blinding condition, while the acute, secondary and juvenile forms often received treatment too late to save vision. Stephen Miller and Redmond Smith, at the High Holborn and City Road branches of Moorfields respectively, became the specialists in this field as it began to modernize, during the 1970s, and provided expert advice to their colleagues and patients when requested to do so, but there was no concerted attempt to channel all cases into specialist clinics. Nor indeed would this have been a practical proposition, before the development of primary care and specialist clinical services in the early 1990s. Even then, the chronic nature of POAG and its long-term management in the old-style general clinics meant that the transition was a gradual process.

The treatment of acute closed angle glaucoma had been transformed by the introduction of a straightforward surgical solution, as early as the mid 19th Century (iridotomy, later to be replaced by peripheral irid-ectomy), which, if undertaken when the intra-ocular pressure had been brought under control beforehand, was usually safe and permanently effective. The juvenile type, causing buphthalmos, was, from early on in his career, the particular interest of Arthur Lister at Moorfields, who developed a highly specialized surgical technique for its treatment, more about which will be considered later. In addition to the three spontaneous forms, there was also a large group of patients with glaucoma secondary to surgical and other forms of trauma, particularly that associated with intracapsular cataract extraction and penetrating injury.

By far and away the most common type, and the cause of blindness in large numbers of older people, POAG was until the 1970s extremely resistant to treatment. Assessment was crude and inaccurate, depend-ing as it did on patients' responses to visual stimuli, which often varied in their strength from one test to another (Lister perimeter and Bjerrum screen) and which were time-consuming and tiring for subject and examiner alike. Topical treatment was limited to preparations of drugs to constrict the pupil and open the drainage angle (e.g. pilo-carpine) or to reduce the production of aqueous fluid (e.g. noradrena-line (Eppy) or a combination of guanethidine and adrenaline (Ganda)), systemic preparations of the carbonic acid anhydrase inhibitor acetazo-lamide (Diamox) and anticholinesterase agents (e.g. ecothiophate iodide (Phospholine Iodide)), all of which had unpleasant side-effects, were sometimes used in extremely refractory cases, while surgical procedures were aimed at creating a permanent drainage fistula by trephining or a modification of this using cautery (Scheie's operation).

It is impossible to tell what great advances Miller and Redmond Smith might have made had they lived and worked in more recent times (**Figure 26**). Both were exceptionally talented surgeons, innovative thinkers and charming and delightful company. Miller was also particularly interested in neuro-ophthalmology and was on the consultant staff of the National Hospital for Nervous Diseases, Queen Square. Through the generosity of a grateful patient, Tommy Frost, he was able to purchase a fundus camera there and used it to examine the optic nerve head, using fluorescein, to detect papilloedema, long before its routine use in retinal vascular disease, while Smith was a brilliant polymath, turning his attention to everything from the functional arrangements of Schlemm's canal to the mathematical calculations for encircling bands for retinal surgery and the use of the former to ensure a perfectly level surface for his tennis court. Both Miller and Smith, perhaps as a result of their broad knowledge and multifarious skills, were generalists at heart and both retained appointments at general hospitals, in addition to their posts at Moorfields – Miller at St George's and Smith at St Mary's (Western Ophthalmic) – while Miller spread his talents even further, with his appointment at Queen Square.

Sir Stephen Miller's extraordinary career is worth recording, and a brief account gleaned from his obituaries will here suffice: Qualifying in 1937, he gained some experience of ophthalmology before the War, which enabled him to nurture both naval and airforce personnel in Malta, where he met

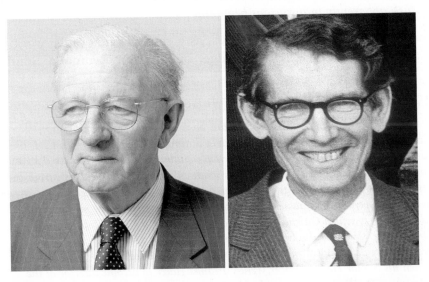

Figure 26 Sir Stephen Miller (*left*) and Mr Redmond Smith (*right*) glaucoma specialists during the 1960s and 1970s, at the High Holborn and City Road branches of the Hospital respectively.

and gained the lifelong support of Keith Lyle, then Air Commodore and Ophthalmologist to the RAF, and ultimately to be his colleague at three hospitals. Following demobilization, he was appointed consultant ophthalmologist in Hull, where he was promised a brand new unit. After six months, however, there was no sign of this promise being fulfilled and he resigned (the new unit finally saw the light of day 21 years later). Lyle advised him to work at Moorfields and the new Institute of Ophthalmology, which he did, and as a registrar at the High Holborn branch of Moorfields, he worked all hours, mastering his specialty. It soon became apparent, however, that there were no jobs to be had in the UK, so he filed papers to go the USA. Sir Stewart Duke-Elder got to hear of this and was horrified, immediately offering him a post at St George's, from which he was soon elevated to the consultant staff.

Subsequent appointments at Moorfields and at the National Hospital for Nervous Diseases, Queen Square established him in the forefront of his profession, and in 1974 he was appointed Surgeon Oculist to the Queen and subsequently rewarded with the honour of a knighthood. In later years he became Hospitaller to the St John's Ophthalmic Hospital in Jerusalem. He also formed a close friendship with a patient, a wealthy industrialist, Tommy Frost, who formed the TFC Frost Trust, funding numerous research projects, including a Chair of Ophthalmology. He was Editor of the British Journal of Ophthalmology *for 10 years, published four textbooks, gave the Doyne Lecture in 1972 and formed the first glaucoma unit in London. All things considered, this was a remarkable career, stemming as it did from such apparently inauspicious beginnings.*

Suddenly, at the end of the 1960s, as a result of innovative work by Cairns and Watson* in Cambridge, building on Redmond Smith's

---

* John Cairns and Peter Watson had both trained as Residents at City Road and then went on to be appointed to consultant posts at Addenbrookes Hospital, Cambridge at the same time. Cairns was a natural wit, with a biting and at times caustic turn of phrase. He did not suffer fools gladly, and was known for the quality of his 'one-liners'. One such was made in response to an enquiry from a visitor to his department as to why he preferred the (new) trabeculectomy operation to Scheie's operation (in which thermocautery was applied to the margin of the sclerotomy), to which Cairns replied: 'I couldn't stand the smell (of the cautery)'. On another occasion, also in response to a visitor, who asked him why he never drank coffee before operating, came the rejoinder: 'Because it keeps me awake'. When his Senior House Officer, Wendy Franks (later to become director of the Glaucoma Service), announced her intention of seeking a training post at Moorfields, he said to her: 'You're interested in the history of ophthalmology, aren't you, Wendy? Well, you'll see plenty of it there!'

ideas about the mechanisms of trabecular outflow, a new and more effective fistulizing operation, trabeculectomy, emerged. This was followed in the 1970s by the introduction of topical beta-blocking agents (timolol) and trials of other methods, involving lasering the trabecular meshwork (laser trabeculoplasty) and insertion of drainage tubes (Molteno tubes), while Redmond Smith tried, imaginatively but with less success, to carry out trabeculotomy, using a fine suture threaded along Schlemm's canal and pulled tight, to achieve a 'cheese-wire' effect. An explosion of technical advance erupted from all this innovative activity, resulting in a range of new drugs, sophisticated methods of assessment and trials of treatment, using laser and surgical technology. Amidst it all came the appointment to the consultant staff at Moorfields, in 1980, of Roger Hitchings, an event that proved to be of importance, not just to Moorfields but also to the management of glaucoma worldwide.

Finishing his residency at Moorfields in 1973, Roger Hitchings was appointed to the consultant staff at Kings College Hospital in 1976 and to the staff of the High Holborn branch of Moorfields in 1980, on the retirement of Sir Stephen Miller. He had already developed a special interest in glaucoma and was not only an excellent surgeon but also the possessor of a keen analytical brain. He set about analysing the outcome of the prevailing methods of treating POAG, including medical management, laser trabeculoplasty and fistulizing surgery, and published the results of this Primary Treatment Trial in a paper that proved to be a defining point of reference in the field. With the retirement of Redmond Smith in 1983 and, in due course of time, the amalgamation of the two branches of the Hospital and the formation of specialist services, together with an expanding outreach programme, Hitchings became the director of the new Glaucoma Service and thereby inherited the largest cohort of glaucoma patients in the Western world.

Meanwhile, during the 1980s, a host of other developments in glaucoma management took place. Some of the most significant of these were advances in visual field testing, first a serious attempt to standardize the visual stimulus and the background against which it was presented to the patient, in the Goldmann perimeter, soon followed by the introduction of computerized instruments, the Friedmann and then the Humphrey, which for the first time brought reproducibility into visual field measurement. These tests were not always simple or quick, and the tiredness and inattention induced by lengthy testing could often neutralize their inherent advantages. A Swedish ophthalmologist, however, came up with a new formula for using the Humphrey (SITA), which reduced the duration of the test to less than half that previously taken. There was also a steady improvement in the quality and range of pressure-lowering drugs.

With the momentous changes in primary and secondary care set in motion at the start of the 1990s, the stage was set for the glaucoma services at Moorfields to mushroom. It was clear that an increase in the number of consultant glaucoma specialists was urgently needed. In 1991 Michael Miller was appointed, soon followed by Peng Tee Khaw, about whom more is related below. Miller, following in the footsteps of his father Sir Stephen, took over the day-to-day administration of the service and oversaw the development of the outreach service at Northwick Park Hospital. He also took office as chairman of the International Glaucoma Association. He set up an outstanding weekly teaching programme at Moorfields, attended by all the glaucoma consultants, as well as junior staff, which stood the test of time. The academic thrust of the service was further strengthened by the appointment of Richard Wormald, who, with his strong epidemiological background, was instrumental in establishing the Cochrane Collaboration.

The appointment of Wendy Franks, an exceptionally practical and well-organized individual with a lightness of touch and wry sense of humour that belied her steely determination, enabled Roger Hitchings to make better use of his time, directing the research effort and future strategy of the Glaucoma Unit. Arriving in 1994, soon after the inception of the specialist services, Franks took over the outreach unit at St Andrew's Bow and in 1996 became Director of the Glaucoma Service, a task for which she was admirably well suited. With the rapid expansion of the outreach programme, the volume of glaucoma work continued to increase relentlessly and further consultant appointments followed, Keith Barton (1995) taking the lead at Barking and Ian Murdoch (1996) in Ealing. Barton set up a much needed subspecialist service in uveitic glaucoma, in collaboration with Carlos Pavesio in the Medical Retina Service. In 2001 Maria Papadopoulos joined the team to complement Khaw's work in paediatric glaucoma and take over from Miller as the clinical lead at Northwick Park, when the latter left Glaucoma to head up the Cataract Service. Ted Garway-Heath was appointed in 2000 on a 50/50 research/clinical contract, with the aim of developing his interest in psychophysical assessment and early detection of optic nerve-head damage, and in 2003 there was further expansion of the service with the appointment of Ananth Viswanathan, also to a 50/50 post, to pursue his research studies on visual field assessment and to take responsibility for the Glaucoma Clinic at St George's Hospital.

The rapid appointments of Papadopoulos, with interests in paediatric glaucoma, Garway-Heath in research into optical imaging and psychophysics, and Viswanathan in visual field testing, reflected not only the increase in clinical workload but also the explosion in research generated by Roger Hitchings' leadership, as the new millennium got under way. Indeed, the high quality of research in glaucoma initiated by Hitchings had been recognized as early as 1993 by Michael Peckham's Research Review Advisory Committee, the Glaucoma Unit being one of only two research teams at Moorfields to be accorded an alpha plus rating. The International Glaucoma Association, founded by Pitts Crick at King's College, was a generous supporter of this research, as also were the Special Trustees and the Friends of Moorfields, all three contributing towards the establishment of the Glaucoma Research Unit, which first occupied a cramped space on the ground floor of the Hospital, wedged between Visual Assessment and Pharmacy, but soon moved to more capacious quarters (1999) in the area on the second floor previously occupied by Parsons Ward.

The continuing excellence of the research programme, including collaborative studies in psychophysics with Fred Fitzke at the Institute, with Professor Gordon Johnson in the Department of Preventive Ophthalmology and with Peng Tee Khaw on wound-healing, soon led to even wider recognition, Hitchings, Fitzke and Khaw all being awarded personal academic chairs. Nor should the efforts of lesser mortals go unrecorded, especially those of Sammy Poinoosawmy, senior glaucoma technician in the unit, whose enthusiastic and diligent work contributed in no small measure to the quality of many studies. Never before had Moorfields boasted so many professors in one department, and as the new millennium opened, there was an air of palpable optimism, in sharp contrast to the view of older surgeons, notably Redmond Smith, who looked upon the results of his labours with a fatalism bordering on despair.

A number of factors other than the introduction of the new tests and treatments contributed to the improved outlook for adult glaucoma patients. The advent of microsurgery had not only enabled more sophisticated methods for the treatment of established POAG, it had also led to great improvements in the surgery of cataract. Previously, many of the most difficult glaucoma cases were those secondary to complications of cataract extraction. The adoption of sophisticated extracapsular surgery, preserving the posterior lens capsule, and later of small-incision surgery, causing minimal interference with the anterior chamber, saw the incidence of secondary glaucoma fall dramatically, while the introduction of safety measures for motorists, as well as improvements in industrial practices, thereby reducing ocular trauma, had a similar though less extravagant impact. Furthermore, the commonest cause of failure in fistulizing surgery, early spontaneous closure of the drainage channel as a result of the natural healing response, was addressed by Khaw's work on wound healing (including a trial of a single sponge application of 5-fluorouracil developed at Moorfields and the Institute to discourage fistula closure, which won an eight-year grant from the Medical Research Council, the largest single grant ever awarded in British clinical ophthalmology).

An entirely new group of pressure-lowering drugs was introduced during the 1990s, the prostaglandin agonists (notably latanaprost), their action based on the effect of prostaglandins increasing aqueous outflow through the uveoscleral channels. Indeed, so effective were they and such was their popularity that in the space of five years the use of trabeculectomy in uncomplicated cases was halved. These agents were found to have few adverse side-effects and soon began to supersede the beta-blockers, particularly in patients with asthma or obstructive airways disease, while alpha-agonists such as brimonidine and iopidine added further sophistication to an already formidable array of drugs.

In the assessment of glaucoma, perhaps the most significant advance, during the 1990s and beyond, apart from the steady improvements made to existing computerized perimetry devices, was the introduction of the Heidelberg Retinal Tomograph and its use to demonstrate the topography of the optic nerve head, a project with which Ted Garway-Heath was much concerned, and one that could lead in the future to objective methods of assessment replacing the traditional subjective method of visual field measurement. Ananth Viswanathan's appointment further strengthened this area of study, his interests in the genetics of glaucoma and in progressor software for visual field testing complementing Garway-Heath's. In its treatment, the introduction of the prostaglandin agonists and development of a topical preparation of acetazolamide were matched by the use of the diode laser, in place of cryotherapy or diathermy, to inhibit the production of aqueous fluid by the ciliary body, while antiscarring agents, such as 5-fluorouracil and mitomycin-C, in conjunction with fistulizing surgery, together with better designs of Molteno-type tubes and plates, transformed the surgical prospect.

Much of the work leading to the greatly improved outlook for patients with glaucoma came from the Glaucoma Unit at Moorfields and it is fair to say that Professor Hitchings and his unit could be considered to lead the world in this field, throughout the 1990s and into the new millennium. Nevertheless, as Ian Murdoch reminded the present author, there is a history, throughout medicine, of new drugs and treatments being hailed and then later discarded, as their defects are discovered, and some of the new anti-glaucoma therapies might in the future suffer a similar fate. To paraphrase Osler: *'Use a new treatment quickly, while it still works'*, or, as another sceptical physician remarked, *'One has only to enter the graveyard of discarded therapies to appreciate the advantage of being in the control group.'*

While perhaps the most obviously brilliant research of the unit emanated from Khaw, Garway-Heath and Hitchings himself, other less glamorous but equally important work, in the field of epidemiology, was done by Murdoch and by Papadopoulos, the latter working with Jugnoo Rahi in the British Ophthalmic Surveillance Unit. As long ago as the 1960s and early 1970s, Professors Perkins and Gloster, at the Institute of Ophthalmology, undertook some notable research work, advancing the epidemiological and theoretical understanding of POAG in the community at large. Ian Murdoch had a strong background in epidemiology, with a Master's degree from the School of Hygiene and Tropical Diseases. He had worked with Barrie Jones in Africa during the mid-1990s and was about to embark on an ambitious study of glaucoma management in Zaire when, due to an escalation of violence there, this was abruptly halted. As a result of this blow to his career plans, he applied for and was appointed to a consultant post at Moorfields, and three years later secured one of the '50/50' research positions, created to encourage high-quality clinical research at the Hospital. He was then able to establish his research base more firmly by joining the Institute's Department of Epidemiology as a Senior Research Fellow. As the lead clinician at the Ealing Outreach Unit, he was in a good position to initiate studies examining the role of optometrists in the detection and referral of patients with suspected POAG, a randomized trial showing that training and interaction with local optometrists doubled the number of new cases of POAG detected. Furthermore, qualitative studies showed that public perceptions and understanding of glaucoma were very limited and a large study was set up to investigate this aspect of the disease, in the Isle of Wight. Nor were Murdoch's research activities confined to the UK; he was involved in a large trial of beta-irradiation of glaucoma filtering blebs (a treatment originally pioneered by Noel Rice in the Paediatric Glaucoma Service) in Africans, funded by the Wellcome Trust, and was also instrumental in pioneering the use of telemedicine. Grand rounds were successfully conducted between Moorfields consultants and colleagues in South Africa, and a link was established between centres in South Africa, Tanzania, Ghana and Gambia, and the Moorfields website.

Not only had there been a transformation in methods of assessment and treatment, but perhaps even more significant were the changes in care brought about as a result of multidisciplinary team working and the introduction of nurse-specialists, who were able to screen for POAG safely and, with structured protocols, to assess patients with POAG and, where appropriate, prescribe for them. Innovations like these, unheard of in former times, but essential if the outcomes of epidemiological studies were to be translated into effective practice, heralded a whole new era of healthcare for the community at large.

Paediatric glaucoma

Prior to the advent of microsurgery, operative procedures on the eye were relatively crude affairs, restricted by the limitations imposed by poor magnification and basic instruments. With the introduction of the operating microscope in the 1960s, however, a whole new range of finer instruments were developed, and consequently a wide range of more sophisticated surgery became possible. One such procedure was goniotomy, the opening up of the congenitally closed angle of the anterior chamber, in children with buphthalmos, a blinding condition, distressing for both the children and their families. Arthur Lister became its foremost exponent in the UK, using a Koeppe contact lens to identify the anterior chamber angle and a fine blade to open it.

> *Peng Tee Khaw records that Lister, a man of the strongest commitment and enormous compassion, hearing about the new method, travelled all the way to San Francisco by sea, via the Panama canal, a journey of some two weeks' duration, to learn it at first hand. At the time of writing, Khaw was still looking after the first patient operated on by Arthur Lister, with pressures still controlled to this day.*

When Lister retired in 1970, Noel Rice, a naturally gifted surgeon, was appointed to replace him and took over this demanding field of surgery, continuing to run the service, in conjunction with a multi-disciplinary team consisting of a paediatrician, Dr Barry Jones, nursing staff, headed by Sister Ero, family support social worker Jackie Howe and play leader Mary Digby, all of whom were equally dedicated to the care and support of these children and their families.

In 1988 Noel Rice became aware of an exceptionally talented young ophthalmologist who had just finished his residency training and been awarded a Wellcome Trust Fellowship to study for a PhD degree on the cell and molecular biology of wound healing. Rice consulted his friend and colleague Arthur Steele regarding the young man's surgical abilities and decided that he would make an excellent choice to take over the paediatric glaucoma surgery, when the time came for him to retire. He arranged for him to attend his operating lists and to examine the children before and after surgery. After spending the next three years researching his PhD thesis, one of them in the USA, the individual concerned, Peng Tee Khaw, returned to the UK in 1992, only to be advised that there was no room for him in the Academic Department at Moorfields. Dismayed by this news and determined to find a job that would allow him to pursue his research interests, he applied for the newly advertised professorial chair at Imperial College, sited at the Western Ophthalmic Hospital. News of this apparent defection subsequently reached the ears of Noel Rice, via the grapevine, much to his alarm, and Khaw was summoned to meet him and explain himself (much, one suspects, to Khaw's own alarm). On hearing the story, however, Rice, who wielded enormous influence in the hospital, asked him to write down what it was that he wanted, to keep him at Moorfields, and then made him an offer he could not refuse, persuading the Hospital to create a full-time consultant post with only two fixed clinical sessions and the rest of the time devoted to research. Only thus did Moorfields retain the services of one of its brightest stars, and the children with paediatric glaucoma their future champion.

Neither Moorfields and the Glaucoma Unit nor the children with glaucoma went unrewarded by this apparently autocratic behaviour, Peng Tee Khaw taking over Rice's work as planned, on the latter's retirement, and displaying a dedication, combined with outstanding intellectual prowess, rarely matched. His advanced surgical thinking, allied with basic scientific knowledge, especially with regard to the treatment of glaucoma with fistulizing operations enhanced by the application of antiscarring agents, produced results, both in adults and children, not previously achieved with safety.

He was joined in 2000 by Maria Papadopoulos, fresh from spending a three-year Fellowship with him in the Glaucoma Unit, during which time she had acquired the necessary surgical and other skills to become a specialist in both adult and paediatric glaucoma. Furthermore, collaboration with Phil Luthert in the Department of Pathology and with Stephen Moss and other scientists in wound-healing and cell biology promised more exciting advances in the future, while the proposed International Children's Eye Centre boded well for the possibilities of improved paediatric research facilities.

Postscript

To the present author and to others of his generation, the pessimistic views of Redmond Smith remain firmly embedded in memory. Talking to the latter as recently as April 2002, his views were little changed. How then, to reconcile them with all the exciting advances made during the last two decades? It seems certain that patients with POAG, although never actually cured of the disease, can now be spared the prospect of blindness for the remainder of their lives. Recent work in the USA confirms this. In the words of Ian Murdoch: *'Our goal is to ensure that every patient will be able to see, until they reach the grave'* – surely a reasonable and optimistic, if pragmatic, goal and one that the Glaucoma Service at Moorfields would be proud to have achieved.

Medical retina

Background

In contrast to surgery for detachment of the retina, which was first introduced in the early part of the 20th Century and was so dramatically successful that it quite soon developed as a specialty in its own right, disorders of the retina not amenable to surgery remained, until much more recently, largely refractory to treatment. The emergence of Medical retina as a recognized specialty did not, as a consequence, happen until very much later, diseases affecting flow in the retinal and choroidal blood vessels, degenerative conditions of Bruch's membrane and the pigment epithelium, and benign tumours and hamartomas of the retinal and choroidal vasculature remaining mysteriously resistant both to scientific interpretation and to rational treatment. Up to the 1960s, apart from irradiation for malignant tumours of the retina in children (retinoblastoma) and choroid in adults (malignant melanoma), which were in any case more often than not treated by enucleation, there was little that could be done for the more common and blinding conditions, such as diabetic retinopathy, that afflicted the retina and its associated tissues. Other disorders, both congenital and acquired, such as retinal telangiectasis, retinal degenerations and retinal vasculitis, were poorly understood, often attracting eponymous titles, such as Coats', Leber's and von Hippel–Lindau disease, and were largely considered untreatable.

In 1961 Novotny and Alvis published a paper describing a new technique for delineating the retinal blood vessels and the flow through them, utilizing intravenous sodium fluorescein. It was found that this agent, when injected into the bloodstream, bound itself to serum albumen, and was, apart from the occasional allergic response, completely harmless. Furthermore, as its name implied, when subjected to light of one wavelength, it fluoresced, emitting light of a different wavelength. Because the dye combined with albumen, it formed a large particle, which could not pass through the walls of normal retinal blood vessels (the cells lining which have 'tight junctions' that are impervious to small molecules). Novotny and Alvis saw the possibility of using it to demonstrate blood-flow and vascular integrity in the ocular fundus. By filtering out the light from the illuminating beam, reflected back from the ocular fundus, only the rays emitted from the fluorescein in the blood vessels (of a different wavelength from the illuminating beam) reached the observer, and a clear image of the blood flowing along the vessels could therefore be both seen and captured on film. Moreover, any dye that leaked out of the vessels could only be doing so through defects in their walls. Thus it was now possible to highlight specifically the retinal blood vessels and the blood within them, thereby demonstrating the integrity or otherwise of their walls, and the quality of flow, and to record this photographically.

Remarkably, the paper that first described the technique was initially rejected by the *American Journal of Ophthalmology*, and was eventually published in a non-ophthalmic journal, *Circulation*. It was there that Colin Dollery, at the Royal Postgraduate Medical School (RPMS), Hammersmith (later Professor of Clinical Pharmacology), who was especially interested in ophthalmology, saw it and recognized its potential importance as an investigative tool, subsequently publishing his own findings in the *British Medical Journal*. The close links between Professor Barrie Jones's unit and the Hammersmith, cemented by David Hill as a senior lecturer working at both Moorfields and the RPMS, then led to collaborative studies between the physicians, led by Professor Russell Fraser, Dollery and Graham Joplin, soon joined by Dr Eva Kohner, at the RPMS, and the ophthalmologists led by Hill and Rolf Blach, plus a number of Wellcome Foundation Research Fellows, including Hung Cheng, Tim Ffytche and Peter Hamilton from Moorfields.

Fluorescein fundus angiography was thus first introduced to the UK by Dollery at the RPMS, who passed the technique onwards; in 1964–65, it was used by Sanders, Bird, Ffytche, Archer and others, under the direction of Sir Stephen Miller, at the National Hospital for Nervous Diseases, Queen Square, for investigating the nature of optic disc swelling; later, David Hill and then Sohan Singh Hayreh used it in the Professorial Unit at Moorfields to define retinal blood flow, and it is they, therefore, who must be credited with its introduction there. The close collaboration between the physicians at the Hammersmith, in particular Graham Joplin, who had been pioneering the use of pituitary ablation for the treatment of florid diabetic retinopathy, with David Hill and the other ophthalmologists from Moorfields, led by Rolf Blach, was to result in the establishment of several landmark studies of diabetic retinopathy, and to the concept of retinal ablation by photocoagulation in its treatment.

Fluorescein fundus angiography (FFA), as it soon became known, transformed the management of medical retinal disease and brought within sight accurate diagnosis and successful treatment of a wide range of conditions affecting the posterior segment. In due course, a miscellany of obscure disorders of the retina and uveal tract, previously lumped together under the umbrella term 'uveitis', or designated by equally obscure eponymynous titles, were recognized as distinct pathological entities, while the application of photocoagulation to ablate leaking blood vessels or destroy abnormal or unwanted tissue rendered them treatable on a rational basis. Accurate retinal diagnosis became a reality, retinal diagnostic clinics quickly springing up to cope with the ever-increasing numbers of patients found to have medical retinal disorders.

A medical retinal revolution at Moorfields

The establishment of FFA at Moorfields, with diabetic patients from the Hammersmith Hospital brought over for investigation and entry into clinical trials of photocoagulation treatment, was soon complemented by the introduction of the other momentous advance in this field, the argon laser. This instrument had first been used by l'Esperance in the USA in 1963, but did not become commercially available in the UK until 1970. In 1971 Moorfields took delivery of its first argon laser, thereby paving the way for the treatment of a wide range of medical retinal disorders, by the most modern and sophisticated method available.

With the technological capability for accurate diagnosis and rational treatment now available, the scene was set, with the return of Alan Bird from the USA, for the development of the fledgling Retinal Diagnostic Department (RDD) at City Road (**Figure 27**, Plate 14). After finishing his residency at the High Holborn branch of Moorfields, Bird had gone to the Bascom Palmer Eye Institute in Miami as a Visiting Fellow in neuro-ophthalmology. Because he had gained some experience of FFA while working at the National Hospital, Queen Square prior to his departure for the US, he was able while there to make himself useful doing fluorescein angiograms when these were required outside normal working hours (and thus developed the close working relationship with Dr Donald Gass that was to cement the foundations of his interest in diseases of the retina). By chance, two weeks after Bird's return to the UK in 1970, Hayreh, who had been doing the fluoresceins at City Road single-handed, was appointed to a senior post in Edinburgh, thereby leaving a void, which Alan Bird was ready to fill. With two cameras and a single stool for the patient, between them, in a corridor of the Unit, Bird and Kulwant Sehmi from the Department of Medical Illustration at the Institute of Ophthalmology established the first true FFA service in the UK, Sehmi taking the colour photographs and Bird injecting fluorescein and taking the angiograms. This was to be a defining moment in the history of Moorfields, Alan Bird going on to establish for himself a worldwide reputation as a clinician scientist in the field of medical retina and genetic eye disease and an equally prestigious position for the RDD at Moorfields.

Meanwhile at the High Holborn branch, Tim Ffytche, who had finished his residency there in 1969, set up a fluorescein service, having learnt the method, like Alan Bird, working under Miller at the National Hospital, Queen Square. This was entirely service-based and continued to be so, treatment being carried out at first using a highly unpredictable ruby laser and later an excellent argon laser. He ran it single handedly, until the arrival of Professor David Hill in 1973, when the Royal Eye Hospital closed and the Royal College of Surgeons Chair of Ophthalmology was transferred to Moorfields, both he and Hill continuing to provide a service at High Holborn after that (with Hill also carrying out research into retinal blood flow), until the transfer to City Road in 1988.

The demand for FFA, from all corners of the Hospital as well as from ophthalmologists nationwide, soon became enormous. A free-standing RDD was formally established at City Road in 1971, with Alan Bird at its head, in the space previously occupied by the old operating theatres on the second floor, the new argon laser being established there and Bird being joined by Peter Hamilton, who had just completed his residency. Thus began one of the most exciting and productive eras in the history of Moorfields and of ophthalmology.

Not only did the beginning of the 1970s see the formal creation of the RDD and introduction of the argon laser, but in addition the collaboration between the physicians at the RPMS and the ophthalmologists at Moorfields was at its height (see **Figure 25**, Plate 13, bottom). In 1971 Peter Hamilton took over from Hung Cheng as Wellcome Fellow, working at both institutions, while Eva Kohner returned from a Fellowship in the USA to join the Hammersmith team. Rolf Blach continued to spearhead the work on diabetic retinopathy, the UK group leading the world in this sphere and undertaking the first randomized controlled clinical trials ever seen in ophthalmology. Meanwhile, Alan Bird, under the aegis of the Professorial Unit, initiated clinical trials in the treatment of macular degeneration, central and branch retinal vein occlusion, macroaneurysm, presumed ocular histoplasmosis syndrome, central serous retinopathy (in conjunction with City University) and optic neuritis, attracting an ever-increasing band of Fellows and Lecturers, from the UK and abroad. It was a golden era of enquiry and advance, and the buzz of excitement and enthusiasm was all-pervasive.

Throughout this heady period, Medical Retina steadily became an established specialty and Bird its acknowledged champion. To suggest, however, that there was anything hierarchical or authoritarian about it would be far from the truth. Indeed, the relationships between the members of the RDD, high and low, were exceptionally informal and friendly. Weekly fluorescein reporting sessions and conferences were held, during which there would be much heckling and banter, mostly of a friendly nature, no member of the team being beyond question or above reproach. Nevertheless, a spirit of excited enquiry and a desire to be first with the answers held sway throughout the decade. The trial of retrobulbar corticosteroids in the treatment of optic neuritis established a precedent, it being the first time that patients were permitted to be referred directly from the Casualty Department to a specialist service for entry into a clinical trial. It was also of special significance, since it involved not only members of the RDD but also the Consultant Neurologist, Dr (later Professor) Ian McDonald and a member of the Optometry Department, Miss Elizabeth Gould.

In May 1975 so strong was the notion of a scientific revolution in the field that it was decided to hold a 'Macular Workshop' (an idea typical of Rolf Blach's fertile brain and Alan Bird's infectious enthusiasm), inviting those interested in the subject, both here and abroad, to participate. Held in the beautiful and tranquil city of Bath, it was a great success, delegates attending from all over Europe, the USA and elsewhere. This event epitomized the spirit of scientific adventure that prevailed during the 1970s in this new field, and those who were privileged to attend would never forget it.

In the year before Alan Bird's arrival, and the setting up of an FFA service, 150 angiograms were performed. In 1970 this figure had increased to 400, by 1971 to 2000, and in 1972 to 4500, a trend that was destined to continue. In 1978 it became necessary to find more space, and the conversion of Edward Ward, no longer needed, owing to reduced duration of bed-occupancy throughout the Hospital, provided a larger area, a location that the RDD was to occupy until the opening in 1986 of the redeveloped lower ground floor.

The development of Medical Retina into a specialty in its own right was not without its difficulties. Ophthalmology was, and to a large extent remains, a surgical specialty. Its practitioners guard their surgical status jealously. Moorfields is no exception to this general rule, and the recognition and acceptance of a non-surgical subspecialty within its hallowed walls did not always receive unconditional support, even when during the 1990s, in terms of new patient referrals and through-put, it became the busiest department in the Hospital, outside A&E and Primary Care. Furthermore, as already described, it started off as a diagnostic service, with a strong research base, the RDD being a department of the Academic Unit, with a full-time clinical academic at its head. In this respect, the Medical Retinal Service was more closely aligned with the Institute of Ophthalmology than any other clinical service, since the departure of Barrie Jones in 1981, and this relation-ship was strengthened further by the appointment of Susan Lightman, an ophthalmologist with outstanding knowledge and expertise in uveitis and systemic diseases affecting the retina and choroid, first to the Duke-Elder Chair and subsequently, in 1993, to the substantive University Professorial Chair of Clinical Ophthalmology. Furthermore, both Rolf Blach and Zdenek Gregor bridged the gap between the medical and surgical disciplines, by working in both the Medical Retina and Surgical Vitreoretinal Services. In addition to its dual role, in terms of clinical and research responsibilities, the number of consultants and the diversity of their interests made it difficult to maintain cohesion. It was largely due to Zden Gregor's dedicated commitment and apparently limitless capacity for hard work as its service director for more than ten years that, in spite of its somewhat incoherent nature, it remained a dynamic and, for the most part, cohesive unit.

Born and raised in Czechoslovakia, Zdenek Gregor came to the UK to study medicine and joined the Medical Retina team in 1975 as a junior clinical assistant. He had decided to do ophthalmology, but at this time had no experience of the subject. He was, in fact, at the level of an SHO. To his utter amazement, he was given sessions at Moorfields in the RDD and within two weeks found himself undertaking FFA and treating parafoveal lesions with the laser. What is more, he also found himself calling the entire staff by their first names, including Alan Bird and Rolf Blach. It was a culture shock, but a pleasant and exciting one. After spending a period of training at the Western Ophthalmic Hospital, he joined the Moorfields residency programme in 1976, and three years later went to the USA on a Fellowship, before returning to a senior lecturer post at City Road. In 1983, on the retirements of Lorimer Fison and Kenneth Wybar, he was appointed to the consultant staff. An excellent surgeon and a prodigious worker, he joined both the Medical Retina and the Surgical Vitreoretinal Services, becoming the director of the former when it became a specialist clinical directorate in 1991. In addition to his clinical duties, both in the NHS and in private practice, he managed to undertake a steady programme of clinical research, a formidable schedule by any standards. He was, further-more, involved in and committed to developments in ophthalmology in Europe and worldwide and as this volume was going to press had been elected to the prestigious posts of President-elect of the Club Jules Gonin and Secretary General of the European Ophthalmological Society. On top of it all, he had taken up (perhaps unsurprisingly) marathon running.

Professor Lightman, who had a strong background in both general medicine and ophthalmology, as well as laboratory science, brought with her unique experience and expertise in the diagnosis and treat-ment of inflammatory eye disease. The strong bias of the Medical Retinal Service towards clinical academic activities was thus consider-ably augmented by her appointment and was explicitly acknowledged by the term Clinical Interface, coined by the Institute to describe the greatly streamlined Department of Clinical Ophthalmology. Indeed, until the emergence of Peng Tee Khaw, the two clinical professors in the Medical Retinal Service accounted for the major part of the research funding of the Hospital, attracting between them some £3 million of research grants, stemming from their work in inflammatory disease and molecular genetics

The impact of Professor Lightman's work, both before her appoint-ment to the Duke-Elder Chair in 1991 and thereafter, was enormous. Not only was there a huge backlog of children and others with devastat-ing ocular inflammatory diseases, such as Still's disease and Behçet's disease, which had previously been virtually untreatable, but the numbers of patients presenting during the 1990s with human immuno-deficiency virus (HIV)-related eye disease increased exponentially. New forms of treatment were developed, including intraocular triamcinolone and subcutaneous interferon-alpha for intractable uveitis, and the use of combination anti-retroviral therapy and intravitreal slow-release depot devices for HIV-related retinitis. The specialist uveitis service soon increased to six clinics per week, in addition to three sessions in the Primary Care Clinic. Large numbers of Fellows, many of them from abroad, came to learn from Professor Lightman's experience and the huge clinical load at Moorfields, and went away with the message that aggressive treatment, early on in the disease process, with immuno-suppressive drugs such as cyclosporin and mycophenolate, as well as the way in which many agents were best administered, could totally alter the accepted prognosis for these patients.

The special interests of Alan Bird veered increasingly towards the genetic basis for ocular disease, particularly with respect to retinitis pigmentosa, an inherited condition causing blindness, and one in which he accumulated, together with Professor Barrie and Dr Marcelle Jay, the largest cohort of affected families in the world. His reputation for linking the scientific basis for ocular disease with its clinical management was unrivalled, as was his ability to put this across, in understandable terms, to clinicians, scientists, patients and the general public. It is certainly the case that Alan Bird's worldwide reputation was in no small part the source of the high profile enjoyed by the Hospital, particularly in Medical Retina, during the 1970s, '80s and '90s, and which attracted large numbers of Fellows from every corner of the globe. Moreover, the large amounts of research funding that he attracted was of enormous benefit to the Hospital, especially after the Culyer Report set out the terms for its allocation in the NHS. Throughout the 1990s and into the first decade of the new millennium, it was obvious to all that Alan Bird had become Moorfields' finest ambassador and a figure of world renown in ophthalmology.

In spite of the heavy accent on research, the Medical Retinal Service continued to undertake an enormous amount of routine clinical work, especially in relation to retinal vascular disease, age-related macular degeneration (ARMD), uveitis and HIV. The successful control of diabetic retinopathy by laser photocoagulation became a routine during the 1980s and 1990s, while the diagnosis and treatment of a wide variety of other retinal vascular disorders evolved during this period. Treatment of ARMD, however, proved to be disappointing, in spite of the introduction of lasers utilizing light of different wavelengths, and the introduction of indocyanine green dye, in addition to fluorescein, to detect subfoveal neovascular membranes. The enhancement of laser beam therapy by the use of verteporfin dye, so-called photodynamic therapy (PDT), was also somewhat disappointing, its greater effectiveness in selected cases being off-set by its high cost (£1000 per vial of dye), which led to the National Institute for Clinical Excellence (NICE, a body set up by New Labour, ostensibly to monitor quality, but in reality to control costs) attempting to restrict its use to a small group of 'classic' cases.

Against these disappointments, there was a big gain, from the patients' point of view, when in the early 1990s it was discovered that retinal holes at the macula, quite common in older people, responded well to surgical treatment, and Gregor, who had retained his surgical interest, was able to spearhead this treatment at Moorfields. Moreover, there was the exciting prospect of a vascular endothelial growth factor

(VEGF) inhibitor that could be injected into the vitreous, to inhibit the growth of choroidal neovascular membranes in ARMD, and a protein kinase C inhibitor that could be given by mouth to reduce diabetic macular oedema. Members of the Medical Retina Service were actively involved in both these trials, Phil Hykin being on the National Advisory Board, and had been asked by the manufacturers of the VEGF inhibitor if they would try this in diabetics too. They were also engaged in the evaluation of intravitreal triamcinolone for diabetic maculopathy, while Zdenek Gregor had demonstrated some benefit to diabetic macular oedema by vitrectomy – an impressive array of clinical research, considering the routine clinical load. The results of treatment with the laser and with gene therapy in other vascular disorders, most notably branch and central retinal vein occlusions, were however, less encouraging, although a trial of radial optic neurotomy by Hykin and David Charteris from the Vitreoretinal Surgical Service showed promise.

The 1990s saw an increase in patient numbers, not only due to the new and better treatments available, but also because of the expansion of the outreach programme. To help manage this increase in activity and to maintain cost-effectiveness, it was decided to invest in a Mobile Unit, fully equipped for routine digital angiography and argon laser photocoagulation, which could be driven to outreach clinics, sparing the need for duplication of expensive equipment (**Figure 28**, Plate 15). This vehicle, custom-built, at a cost of £200 000, was largely the brainchild of the Chief Nurse, Roslyn Emblin, and was supported financially by members of the clinical staff. The project was driven forward by Christine Miles, Director of Operations, and was inaugurated in 1998* and immediately put into service.

Its use proved to be limited, however, by the most mundane of considerations, such as how close to the ophthalmic out-patient clinic it could be brought. Its large size restricted its manoeuvrability and hence it could not be driven close enough to some of the outreach clinics to enable it to be used. Nevertheless, its use at Ealing, where the

---

* *Not without incident. Just before the 'launch', by Countess Jay, the Minister of Health, it inadvertently struck a lamp-post whilst reversing, resulting in a large and very obvious dent in the nearside rear bodywork, which seriously spoilt its good looks and which could not possibly be repaired in the short time available. There was much consternation amongst senior staff, until the Operations Manager, Christine Miles, hit on the bright idea of attaching coloured balloons to the affected area, thereby completely camouflaging the damage as well as adding a festive touch to the occasion.*

local population was found to have an incidence of diabetes mellitus in excess of 10%, proved to be of enormous benefit.

To cope with the increased workload, and to compensate for the retirements of Rolf Blach, Tim Ffytche and Peter Hamilton, further consultant appointments were made. Carlos Pavesio, who had developed a special interest and expertise in uveitis, was appointed to add an extra dimension to the management of patients benefiting from the enormous improvements in knowledge and expertise in this area, while Phil Hykin and Jonathan Dowler were both soon engaged in the day to day management of retinal vascular disease, especially diabetic retinopathy (PDR), and ARMD, in addition to commitments in the outreach units, which included screening for PDR. The complement and expertise of the service were further enhanced by the arrival of Andrew Webster, a clinical academic with a strong research background in the genetics of hereditary retinal disease, to join Alan Bird in this sphere of activity, as well as being engaged in a Medical Research Council sponsored trial of phenotyping in ARMD, and by Catherine Egan in diabetic screening. The Hospital's low profile in this important area had for some time been a source of disquiet, while the heavy commitment of the existing staff, especially Phil Hykin, made it difficult to achieve more. Egan's appointment in 2002 and the commitment by the Trust to setting up sophisticated systems for photographic screening for diabetic retinopathy were welcome steps in this direction.

To enhance the research potential of the service, a further 50/50 consultant post was created. This was initially filled by an excellent candidate, who was suddenly awarded a huge grant by the Medical Research Council to go off and carry out research elsewhere. The post thus fell vacant again almost immediately, to be taken in October 2003 by Adnan Tufail, whose special interest lay in age-related macular degeneration.

Ocular oncology
Since the time of Henry Stallard, Moorfields had a close association with St Bartholomew's Hospital (Barts) in the field of ocular oncology, in particular the treatment of retinoblastoma, a genetically determined, frequently hereditary, malignant tumour of the retina affecting children. When Stallard retired in 1966, his place was taken by Michael Bedford, a very different character from his distinguished predecessor. Bedford was a competent and conscientious surgeon, but did little to advance the subspecialty before retiring in 1981 on the grounds of ill-health. A difficult interregnum ensued on his abrupt departure. There

was no obvious successor, in a highly specialist field of great importance and clinical need. In the event, after a period of more than a year,
John Hungerford, formerly a Resident at City Road and then a senior
registrar at University College Hospital, was appointed in 1983 to the
joint post of senior lecturer at Moorfields (four sessions) and
consultant ophthalmologist at Barts (seven sessions), the Moorfields
component of the post being strictly for the purpose of running an
ocular oncology service.

The situation was somewhat bizarre. As Hungerford himself related
to the present author, he had no special experience or expertise in
oncology whatsoever, and recalled that on his appointment, he asked if
he should immediately set off on a tour of centres in the USA to learn
about it. *'No', was the response, 'we shall look a laughing stock, if you do
that. Get stuck in and learn as you go along!'*

Such was the somewhat inauspicious start to a distinguished career
in ocular oncology. However, to his unalloyed credit, Hungerford overcame this unfavourable beginning with courage and commitment, to
become a world leader in the field. Indeed, as he later confided, he had
one supreme advantage over his expert contemporaries – an open
mind, in a specialty torn between numerous supposedly best treatments, each promoted by a different centre, without sufficient evidence
of any one being, overall, more efficient than another. He did indeed
'learn on the job' and was soon in a position to go to the USA and see
for himself the diversity of methods, returning to devise a new approach
based on stratification and rationalization of the available technology,
based on what he had seen. Collaborating with two colleagues at Barts,
Nick Plowman, an oncologist and Judith Kingston, a paediatric
oncologist, both of whom were appointed at about the same time, he
set out to modernize the treatment of retinoblastoma, malignant
melanoma and conjunctival melanosis, the most numerous malignancies that came his way.

Low-energy plaques, incorporating iodine-125 and ruthenium-106,
replaced cobalt, irradiation techniques sparing the crystalline lens
supplanted methods causing huge damage to the external ocular
tissues, and later were themselves superseded by chemotherapy, and a
whole new raft of treatments was tried and tested. Ophthalmologists
who had previously treated the commoner tumours such as melanomas
themselves, often by enucleation, referred cases to Hungerford, as did
those in doubt about differentiating between malignancy and other
benign conditions mimicking it, and his practice soon increased from
1000 to 5000 new cases per year. Nevertheless, where retinoblastoma
was concerned, there was a fall in numbers for two reasons: first, a new

centre for childhood malignancies was opened in Birmingham, and secondly, new policies laid down by the Royal Colleges of Paediatrics and Ophthalmologists relating to their treatment deemed Moorfields to be unsuitable for children. Paradoxically, too, the change from irradiation to chemotherapy for advanced disease, caused a shift in practice from the ophthalmologists to the oncologists.

Other methods of treatment were also tried by Hungerford, including local resection, a technically challenging method first undertaken by Stallard, which proved to have unacceptable complications. An innovative, but in the end flawed, concept of using proton-beam therapy, enabled by a £2m grant to modify equipment at the Clatterbridge unit , also had to be abandoned, due to serious side-effects, and the introduction of the gamma knife had similar results. In the end it seemed that the 'softer' methods were the most promising, including, latterly, photodynamic therapy for choroidal haemangiomata. Nor should it be forgotten that Hungerford and co-workers were the first to isolate the retinoblastoma gene locus and use it in 1987 in the first example of genetic exclusion, an achievement published in the *Lancet* that year.

For the future it seemed likely that, as a result of changes in policy nationally, arising from scandals in paediatric and pathology services at Bristol and Alder Hey during the dying days of the 1990s, Moorfields would lose its paediatric surgical practice to the 'children-friendly' Royal London Hospital or to the Hospital for Sick Children, Great Ormond Street, and that the trend towards chemotherapy would swing things increasingly in the direction of the oncologists. Collaborative studies between John Hungerford and Ian Cree, formerly pathologist at the Institute of Ophthalmology, on micrometastases and delayed tumour expression, could lead to significant advances in the field of ocular oncology. Whether, when the former retired, Moorfields would retain its position in the vanguard of scientific and clinical progress remained to be seen.

Pathology services

Prior to the upheavals that took place in the early 1990s, the Pathology Department at the Institute formed an important bridge between basic science at the Institute and clinical practice at the Hospital. Norman Ashton was an excellent teacher and so were his staff. While Alec Garner, his successor, took great pains to forge strong links with the Hospital. In the 1960s and 1970s Residents spent a period of three months of study in the department, learning the pathological appearances of gross disease specimens as well as the microscopic details in histopathological slides. Not only did Ashton himself take part in teaching, so too did his senior associates, Alec Garner, John Harry and Gwyn Morgan.

During the 1980s, after Garner took over as head of the department, there were regular informal reviews of recent pathology specimens for the benefit of Residents, as well as 'hands-on' training of overseas visitors. There were also monthly clinicopathological conferences, and the Pathology Department participated actively in the weekly orbital clinics with John Wright and Glyn Lloyd. The move from Judd Street to Cayton Street, immediately adjacent to the Hospital, in 1980 further strengthened this close relationship, although the relentless reduction in financial support, as a result of the Thatcher government's policies towards research, were already beginning to tell. In 1981 Morgan took early retirement and in 1984 Harry left to take up a senior post in Birmingham.

Meanwhile, the department provided a comprehensive diagnostic service for the hospital, including haematology, biochemistry and microbiology, and in the early 1970s a diagnostic immunology service was available, not only to Moorfields but also to other units nationwide. As time went on, there was an increased emphasis on functional as against purely descriptive anatomical pathology, Ian Grierson and Paul Hiscott looking at such things as the behaviour of ocular scar tissue in glaucoma and the composition and action of epiretinal membranes associated with complicated retinal detachments. There was also a gradual transition from the use of animal experimentation to cell culture as a research tool, while the employment of transmission electron microscopy increased and scanning electron microscopy came in.

Nevertheless, as the 1980s progressed, there was a steady attrition, staffing levels falling from eight at the beginning of the decade to five by its end, and as the 1990s began, there was, as described in the section of this volume dealing with events at the Institute of Ophthalmology (see Part 3), increasing pressure to rationalize services. Indeed, the move of the remaining departments from Judd Street to the island site and their restructuring in 1991, far from adding support to clinically related pathology services, signalled their demise in favour of pure research activities, while Grierson and Hiscott left for Liverpool and Alison McCartney for St Thomas'.

In many respects, this change in philosophy heralded a brave new world of exciting scientific discovery, and the fresh direction boded well for the future of ophthalmic pathology. The new professor on Alec Garner's retirement in 1993, Phil Luthert, brought with him entirely different expertise, in tune with modern developments. Ian Cree joined the department and proved to be an excellent teacher, as well as researcher, but his primary interests were in oncology and it was not long before he left for a professorial chair in Southampton. The Hospital was placed in a difficult position, however, depending as it did on a comprehensive pathology service for its patients, and had to look carefully at the financial and other implications of retaining a broadly based service. In the event, clinical diagnostic pathology services other than histopathology and microbiology were, from 1993 onwards, discontinued from the Institute and were bought in by Moorfields from other hospitals in London – a sad if inevitable reflection on the changed nature of the Hospital/Institute relationship, which Garner had tried so hard to preserve. So far as microbiology was concerned, however, John Peacock, the senior medical laboratory scientific officer, had been in post for more than 30 years and continued to provide a comprehensive and invaluable service. He was supported, until his early retirement on health grounds, by Melville Matheson, while both Rosalind Hart and Bob Alexander had served as technical staff for longer than twenty years.

Physicians

Background

Single-specialty hospitals such as Moorfields have always, with some justification, attracted criticism on account of their perceived inclination to treat their patients as interesting examples of esoteric pathology, rather than as complete human beings, the more general aspects of their condition, as a result, being either neglected or ignored altogether. In Moorfields' case, this might apply to patients with many eye conditions commonly associated with systemic disease, in particular hypertension and diabetes, which are common in Western society. In recognition of this inherent weakness, the Hospital has always had on its consultant staff physicians of the highest calibre, able to provide expert advice and care for patients so afflicted. Nevertheless, over the years, it became clear that so many of the disorders suffered by patients with eye disease were neurological in origin that the physicians appointed to the Hospital were more and more commonly those with a special interest in neurology. By the 1970s, although Christopher Earl's assistant at High Holborn, Dr Stephen Llewellyn-Smith (a consultant physician at a district general hospital elsewhere) and Dr Gavey at City Road provided general medical expertise, two out of the three consultant physicians at City Road, and the single consultant at the High Holborn branch were all neurologists.

This trend notwithstanding, when Dr Gavey retired from City Road in 1976, his place was taken by Dr David Galton from St Bartholomew's Hospital, who had a special interest in prothrombotic lipid disorders, diabetes, hypertension, hypercholesterolaemia and hypertriglyceridaemia, all of which predisposed patients to vascular occlusive disease affecting the retina and optic nerve. Galton was academically brilliant and wrote and published extensively. He was comfortable in the role of physician/oculist and enjoyed working at Moorfields. When the Hospital became a Trust, however, the situation changed, the management, led by Bob Cooling, demanding higher throughput of patients and recommending that he refer them back to their GPs for management. This he was reluctant to do, knowing that many GPs were not conversant with the complexities of blood lipid and glucose abnormalities and had little time to spend on their treatment and management, and he refused to comply. The situation deteriorated to such an extent that he threatened to take the Trust to court, but in the event the Hospital backed down and the clinic continued until David Galton retired in 2002. From that time onwards, however, no general physician was appointed and the shape of the medical services began to look very different.

There were two main reasons for this change in direction: first the progressive reduction in in-patient stay and the shift to day-case surgery and secondly, as a consequence of that change, the much greater involvement of GPs in the general management of their patients, while they were undergoing ocular treatment. Furthermore, the increasing sophistication of ophthalmic diagnosis and pathology called for neuro-ophthalmologists as well as ophthalmic neurologists (something which had long been recognized by the National Hospital for Nervous Diseases – now the National Hospital for Neurology and Neurosurgery – Queen Square, with the appointment there of Michael Sanders), and in 1994 the first neuro-ophthalmologist at Moorfields, Paul Riordan-Eva, was appointed.

The strength and depth of expertise in neurology at Moorfields was always outstanding. In 1960 Dr Christopher Earl, already on the staff of the hospital at Queen Square, was appointed to the High Holborn branch to replace Dr Frank Elliot on the latter's decision to accept an appointment in Philadelphia. A quiet unassuming man, with a wry sense of humour and great personal charm masking a razor-sharp intellect, Earl served the Hospital for close on 30 years, throughout that time teaching and inspiring a whole generation of ophthalmologists emerging from High Holborn, including Desmond Archer, Alan Bird and Michael Sanders, all of whom were to go on to be towering figures in ophthalmology. He also carried out clinical research at Moorfields, publishing amongst others papers on retrobulbar neuritis and the results of surgical intervention in cases of chiasmal compression.

On the retirement of Dr SP Meadows and Dr Simon Behrman, in 1968–69, Dr Ralph Ross-Russell and Dr Ian McDonald were appointed at the City Road branch, the former jointly with St Thomas' Hospital, and the latter with the National Hospital, Queen Square. Ross-Russell had a special interest in vascular disease and was influential in describing the characteristics of retinal emboli. Dr (later Professor) McDonald had established a worldwide reputation for his pioneering work on the mechanisms involved in demyelinating disease and its treatment, a large proportion presenting as optic neuritis with visual loss. They worked well together, each running a separate out-patient clinic of their own, as well as a combined one.

McDonald recalled being told by his predecessor, on his appointment to the staff, that the surgeons would treat him and his medical colleagues just like a taxi rank: 'If one doesn't come, simply call another!'

Ian McDonald held an out-patient clinic on Wednesdays during which he would see tumour cases involving the orbit and optic nerve, referred by John Wright, who would see them with Glyn Lloyd (and later Ivan Moseley) in the orbital clinic the same afternoon. There, they would be investigated by orbital venography, air orbitography and later by ultrasound, until the introduction of computed tomography (CT) scanning at Queen Square in 1973 transformed the diagnostic process and rendered the previous methods obsolete. This collaboration produced an unparalleled series of more than 2000 cases, during a period stretching over 20 years. The investigation of demyelinating disease, although aided greatly by electrophysiological studies, was more problematic, until the introduction of magnetic resonance imaging (MRI) transformed this too, the role of both these modalities in this field being first established in collaborative projects between Moorfields and the National Hospital, Queen Square.

Contrary to previous practice, the neurologists were happy, when they considered it appropriate, to investigate and treat their Moorfields patients on site, rather than taking them over to Queen Square or St Thomas'. They were also keen to undertake clinical research projects at Moorfields. Notable amongst these were the seminal studies undertaken on treatment of optic neuritis by intra-orbital steroid injection, carried out by McDonald, in conjunction with the Retinal Diagnostic and Optometry Departments, and the work done by Ross-Russell on intravascular retinal emboli. In the midst of this, however, they and Galton undertook a considerable amount of general work, seeing and looking after a large number of patients, referred by the house staff and anaesthetists.

Earl retired in 1987, and, in view of the imminent closure of the High Holborn branch, it was decided to appoint a locum physician there in his place. This was an obvious choice, as Gordon Plant had been work-ing at Moorfields, in a part-time capacity, since 1984, as clinical assistant and then registrar, to the physicians' clinic, together with a research post at Cambridge and clinical sessions at The National Hospital, Queen Square. When the branches finally amalgamated in 1988, he went off to the USA on a research fellowship, finally returning in January 1991 to a substantive consultant post jointly between St Thomas', Queen Square and Moorfields.

As outlined above, the emphasis on neuro-ophthalmology grew stronger during the 1990s, the appointment of Paul Riordan-Eva pointing to the transition towards a department of neuro-ophthal-mology. When first Ross-Russell and then McDonald retired, no attempt was made to replace them, Plant taking over their sessions. Riordan-Eva's early departure in 1996, due to ill-health, did nothing to halt the process, and in 1997 James Acheson, who was already on the consultant staff at the Western Eye Hospital, left there to take over as consultant neuro-ophthalmologist jointly between Queen Square and Moorfields. Unlike his predecessor, Acheson had surgical sessions in the Strabismus and Paediatric service, and soon after the beginning of the new century the Department of Neuro-ophthalmol-ogy was subsumed into that service, where it now found itself more comfortably at home.

Thus it can be seen that during the 40 years under present review, the role of the physician at Moorfields underwent a transfor-mation. Contrary to what might appear to be the case, however, this role had, for a number of reasons, been made stronger rather than weaker. First, Gordon Plant worked at a large general teaching hos-pital (St Thomas'), and at both a specialist neurological institution (the National Hospital, Queen Square) and a specialist ophthalmo-logical institution (Moorfields), entailing a 10-session commitment to general and ophthalmic neurology, with clinical exposure to neuro-ophthalmology unrivalled anywhere in the world (fully half of his sessions were in ophthalmic departments). Secondly, the close working relationship between him and James Acheson, both at Moorfields and Queen Square, added a new dimension to the service he was able to provide, while the increased commitment at Moorfields allowed him to focus more fully on the complex problems referred to him there.

Furthermore, because the pattern of referrals had altered, due to changes in ophthalmic practice, there had been a move away from long-term management of general medical problems and a much greater focus on neuro-ophthalmological disorders. Where formerly patients were referred by the house staff and anaesthetists for medical opinions and management, particularly assessment of fitness for surgery, now the preponderance of surgery under local anaesthesia and the trend towards pre-assessment clinics and day-case surgery had altered this entirely, while the long-term management of medical disease was increasingly undertaken outside Moorfields. On the other side of the coin, the physicians found themselves closer to the front line when it came to the referral of patients from other out-patient clinics. General ophthalmic clinics, where patients were always seen by senior members of the ophthalmic staff and serious ocular conditions diagnosed or excluded before they arrived, were now a thing of the past. The patients coming to the physicians' clinics might have only been seen by less experienced staff, meaning that patients might now be sent to the physicians without comprehensive ophthalmological screening beforehand.

This realignment of interests, with increased focus on specialist neuro-ophthalmological conditions, to the comparative exclusion of general medicine, had intensified the need, since Professor McDonald's departure, for improved research facilities and specialist teaching. Multiple sclerosis remained one of the chief subjects for this research, with early diagnosis, based on a single MRI scan and the McDonald criteria, and treatment trials of disease-modifying agents such as interferon-beta being the foremost objectives. The appointment of two Fellows, their time divided between Queen Square and Moorfields, went some way towards satisfying these demands, teaching and training being second to none, while the Research and Development funding was the highest for any department in the Hospital and a research review in 2000 rated the department highly. The ultimate goal might be the establishment of an academic department of neuro-ophthalmology based across the two institutions. In any event, even if the Hospital no longer had a broadly based medical ophthalmologist on its staff, the future of neuro-ophthalmology at Moorfields seemed assured.

The Diagnostic Clinic
The recognition in the 1960s of an incontrovertible link between venereal and ocular infections, demonstrated by Barrie Jones' work

on *Chlamydia* and trachoma inclusion conjunctivitis (TRIC), provided scientific proof of the underlying cause of ophthalmia neona-
torum and paratrachoma. In recognition of its importance,
Moorfields had long had on its staff a consultant specializing in
venereal diseases. In 1964 Dr Eric Dunlop, consultant venereologist
at the London (later the Royal London) Hospital, joined the
Moorfields staff in a part-time capacity, and formed a close relationship with Barrie Jones, working with him in close harmony for many
years in a highly productive collaboration. They were the first to
identify chlamydial infection as an important cause of genital infections and complications, while Dunlop's work on penicillin levels in
the cerebrospinal fluid formed the basis of neurosyphilis treatment
in the UK. In 1985, following Dunlop's retirement, Dr Beng Goh
was appointed to both Moorfields and the Royal London Hospital
in his stead.

Increasing sexual freedom and activity, especially amongst the
young, and the changes in social interaction across London from the
1950s onwards both contributed to alterations in the pattern of
venereal disease as the 20th Century drew to a close. Beng Goh's
commitment to Moorfields became steadily broader, his role gradually
encompassing the whole gamut of what was now termed 'sexual
health', ranging from prevention and management of sexually transmitted infections to advising on contraception and the management of
erectile dysfunction. The advent of HIV and the AIDS epidemic coincided with his appointment, but much of the ocular disease associated
with it became the province of Susan Lightman and Carlos Pavesio,
both establishing their positions as leading authorities on HIV infection
involving the eye. Moreover, not only was HIV a major cause of ocular
venereal disease during the latter part of the 20th Century, but this
epoch also saw the incidence of other sexually transmitted viral infections, such as genital warts and herpes, as well as more traditional infections such as syphilis, increase alarmingly. It led to a wider and wider
spectrum of problems being seen in the Diagnostic Clinic, Goh collaborating with Mala Viswalingam in the External Disease Service, their
weekly clinics coinciding to provide a user-friendly service. Conditions
such as chlamydial and gonoccocal eye infections, Reiter's disease,
pediculosis of the lashes, herpes simplex keratoconjunctivitis and mol-
luscum contagiosum of the eyelids could all be markers of sexually
transmitted and HIV infection. Close collaboration between the
venereologist and the external eye-disease specialists, to facilitate contact tracing, was therefore essential if further spread of these potentially
devastating conditions was to be prevented.

Strabismus, paediatrics and neuro-ophthalmology

Background

Although, until quite recently, the Orthoptic Department traditionally had consultant surgeons specializing in disorders of ocular motility, as its Director and Deputy Director, until the early 1970s strabismus and other disorders of ocular motility, like most sub-specialties of ophthalmology, came within the province of all members of the consultant staff. In 1971, however, Peter Fells, at that time a senior lecturer in the Department of Clinical Ophthalmology, initiated a 'squint pool', into which all cases of strabismus were entered, thereby ensuring that the Residents at the City Road branch of the Hospital saw and operated on as many cases as possible, under his expert guidance and supervision. His subsequent appointment to the consultant staff, and as director of the Orthoptic Department, in 1973 brought about a significant change in policy, most cases of strabismus at City Road from then on being referred to him.

Fells had the distinction not only of being one of the foremost authorities on disorders of ocular motility and President of the European Strabismological Association, but also of being the first ophthalmologist to have been awarded a Fellowship by the Harkness Foundation, to go to Columbia University, New York to study disorders of ocular movements. On his return from the USA, he joined the Professorial Unit as a lecturer, where he also became interested in orbital surgery, particularly that associated with thyroid disease and orbital trauma, interests that he continued to pursue until his retirement. In 1974 he set up the first thyroid eye clinic, in which patients were seen by an ophthalmologist and physician together. He also worked closely with the ENT surgeon to the Hospital, Brian Pickard. These were unique examples of cross-specialty collaboration. His chief interest was in strabismus, however, as evidenced by his Editorship of the *Proceedings of the International Strabismological Association*.

Meanwhile, in 1968, on the retirement of Keith Lyle, a major figure in the world of strabismology, Kenneth Wybar had taken over as Director of the Orthoptic Department at the High Holborn branch of the Hospital. Wybar, a man of very considerable intellect, as well as great energy, co-wrote Volume V of Duke-Elder's *System of Ophthalmology*. He spread himself rather thinly, however, working at Moorfields, Great Ormond Street, the Royal Marsden Hospital and in private practice. On his retirement in 1986, John Lee, recently returned from a year as a Fellow with John Flynn in Miami, studying the latest developments in the field of oculomotor disorders, was appointed to the staff at High Holborn.

A dynamic personality with a formidable intellect, biting wit and often iconoclastic and irreverent views, Lee was to be a huge asset to the Hospital. Not only did he later lead the sub-specialty with verve and dynamism but he was also destined to play a major part in the development of medical education at Moorfields. From 1987 to 1992 he was Clinical Sub-Dean, before, on the termination of the Dean's role at the Institute, this post too was abolished, and a Surgical Tutor (the present author) was appointed to oversee medical education in the Hospital. He also contributed to the academic activities of the Oxford Congress, became President of the Ophthalmological Section of the Royal Society of Medicine, and for many years organized the annual scientific meeting for Moorfields Alumni, while, finally, in 1997 he became Director of Education for the Trust.

The Orthoptic Departments

The field of orthoptics has a long and distinguished history, the first School and Department of Clinical Orthoptics in the UK being opened in 1930 at the Royal Westminster Ophthalmic Hospital (later to become the High Holborn branch of Moorfields) by Mary Maddox, known worldwide as the First Orthoptist. In 1932 a second department was opened, this time at the Central London Ophthalmic Hospital, under the direction of Sheila Mayou, the first ever recipient of a Certificate of Proficiency in Orthoptics. At the inception of the NHS in 1948, when the Central London Ophthalmic became the Institute of Ophthalmology, Miss Mayou and the School moved to City Road, the two schools remaining independent until 1981. Principal orthoptists during this time included, among others, Pam Dowler, Sylvia Jackson, Barbara Lee and Betty Gosnell. In 1981 the High Holborn school under the direction of Barbara Lee, and the City Road school under Sheila Mayou (later Betty Gosnell), were amalgamated into a new joint Orthoptic School and Clinical Department under the direction of Miss Lee and Mr Peter Fells.

In 1984 Miss Katherine Swale took over as Principal of the School, being succeeded in 1989 by Mrs Ann McIntyre, Peter Fells remaining as Medical Director throughout. The hospital-based orthoptic training scheme came to an end in 1994, however, when, in tune with trends in education, teaching and training, education in orthoptics was transferred to the Universities of Sheffield, Liverpool and Glasgow. The University of London apparently demonstrated little enthusiasm for this field of study, and by the time it realized its mistake, attempts to start a School of Orthoptics, at University College, came to nought, through lack of funds, a problem common to most of the professions allied to medicine. By dint of the imaginative thinking, skilful negotiation, and goodwill of Geoff Woodward, Head of Optical Science at the City University, however, the Orthoptic Department at City Road was able to take over the teaching of binocular function there, and the teaching activities and emoluments of the orthoptic staff were, in spite of the closure of the school, thereby maintained (**Figures 29 and 30,** Plate 16).

On the amalgamation of the two branches of Moorfields in 1988, John Lee joined Peter Fells at City Road and, when the specialist clinical services were formally inaugurated in 1991, they formed the Strabismus and Ocular Motility Service, with John Lee as its director. The increased workload, resulting from referral of all strabismus cases and as a consequence of outreach developments, was somewhat offset by a gradual reduction in the numbers of children requiring squint surgery, partly as a result of improved rates of detection, and at an earlier age than was formerly the case, and partly because of a more conservative approach to children with incurable deviations of minor degree. On the other hand, treatment of adult strabismus markedly increased, because, in common with other disfiguring or unsightly conditions (to which reference has already been made, in relation to oculoplastic surgery), in the new, enlightened social environment, elderly people were no longer expected to just 'put up and shut up'.

The workload certainly continued to increase overall, and in 1995 a further consultant appointment was made, Gillian Adams joining the service. In 1996 Peter Fells retired and John Sloper took his place, Miss Adams taking over as consultant lead for the Orthoptic Department, now under the direction of Ann McIntyre, and James Acheson enrolling with the service in 1999 on his appointment as neuro-ophthalmologist. Meanwhile, the service maintained its high profile nationally, many patients being referred to Moorfields for second opinions, while John Lee was elected President of the International Strabismological Association and founded and led the British Isles Strabismological Association.

The culture, particularly vis-à-vis the orthoptic service, changed markedly over the years, as was perhaps evident from the change in overall command, from consultant surgeon to orthoptist. The relationship between the surgeons and orthoptists became more and more that of a partnership, and the orthoptic staff began to play an increasingly important role in scientific research. In 1967 the first orthoptic research post was established, with funding from the Friends of Moorfields, and Rosemary Watts was the first to fill this position. This post subsequently became part of the orthoptic establishment and Watts' successor was

Barbara Dulley, to be followed by Liz Dell, Bernadette McCarry, Louise Garnham, Linda Kousoulides and Emma Dawson. Ann McIntyre, Louise Garnham and others frequently presented their work and published scientific papers alongside their medical colleagues. The old notion that orthoptists were the handmaidens of the ophthalmic surgeons had once and for all been consigned to the dustbin of history. (*The present author can remember a senior member of the consultant staff commenting, many years earlier, 'orthoptists are just nurses who don't want to get their hands dirty', while a former Resident was reputed to have said that to be an orthoptist was 'a phase in the life of a middle-class girl' – both comments reflecting the chauvinism of a bygone era.*)

Improvements in the early detection of amblyopia and compliance with treatment led to a marked fall in its incidence, although the problem of successfully treating it once established remained as obstinate as ever. This was in spite of flights of fancy, such as the (Cambridge) CAM instrument for stimulating the visual cortex or even the advanced neuroscientific investigations of Professor Sillito and others into the plasticity of its behaviour. Early detection and simple patching were still the mainstay of its management. Nevertheless, in 2003 Adams and Sloper noted that there was an increasing trend towards early squint surgery in young children and an increase in demand for strabismus surgery in elderly patients.

Advances in neither surgical nor medical techniques are particular features of strabismus surgery, the methods of treatment having changed little since the first operation for squint in 1839. Two notable improvements did nevertheless occur during the period under review. These were, first, enormously improved suture materials, especially polyglycolic acid (Dexon) instead of catgut, and secondly the use of adjustable sutures and botulinum toxin for adult squints, introduced by Jampolsky and Scott respectively – techniques that John Lee brought back to Moorfields in 1982 after visiting San Francisco. Perhaps the most significant change in this area of practice, however, has been the approach to the treatment of children. Formerly, it was not uncommon for children to be seen in adult clinics, accommodated on adult wards and operated on adult lists. In the 1980s and 1990s this gradually came to be regarded as being no longer acceptable. It was recognized that children, certainly those under the age of 10 years, as well as being emotionally and psychologically immature, react quite differently to a wide range of drugs and other treatments, and that their clinical management must therefore be undertaken quite separately from that of adults. In the NHS Plan (2000) the National Service Framework for children required hospitals to provide child-friendly services, including dedicated children's units, and that all staff who dealt with children be appropriately trained.

The appointments of Gillian Adams, with a special interest in paediatric strabismus, and of highly trained paediatric anaesthetists were evidence of this change in attitude, while the proposed development of an International Children's Eye Centre was set to bring further advances in that direction. Indeed, the appointment of Tony Moore to the Duke-Elder Chair and his position as the academic lead in paediatrics, coupled with Dr Alison Salt's joint post with Great Ormond Street, signalled a marked shift towards a broader stance in the paediatric services at Moorfields.

Children's Department

The Hospital first acknowledged its increasing responsibility for children with eye disease in 1975, when it decided to seek the services of a paediatrician. Barry Jones was a young physician seeking an appointment at a children's hospital, and applied for the sessional post at Moorfields in the hope of obtaining the job he really wanted, the linked appointment at the Queen Elizabeth Hospital for Children in Hackney. As he was later to admit, so far as he was concerned at that time, ophthalmology was 'two diseases and three operations'. Ironically, however, although he was successful in achieving his stated ambition, he became, in due course of time, increasingly interested and involved in the ophthalmic side of the post, working closely with the ophthalmologists at Moorfields with particular interests in paediatric eye disorders, ranging from genetic disease to hysterical blindness. Indeed, of the latter, he went on to collect by far the largest series of cases (over 400) in the world.

> *Barry Jones told the author that when he was first appointed to the post at Moorfields, like Ian McDonald (see above), he received a warning: 'Watch out, you'll have trouble with the surgeons'. In the event, however, he never found this to be the case.*

He soon set up joint clinics, with Barrie Jay in genetics and with Richard Collin in microphthalmos and anophthalmos, and worked especially closely with Noel Rice in the management of children with buphthalmos.

The Paediatric Service went from strength to strength, with the appointment of a family support social worker Jackie Howe (later Martin), and play-leader Mary Digby funded by the generosity of the Friends of Moorfields, contributing in no small part to the enormous progress in the rehabilitation of visually impaired children, made nationwide since 1975. Indeed, the Friends were always a mainstay of financial support and encouragement to Barry Jones and the unit, funding the purchase of items of equipment, as well as Mary's salary, to bring the care and comfort of the children and their families up to the standards of a more compassionate and enlightened world.

The prevailing spirit was best summed up, perhaps, when a child, asked what he would like for his birthday treat, replied: 'Oh, a party in the play-room at Moorfields'.

The ward sister, Sister Ero, was the first nurse at Moorfields to have undergone full paediatric training, and was a trenchantly strong personality. Relations between Ero and Digby were, in particular, never easy, while anxious, distraught parents could sometimes be threatening to the nursing staff, but Barry Jones had a profoundly unifying influence, and in spite of their strongly individual personalities, they all managed to work well as a team, drawing inspiration from each other, so that the sum of their individual parts was greater than the expected whole.

Dr Barry Jones, seeing a baby boy in the ward, one day, apparently unclaimed, after recovery from cataract surgery, famously remarked 'If someone doesn't take that baby away before this week-end, then I shall have to' – they didn't and so he did, adding him to his already large family.

Noel Rice, too, was particularly influential in establishing and maintaining the ethos of the Paediatric Department, setting an example of practical, supportive care of the children with paediatric glaucoma, as well as compassion and understanding for their parents.

The (new) Paediatric Service
The rapidly emerging trend during the 1990s and into the new millennium, towards the complete separation of children's services from those of adults, in all fields of medicine, hastened by public alarm arising from scandals in the media, demanded a positive response from Moorfields. In 2001 moves were made to form a separate specialist Paediatric Service, with Professor Tony Moore at its head, from what had, up to that time (albeit shared to a lesser degree by the other specialist services), been chiefly the responsibility of the Strabismus and Paediatric Service (see below). In April 2003 this new service became a free-standing reality with responsibility for all children at Moorfields. Dealing with more than 20 000 children annually, it not only straddled all of Moorfields, but also formed a strong link with the Hospital for Sick Children at Great Ormond Street (GOS), all the

consultant ophthalmologists there having honorary contracts with Moorfields and sharing an on-call rota. The service now comprised not only the ophthalmologists, Moore, Alison Davies and those at GOS, and Dr Alison Salt, consultant paediatrician between the two, but also a consultant representative from each of the core specialist services at Moorfields.

While Professor Moore's special interests lay in the field of ocular genetics, Alison Davies was a paediatric ophthalmologist, appointed in August 2003 jointly with the Mayday Hospital Croydon, to take responsibility for children in A&E and Primary Care at Moorfields. With Salt's joint appointment with GOS, Moore's honorary contract there and the GOS consultants' appointments at Moorfields likewise, the new Paediatric Service was now part of a joint department between the two hospitals and promised to be very strong indeed. Ties with the Institute of Child Health, including the appointment of Jugnoo Rahi, paediatric ophthalmic epidemiologist, as a senior lecturer and Robin Ali as ocular gene therapist, promised well for future research. Furthermore, the appointment of architects and production of plans for the construction of the new International Children's Eye Centre, for which nearly £10m had already been pledged, made the prospects for the future brighter still.

Operations on children, which now totalled more than 1500 per year, were from this time onwards undertaken in two of the eight operating theatres specially designated and equipped for the purpose and anaesthetics were given only by anaesthetists with wide paediatric experience. The completion of the International Children's Eye Centre, projected for 2007, would provide completely separate clinic space and other out-patient facilities for children, as well as space for research.

Neuro-ophthalmology

The increasingly close relationship between ophthalmology and neurology has already been noted, as has the enormous change in outlook and emphasis during the past 30 years. The appointment to the consultant staff of two neurologists at the close of the 1960s, making a total of three out of the four physicians, reflected this. In 1994, however, Moorfields took the step of appointing a fully trained ophthalmologist, accredited by the Royal College of Ophthalmologists, Paul Riordan-Eva, to a joint post with the National Hospital, Queen Square and the Institute of Neurology. This was the first time such a post had been created and it was warmly welcomed by both institutions. Riordan-Eva was an outstanding candidate and it was a very popular appointment. He was soon inundated with work, both at

Moorfields and at Queen Square, where he also had research sessions. Sadly, however, serious ill-health supervened and he was unable to sustain this high level of activity, a situation that the Trust could not afford to accept, and which led, in 1996, to his resignation.

His place was taken by James Acheson, who was similarly qualified for the joint post, but elected to continue with his surgical sessions. He was already a member of the consultant staff at the Western Ophthalmic Hospital, so it was not possible for him to start at Moorfields until 1999. With a special interest in teaching, Acheson also took on the role of Training Programme Director for the North Thames Region, on the present author's retirement from the staff of the Hospital, in January 2000. Because of the special interests and expertise in treatment of disorders of ocular motility, with surgery and botulinum toxin injection, which he had developed before his appointment at Moorfields, Acheson seemed to fit best into the Strabismus and Paediatric Service. As he readily admitted, however, the place of a neuro-ophthalmologist in the general scheme of a single-specialty hospital like Moorfields was a slightly uncomfortable one, and future developments such as the changing attitude to paediatric care and the construction of the International Children's Eye Centre could alter the position completely. Furthermore, it would be difficult, when the time came to do so, for an ophthalmologist without previous experience of neuro-ophthalmology to step into his shoes. As it was, things worked well. Acheson combined easily with Gordon Plant, consultant neurologist to the Hospital, and was happy to share his expertise across adjacent disciplines. It was nevertheless quite easy for his patients to 'get lost' in the maelstrom of referrals to other services and hospitals, so that the quantity and value of his contribution could readily be obscured. In 2003, with the secession of the Paediatric Services, the neuro-ophthalmologists joined with the strabismologists to form the Strabismus and Neuro-ophthalmology Service.

Vitreoretinal surgery
Background

Of all the conditions afflicting the human eye, none has been more successfully brought within the scope of surgical treatment than retinal detachment. At the beginning of the 20th Century, there was no effective treatment for this disorder whatsoever, and if both eyes were involved, as was quite commonly the case, the patient thus afflicted was rendered completely blind. During the first half of the 20th Century, due to the imagination, courage and self-belief of one man, all this changed. Jules Gonin, a Swiss ophthalmologist, foresaw that detachment of the retina was caused by breaks in its integrity, usually in the periphery, and that, if one could close and seal these, it could be re-attached. He devised an operation for doing so, which entailed puncturing the sclera under the detached retina, thereby releasing the subretinal fluid, and applying a red-hot cautery to the eye-wall to create an inflammatory reaction that would cause adhesion between it and the retina.

This simple (and rather crude) procedure was effective in more than 50% of cases, thereby demonstrating that retinal detachment was a treatable condition and setting in train a series of advances in surgical method that have continued to the time of writing. As thermal cautery was overtaken by electrocautery, electrocautery by diathermy, diathermy by cryotherapy, and scleral buckling by vitrectomy and gas injection, through the years, retinal reattachment surgery grew ever more sophisticated and reliable. Furthermore, major advances in method and instrumentation, in particular that of vitrectomy, have spawned the development of techniques applicable to the treatment of a wide range of intra-ocular pathology other than retinal detachment. Thus did Gonin's momentous leap span a huge and previously unbridgeable void in the understanding of and ability to treat a wide variety of previously blinding eye disorders.

In common with much of the scientific world of 100 years ago, news did not travel fast, nor, as today, was there always an instantaneous desire or capacity to embrace new concepts, or to apply them. As a consequence, it was 10 years after Gonin first published his ideas and reported a series of successful cases before the first retinal reattachment operation was performed at Moorfields (in 1929), by Sir William Lister. His assistant at the operation was C Dee Shapland, an up-and-coming young surgeon, who subsequently became the doyen of British retinal surgery in the 1930s and 1940s. There were to be a great many changes, in both method and instrumentation, devised by European and American ophthalmologists, during the next 20 years (including Shapland's own innovation of lamellar scleral resection), most of them of relatively minor importance, but nevertheless leading to gradually improving results.

Shortly after the Second World War, however, a young Belgian ophthalmologist, Charles Schepens, made a notable advance. Schepens realized that the limitations imposed by the use of the monocular ophthalmoscope were a major obstacle to progress in retinal reattachment surgery and that a binocular instrument would be much better for detecting small peripheral breaks. Although the binocular ophthalmoscope had been invented (by Girard Teulon) only 10 years after the monocular one (by Helmholtz in 1851), it was unwieldy and difficult to use in its original form. Schepens modified it so that it could be worn on the head, thus leaving the hands free to hold the condensing lens, thereby giving it great flexibility. He decided to go west and, taking his idea with him, came to London, seeking an appointment at Moorfields, where, for reasons that are unclear, his overtures were rejected. Moving on to the USA, in 1947, he demonstrated his new instrument at the American Academy Meeting and was soon appointed to the staff of the Massachusetts Eye and Ear Infirmary, rapidly becoming the doyen of retinal surgery in the USA and dominating the field worldwide for many years thereafter. Other seminal contributions to the advancement of retinal reattachment surgery during the 1950s included the 'non-drainage' procedure, devised by Custodis, and the introduction of cryotherapy by Lincoff (and Amoils) and of photocoagulation by Meyer-Schwickerath.

The xenon arc photocoagulator (nicknamed 'jumbo' on account of its similarity to an elephant in both appearance and size) was a major advance in other respects, especially pan-retinal photocoagulation (PRP) for diabetic retinopathy, and was soon used by many surgeons for this purpose. It was not easy to use, however, and over-treatment was easily done. A very senior consultant undertaking PRP with it for the first time did so with consider-able gusto watched by his Resident, an engagingly frank and outspoken Canadian, and then stood back with some pride saying, 'Well, my boy, have a look and tell me what you think'. The young man peered into the eye and then stood up, exclaiming 'Gad, Sir, it looks like Dresden after the bomb-ing!' – a comment that failed to be warmly appreciated.

Most surgeons in the UK, including those at Moorfields, were slow to grasp the importance of Schepens's innovation, continuing to under-take retinal surgery using the monocular direct or indirect ophthalmo-scope as before, although Schepens and others in the USA began to obtain and publish greatly improved results, especially in aphakic eyes with small peripheral retinal breaks. One up-and-coming young English ophthalmologist, however, Lorimer Fison, had different ideas, and saw the wisdom of Schepens' method and that the future of successful retinal reattachment surgery lay in being able to identify small breaks, such that very few cases were not amenable to successful treatment.

Because retinal surgery was extravagant, both in terms of operating time and bed-occupancy, Moorfields had given Shapland his own Unit, with its own operating theatre and a considerable number of beds, at the Highgate Annexe of the Hospital. Fison became Shapland's assistant there and, by dint of travelling to the USA, to see and learn for himself binocular indirect ophthalmoscopy and other techniques such as scleral indentation, from Schepens and others, was soon able to acquire and bring back to the UK his unique knowledge and expertise in retinal surgery. On Frank Law's retirement from Moorfields in 1962, Fison was appointed to the consultant staff and succeeded Shapland as retinal surgeon to the City Road branch of the Hospital, this being the first example of a truly specialist appointment.

Development of retinal surgery at Moorfields

The development of retinal surgery during the 1960s and 1970s proceeded rather differently at the two branches of the Hospital. There were a number of reasons for this, the most cogent being the approach to indirect ophthalmoscopy. When Lorimer Fison returned from the USA in the late 1950s, he had brought with him not only the knowledge and skills that he had learnt there, but also a burning desire to emulate or even outshine Schepens and his group. To this end, he set about designing his own head-mounted binocular ophthalmoscope and persuaded the foremost ophthalmic instrument makers in London, Keelers, to cooperate with him in developing and marketing it. This they did, with great success, the Fison Indirect Ophthalmoscope (or 'hattie', as he preferred to call it) becoming the standard instrument in the UK, used by every ophthalmic surgeon. At the City Road branch of Moorfields, as a result of Fison's single-minded approach, Residents spent several months at a time totally immersed in retinal detachment surgery, staying overnight in the Retinal Unit at Highgate and supervising the care of large numbers of patients with retinal detachments, many of them complicated cases.

At the High Holborn branch, retinal surgery was, at least until the arrival of David Hill (after the closure of the Royal Eye Hospital), the province of James Hudson and, to a lesser extent, Barrie Jay. Five years Lorimer Fison's senior, Hudson was a meticulous and painstaking surgeon (he is reputed to have not infrequently been dissatisfied with the appearance of the retina, after several hours of surgery, and started the operation all over again), who used the monocular direct ophthalmoscope, with consummate skill, but was never really at home with the binocular instrument, a considerable disadvantage. He nevertheless encouraged and inspired his juniors, several of whom took up retinal surgery, including Barrie Jay and Jack Kanski, amongst others, and then taught and promoted the modern methods and latest techniques to generations of Moorfields Residents. In other respects he was a formidable operator too, developing a wide network of powerful connections and raising large sums of money for the Hospital. Both the Hayward Foundation's generous funding of the City Road operating theatres and that from the Francis and Renee Hock Foundation, to finance retinal Fellowships, were the results of Hudson's entrepreneurial skills, and he also counted high-ranking diplomats and cabinet ministers amongst his friends. He was awarded the CBE, while amongst his other distinctions he, like Lorimer Fison, served as President of the Ophthalmological Society of the UK, precursor of the Royal College of Ophthamologists (**Figure 31**).

Retinal out-patient clinics were established at both branches of the Hospital, and the standards of retinal detachment repair were as high as those anywhere in the world. When the Duke of Windsor, formerly King Edward VIII, developed a retinal detachment, both Hudson and Fison were called in and combined their skills in its successful repair. Meanwhile, John Scott, who had learnt retinal reattachment surgery as a Resident under Fison at City Road, was appointed to a consultant post in Cambridge in 1967, and soon afterwards began to pioneer special techniques for the treatment of complicated detachments, using silicone fluids, a technique that had first been used by Paul Cibis in the USA. The method was bitterly opposed by the Schepens group, so that after Cibis's untimely death in 1965, it was virtually abandoned in the USA until many years

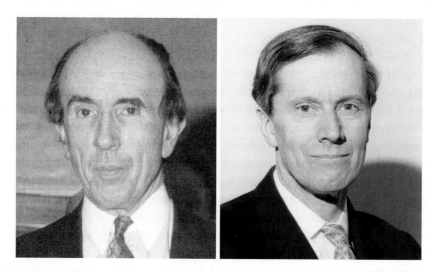

Figure 31   Mr James ('Jimmy') Hudson (*left*) and Mr Lorimer Fison (*right*), retinal surgeons during the 1960s and 1970s, at the High Holborn and City Road branches of the Hospital respectively.

later. As a result of Scott's imagination, drive and single-minded determination, however, it was practised with considerable success in the UK, by him, the present author and others, at Moorfields and elsewhere, soon becoming an established method of treating otherwise hopeless cases.

The dawn of vitreoretinal surgery

If the 1950s had been a decade of consolidation and promotion of good practice in retinal surgery, mostly devoted to the development and refinement of techniques established during the course of the preceding decades, the 1960s and 1970s saw an explosion of technology. By the mid-1960s, diathermy was already being supplanted by cryotherapy, silastic sponges and silicone bands were replacing polyviol plombs and supramid sutures, and photocoagulation had joined the armamentarium. In 1968, however, an event took place that was to entirely reshape the world retinal surgery. David Kasner, an ophthalmologist working at the Bascom Palmer Eye Institute in Miami, carried out removal of the vitreous, in a case of primary amyloidosis, using what is known as the 'open-sky' method. It was a crude and hazardous operation, but was, notwithstanding, successful. A colleague working at the Bascom Palmer, Robert Machemer, although impressed by the result of the operation, was appalled by the method, and sought to refine it, leading, two years later, to the development of a sophisticated technique, using custom-built microsurgical instrumentation via the pars plana, so-called closed vitrectomy.

The pars plana approach had previously been described by surgeons in the UK in 1969, and was the topic of a paper by James Hudson, discussed by Ian Duguid, Giles Romanes and others at the Annual Meeting of the Ophthalmological Society of the UK. Duguid described how he had himself done more than 25 such operations, but the technique had not progressed beyond the point of using manual excision of the vitreous with swabs, scissors and (sometimes) cryoprobe. The new method of treatment not only transformed the surgery of retinal detachments, but also introduced a whole range of new options in the management of other intraocular conditions, ranging from diabetic retinopathy to severe ocular trauma. The most exciting and innovative era in retinal surgery since Gonin's original discovery had arrived.

Retinal surgery at the City Road branch of Moorfields was, prior to 1974, conducted at the Highgate Annexe of the Hospital, whence it had been consigned in the late 1950s during Shapland's reign. The secluded atmosphere and pleasant surroundings were very conducive to total immersion in the subject and were ideal for teaching the complex disciplines required. Generations of Residents benefited from this seclusion and from Fison's dedication and teaching. Furthermore, the proximity of Kenwood House, a national treasure, with splendid grounds and good conference facilities, enabled him in conjunction with Rolf Blach and others, to hold symposia there of the highest quality. Lorimer Fison had a special ability, over and above that of surgical expertise, not only to encourage and inspire his juniors but also to leave them alone, when they most needed it, to develop their own special interests. He was not afraid to delegate and entrust to them difficult and challenging tasks. Thus it was that in 1973, when closed vitrectomy had been firmly established in the USA by Machemer, two of Fison's junior surgeons (the present author and Stuart Saunders) were dispatched to Miami to learn the new technique and to bring back a vitrectomy instrument for use at Moorfields.

> *Red-tape was not as sticky as it is today, nor security as tight, and the present author was able to obtain one of the vitrectomy instruments (the Vitreous Infusion Suction Cutter or VISC VII) for Moorfields, without having to actually pay for it, and bring it back in his overnight bag without declaring it at Customs. The instrument was therefore neither paid for nor in the possession of its rightful owners. On arrival home from Heathrow Airport by taxi, he left his bag on the pavement outside the house. An hour or so later, a neighbour kindly brought in the bag containing the instrument and returned it without mishap, a somewhat uncertain beginning to vitrectomy in the UK and one that might otherwise have proved both costly and embarrassing!*

From then on, vitrectomy became an increasingly important part of the retinal surgical armamentarium at Moorfields and throughout the world, and vitreoretinal surgery was increasingly used in the treatment of complicated retinal detachments, proliferative diabetic eye disease, penetrating ocular trauma and a host of other, less common conditions affecting the posterior segment.

Rolf Blach, who was already a long-established consultant at the Hospital, was one of the first to use the new machine at City Road, and was soon joined by David McLeod, while Leaver and Saunders were followed by Bob Cooling and later by Zdenek Gregor, when he returned from a Fellowship in the USA. Although Saunders soon departed to seek his fortune in Australia, the other four were subsequently appointed to the Moorfields consultant staff. At the High Holborn branch of the Hospital, Hudson encouraged Jack Kanski, who was already a consultant elsewhere, but worked part-time in the Retinal Unit, to start vitrectomy there, and this he successfully did, at first using the method in the treatment of patients with chronic uveitis and complicated cataract. Other members of Hudson's unit also took it up, including James Govan and James Ramsay, and encouraged its use when they too were appointed to consultant posts in various parts of the country.

During the second half of the 1970s, the retinal units at both branches of Moorfields espoused and developed new vitrectomy techniques, throughout the 1980s combining vitrectomy with the injection of intra-ocular silicone oil and expanding gases. Increasingly sophisticated instrumentation rapidly became available, enabling bimanual microsurgical manipulation of intra-ocular tissues, intra-ocular delivery of photocoagulation, and the application of gas and silicone oil to the closure of retinal breaks. Conventional surgery, using scleral buckles for straightforward cases of retinal detachment, gave way during the 1990s to internal tamponade with air and expanding gases, while complicated cases were managed with intra-ocular membrane dissection and tamponade with long-acting gases and silicone oil. Advanced proliferative diabetic retinopathy was similarly amenable to bimanual dissection, intra-operative laser photocoagulation and, where necessary, internal tamponade with gases or silicone oil.

One consequence of this explosive diversification and expansion of vitreoretinal surgical technology was the need for increased manpower. At the High Holborn branch, Professor David Hill had joined the consultant staff in 1973, bringing with him expertise in the treatment of both medical and surgical retinal disorders. Nevertheless, he did not undertake surgery in complicated cases and much of his time was devoted to research into the regulation of retinal blood flow, work that he had already been pursuing for some years, in his capacity as the Royal College of Surgeons Professor of Ophthalmology. The consultant staff of James Hudson's unit had been increased in 1969 by the appointment of Barrie Jay, but he was already on the staff of the London Hospital, so this was a part-time post and he did not, in any case, get involved in the new technology. Jack Kanski continued to work in the unit part-time and, with David Watson, James Ramsay, James Govan and others, developed vitreous surgery at the High Holborn branch, but none of them were consultants at Moorfields and it was not until the present author's appointment, following Hudson's retirement in 1981, that vitreoretinal surgery was represented there at consultant level.

In 1975 it had become clear that the ultrasound equipment, newly acquired by John Wright to investigate orbital disease, was more suited to the definition and diagnosis of intra-ocular disorders than to those of the orbit, and David McLeod, just having completed his residency, was assigned to work alongside the ultrasound physicist, Marie Restori, exploring the possibilities of its use in vitreoretinal investigation. As Lorimer Fison had elected not to take part in vitrectomy himself, there was a clear need for a consultant specializing in both vitreoretinal surgery and the use of ultrasound in this field. In October 1977 McLeod was appointed to the consultant staff at City Road, joining Fison in the Retinal Unit and working with the present author and Rolf Blach in developing vitreoretinal surgery at City Road. With the future amalgamation already decided, there was close cooperation and inter-action between the vitreoretinal surgeons at the two branches from this time on, all of them, while remaining clinically autonomous, working together in a joint Vitreous Clinic.

It was an exciting time. The Vitreous Clinic rapidly became very busy and the number of cases deemed suitable for vitrectomy escalated. Nevertheless, only what would now be considered the most straight-forward cases were accepted at first for surgery. Even simple vitreous haemorrhages were a challenge, as the instrumentation, especially intra-ocular illumination and microscopy viewing systems, was rela-tively crude. To complicate matters further, there was no means of car-rying out intra-operative photocoagulation, membrane peeling was hazardous, delamination and en-bloc dissection had not yet been thought of, and the combined use of intra-ocular gases and silicone oil with vitrectomy was a new and untried adventure. The team learned rapidly and visited centres in the USA and around the world, sharing experiences and absorbing knowledge like sponges.

The VISC VII instrument was soon superseded at Moorfields by the Douvas Rotoextractor* and the Rotoextractor by Gholam

---

* *The Rotoextractor had been designed, as its name suggests, for small-incision removal of cataracts, but Nick Douvas quickly saw the opening in vitreous surgery and modified his ideas accordingly. Small in stature, and distinguished by a particularly obvious toupee, he was a delightful, roguish entrepreneur. He lived and had his clinic in Port Huron, on the banks of the Great Lake, not far from the Canadian border, and his wife Arlene was his helpmeet, surgical assistant, scrub-nurse and devoted business partner. So worried was he that his design might be copied by his American colleagues that during a conference in the USA he took the precaution of demonstrating his new vitrectomy instrument to the present author in the privacy of the Gentlemens' Rest Rooms!*

Peyman's disposable cutter, all of them bulky multifunction instruments.

*At the first of Robert Machemer's Vitrectomy Workshops, held each year from the early 1970s onwards, in Vail, Colorado, Douvas read a paper. These meetings were extremely informal, the scientific sessions taking place from seven to nine o'clock in the morning, when the ski-lifts opened, and from six o'clock in the evenings, when they closed, but they were in deadly earnest. There were only about 20 of us there, all but two (Klaus Heimann from Cologne and the present author) Americans, and everyone was learning. On this occasion Jackson Coleman from Cornell University New York, asked Douvas: 'Hey, Nick where **is** this Port Huron? – it must be the end of the earth' Nick Douvas bridled at this and replied 'Oh no it most certainly isn't', to which came the retort 'Well, you must be able to **see** it from there!'*

Then, in the mid-1970s, the common gauge system devised by Conor O'Malley in San Jose California was introduced. This new technology, combined with Steve Charles' innovative surgical techniques, transformed the flexibility and adaptability of closed vitrectomy techniques and set the unit on the path of more sophisticated surgery, especially using vitrectomy combined with intra-operative photocoagulation, intra-ocular fluid/gas exchange, fluid/silicone oil exchange and the dissection of epiretinal membranes. Advanced proliferative diabetic retinopathy, retinal detachments complicated by proliferative retinopathy and giant retinal tears, as well as cases of severe intra-ocular trauma, all became amenable to successful treatment. Vitreoretinal surgery was suddenly the most exciting and challenging field in ophthalmology, McLeod leading the way in diabetic retinopathy, Leaver in giant retinal tears, Cooling in trauma and Gregor in the surgery of epimacular membranes and macular holes, and all of them achieving increasingly good results in the treatment of complicated cases of retinal detachment.

Special mention must be made here of the immense contribution to the Moorfields Surgical Vitreoretinal Unit made by Graham Nunn, vitreoretinal surgical technician extraordinaire. Talent-spotted by David McLeod in 1980 at the High Holborn branch, where he was working as a theatre porter, he went on to become a vital part of the Vitreoretinal Surgical Service. Nunn developed great technical knowledge and skill, which was allied with an obsessive personality, offset by charm and a powerful sense of humour. He did not suffer fools gladly (on one occasion, when exasperated by the conduct of one of his colleagues in the operating theatres, nearly

breaking his wrist by beating his fist against an immovable object!), but
successfully passed on his skills to generations of nurses who were willing to
learn. The development of the Vitreoretinal Service at Moorfields owed no
small part of its success to Graham Nunn's dedicated service and all-
embracing common sense.

By the end of the 1980s, the world of retinal surgery had been entirely
transformed, and during the 1990s, further refinements in vitreoretinal
surgery rendered even macular holes and subretinal pathology
amenable to surgical treatment, although the latter yielded positive
benefits in only a minority of cases. The beginning of the 21st Century
saw more than 50% of retinal detachments at Moorfields being treated
by vitrectomy methods, with overall surgical success in more than 90%
of cases, similar success in the treatment of giant retinal tears, and
successful trials of a 'cocktail' of drugs in the treatment of proliferative
vitreoretinopathy. The combination of improved methods of surgery,
with chemotherapy to combat retinal scarring in eyes most susceptible
to it, was set to make a major impact on outcomes in these complex
cases. There was a 25% increase in throughput in the space of only four
years, due to a rise in both elective and emergency cases, partly because
Moorfields was still the only vitreoretinal unit in the UK providing a
service 24 hours a day, seven days a week. Regular clinical audit showed
a steadily rising success rate for surgery, with consultants and Fellows
operating together in the most complex cases. Furthermore, the BIOM
(Binocular Indirect Operating Microscope) had made a big impact,
both because it enabled better surgical access and because it obviated
the need for an assistant, an important factor in the context of reduced
doctors' working hours.

The enormous increase in volume of retinal surgery generated by the
new and successful methods, coupled with the need to offer a service to
the community in outreach clinics, led to further consultant appointments after the amalgamation of the two branches and the entry of
Moorfields into the so-called 'marketplace' devised by the Thatcher
government. In 1988 David McLeod left Moorfields to take up the
Professorial Chair in Manchester, and for a time after the amalgamation the consultant numbers dropped. In 1994, however, Bill Aylward,
previously a Resident and Fellow at Moorfields and subsequently a
Visiting Fellow at the Bascom Palmer Eye Institute in Miami, joined
the vitreoretinal surgical team and also established a Moorfields
surgical vitreoretinal service at St George's Hospital Tooting, while
Paul Sullivan was appointed in 1996, and did the same at Watford
General Hospital, and David Charteris in 1998 at the Mayday Hospital

Croydon. Not only were these three consultants excellent vitreoretinal surgeons, but Aylward also brought with him special expertise in information technology, Sullivan in teaching and Charteris in research. Meanwhile, 1995 saw the retirement of Rolf Blach and 2000 that of the present author, Sullivan taking over as service director and Eric Ezra joining the staff in 2001 and taking over the service at St George's. Ezra had been responsible, with Gregor, for much of the important progress in surgery of macular holes, as well as work on the surgical management of advanced proliferative diabetic retinopathy, but he was also a superb surgeon, equally at home in the anterior segment.

In 2002, when Bob Cooling stepped down as Medical Director of the Trust, Bill Aylward took on this onerous and vital responsibility, while June 2003 saw Cooling's retirement from the staff of Moorfields, after playing a long and remarkable part in its history. His place on the vitreoretinal team was taken by Lyndon da Cruz, who had been a Fellow in Australia before coming to Moorfields, and who was another outstanding surgeon appointed on a 50/50 contract, to boost the research impact of the service in the new millennium, especially in the field of submacular surgery. It was the encouraging results of the multicentre study of low-molecular-weight heparin, combined with 5-fluorouracil in the prevention of proliferative retinopathy, however, that above all else were most likely to dominate the Vitreoretinal Service's activities in the future.

CHAPTER 3

Nursing Services

Background

Socioeconomic and technical developments in medicine during the past 40 years have totally changed the face of nursing practice. Until the early 1960s, hospital medicine adhered to a strict hierarchical format, everyone, from the most senior to the most junior doctor, nurse, porter and domestic, knowing their place. It was an oligarchical world of its own, little affected by the wider changes in society at large, consultant surgeons wielding absolute power and senior nursing staff, in their own domain, doing likewise. Consultants often behaved like gods, while hospital matrons were usually queenly figures. The nursing hierarchy was divided, broadly speaking, into two distinct categories: the senior elite consisting of ward sisters and above, and the others – staff nurses down to nurses in training – being generally much younger and comparatively inexperienced. Most of the ward sisters and other seniors were unmarried, their lives totally devoted to the service of their patients and the practice of medicine. Marriage generally meant leaving the profession, so the few who occupied senior positions were usually much older and more experienced than their juniors and their authority was consequently absolute. Nursing was considered to be one of the most honourable and respected professions to which a young woman could aspire (male nurses were a comparative rarity, outside the staff of mental institutions), and the low pay and strict discipline were not at that time considered inimical.

Even in the wider world outside hospital life, professional pride, autonomy and standing in medicine were enormous, and the present author recalls the occasion in the mid 1960s, when his father-in-law, a popular and respected general practitioner in a provincial town, emerged from evening surgery visibly shaken and upset, when for the first time, a patient had dared to question his diagnosis and proposed management.

Just as the 'swinging sixties' changed the face of industrial relations, the Trade Unions challenging the authority of Government, and workers their bosses, so the medical world saw the first glimmerings of a more liberal way of life. In the nursing profession it began to be accepted that it was possible for senior nurses to have a life outside the hospital walls and still remain dedicated to the care of their patients, and it was not long before many of the archaic principles and traditions of the past were swept away. Harold Wilson's 'technological revolution' and the sharp upturn in economic fortunes that followed the austere and rather dreary 1950s were largely responsible for this sea change in social culture. In medicine the rapid development of new, more sophisticated treatments – pharmaceutical, radiological and surgical – as well as methods of diagnosis and assessment, caused havoc amongst the traditional practices of the past. This was probably at least as true in ophthalmology as in any other branch of medicine, and its effect was felt at Moorfields within a very short space of time.

Not only did the nursing itself become more technical, but also patients stayed in the hospital for shorter and shorter periods, and were discharged and taught to manage their own postoperative care. Nurses were therefore required to understand and explain to patients the importance and implications of their treatment, to a degree and at a speed previously unknown. By the year 2003, with around 80 beds at City Road, instead of more than three times that number spread over the two branches as was previously the case, and with 10 community eye service Outreach Units, not to mention the new Diagnostic Treatment Centres, the distribution and working practices of the nursing staff had, in the space of less than 30 years, been completely transformed.

When Margaret Mackellar retired after 28 years as Matron in July 1970, her replacement, Marion Tickner, although a paragon of the highest standards of nursing care, was not a great champion of modernization and continued to steer a steady course through well-charted waters.

> *Her conservative attitude is perhaps well illustrated by the story of her greeting the Casualty Sister at the High Holborn branch of the Hospital when she first arrived (and finding her as was her wont, sleeves rolled up, busy in the department), with: 'Sister, put those sleeves down, please'.*

Unsurprisingly, therefore, in spite of the enormous advances in ophthalmology during the 1970s, and efforts to encourage a more modern approach, her tenure led to little in the way of major changes in nursing practices at Moorfields.

Thirteen years later, with the appointment of a new Matron, the Hospital saw the opportunity to usher in a change of culture, and grasped it eagerly. To the horror and dismay of the nursing hierarchy, the appointments panel were bold enough to choose not only a candidate with considerable management experience (she had been head of nurse recruitment and student personnel at St Thomas' Hospital and had managed the International Department at the Royal College of Nursing for seven years), but one who had little experience of ophthalmology and did not possess the Ophthalmic Nursing Diploma (OND). Such was the sense of outrage amongst the senior nurses at Moorfields at this break with long-established tradition that they initially threatened to resign, en bloc, if the appointment was confirmed. Suffice it to say that this was, fortunately, a threat that they did not, in the event, carry out.

Roslyn Emblin's tenure as Matron (officially titled Chief Nurse) was marked by momentous changes, not only as a result of the redevelopment of the Hospital and the amalgamation of its two branches, but also because of the huge changes in clinical practice brought about by innovations in surgical and other therapeutic methods (**Figure 32, Plate 17**). Coming on top of the cultural changes to which allusion has been made, these caused the role of the ophthalmic nurse to become unrecognizable from that of yesteryear. As soon as she arrived, it was clear to Emblin that the Ophthalmic Nursing Board (ONB) had become outdated, lying as it uniquely did outside the professional statutory regulatory framework of the English National Board for Nursing, Midwifery and Health Visiting (the ENB), so that its qualification, the Ophthalmic Nursing Diploma (the OND), was not recognized on the same footing as other specialist nursing qualifications. Using her contacts and experience nationally, in addition to her management and communication skills, she was able to bring the ophthalmic nursing qualification into line, rewriting the curriculum, disbanding the ONB and slowly building on the foundation of these changes, modernizing ophthalmic nursing education at Moorfields.

In the 1990s this modernization was taken a step further, when the Moorfields School of Nursing became part of a university education for ophthalmic nurses, provided by Thames Valley University. Ophthalmic nurses were able henceforth to gain a university diploma recognized by the ENB and then go on to undertake specialist modules in different aspects of ophthalmic care, including health promotion, teaching, counselling and research, leading to a Bachelor's or Master's degree or even, with a much greater commitment to research, towards the award of a PhD.

On the shopfloor, there was a pressing need to modernize the system for coordinating clinical decisions made in the out-patient department, with procedures for admission, operation and discharge. The rapidly evolving changes in surgical technique in the 1980s, particularly in cataract surgery, meant that pre-admission assessment was necessary.

Such was the rapid cascade of admission, surgery and discharge that it was of paramount importance to ensure that there was close coordination between patient, referring doctor, anaesthetist, surgeon, and ward and operating theatre staff. No longer was there the luxury of hours or even days with the patient in hospital, prior to and after operation, during which doctors, nurses and others could coordinate events. Things could go badly awry if there was any slip-up between one event and the next. To address this problem, the new post of Patient-Care Coordinator was introduced, senior nurses beginning to act, for the first time, as nurse-practitioners, carrying out assessments, counselling and explaining to patients, and ensuring that admission procedures were correct, beds available and that GPs, surgeons and in-patient staff were kept fully informed.

This was the first stage in a patient information project aimed not only at enhancing the quality of patient care but also at modernizing and extending the roles of the nurses. A series of explanatory booklets for patients were written by nursing staff, touch-screen computers providing information were positioned in the Out-Patient Department at City Road and in the Community Outreach Units, and a telephone helpline, Moorfields Direct, soon followed (see below). These initiatives were generously supported by the Friends of Moorfields, as was the development of another nursing initiative, the Patient Hostel, which provided self-caring overnight accommodation for patients who lived too far away to get home on the day of surgery.

Meanwhile, gradual changes on the wards enabled senior nurses to develop clinical skills previously limited to doctors, and with the help of sympathetic clinicians, a core of skilled nurse-practitioners emerged. Establishment of the Primary Care Clinic in 1986 and the modernization of the A&E Department, followed in the early 1990s by the development of the Community Eye Service Outreach Units, inevitably led to increasing demands for highly trained nurse-practitioners. These were needed not only to support the existing complement of clinical assistants but also to replace them, as their numbers dwindled, opportunities opening up thereby, for specialist nurse-practitioners in glaucoma, medical retina and other specialties. By virtue of its modernized approach to nursing education, Moorfields was able to offer specialized courses, in addition to the university curriculum, and so maintain its leading position in innovative teaching practices and training (**Figure 33**, Plate 17).

Not everything advanced as quickly or as progressively as some might have wished. It was perceived in some quarters that a small team of close associates maintained too firm a control over the nursing body, with limited opportunities for wider devolvement of managerial power and freedom of action amongst the more junior nursing staff. This notwithstanding, the senior nursing management team was a well-coordinated and effective group and the Chief Nurse was ably assisted by her 'right-hand man' Ann Hughes (officially styled Director of Nursing Services), whose down-to-earth, hands-on approach to nursing management was an invaluable resource and was key to maintaining good relations with other members of staff. Her somewhat authoritarian style of management may have been influenced by Roslyn Emblin's appointment as Deputy General Manager and later Deputy Chief Executive, posts that at that time embodied the role of director of personnel. Even when Ian Balmer introduced the new post of Director of Personnel, to bring the management structure into line with modern practice, on the assumption of Trust status in 1994, the new Director, Ken Gold, was not given the opportunity to assume responsibility for nursing personnel and recruitment. Mary Ryan (Director of Nursing Education and Personnel), who had a Master's degree in Human Resource Management, retaining this function.

Nevertheless, key changes in nursing culture gradually took place in all sorts of areas, orchestrated by Emblin and largely driven by Hughes, ably supported by her Assistant Nursing Directors, Lyn Heywood in the Out-Patient Department and, in turn, Linda Mepham, Sue Humphreys and Joyce Morrin in the operating theatres. It was not until the Hospital's management was totally restructured, however, with the introduction of tridivisional lines of command, that the traditional style of nursing hegemony was finally disbanded. This perceived weakness apart, by the time she left, Roslyn Emblin had made a huge impact in the field of nursing education, her legacy the evolution of a new breed of ophthalmic nurses, possessed of a wide range of skills hitherto unknown, and able to market their professional expertise worldwide, with confidence and pride.

Apart from the nurse-practitioners in primary care, glaucoma, medical retina and other specialist areas, in the mid-1990s senior nurses were introduced into the specialist services when these became free-standing directorates. The Service Sister was a unique concept embodying the roles of manager, nurse and researcher in varying degrees, at the discretion of the individual herself and the director of the specialist service group. They were encouraged to develop their roles as they saw fit, some as managers and organizers, some as nurse-clinicians, in the out-patient clinics or operating theatres, and others in the field of clinical audit and research, largely depending on the differing needs of the patients in the different specialist services. Seven nursing sisters were appointed, to the Adnexal (Sophie Lewis), Cataract (Carmel King), Corneal and External Disease (Patricia Maddison), Glaucoma (Chris Smith), Medical Retina (Kate Rumble), Strabismus and Paediatric (Anita Aubrey) and Vitreoretinal Surgical (Catherine Bankes) Services, several of whom remained in post for many years, finding their jobs exciting, challenging and satisfying. Not only were they free to define and develop their own particular role within the service, they were also able to train others, in some cases further advancing and expanding the roles of emerging nurse-practitioners throughout the Trust. The understated introduction of these posts somewhat obscured their significance, for, contrary to former practice, where promotion above ward sister meant abandoning direct patient-care, here for the first time, was an opportunity for senior nurses to assume an enhanced range of managerial responsibilities and autonomy whilst remaining firmly within the clinical arena. The evolution of such an increasingly important group of skilled professionals was further enhanced by the provision of a skills laboratory, in space previously occupied by the practical classroom in the School of Nursing, and the opportunity was taken to combine this with a similar facility for junior ophthalmologists.

Moorfields Direct

In line with the government's drive towards greater patient involvement with, and accessibility to, medical services, in 1988 Moorfields set up its own telephone helpline (**Figure 34**, Plate 18). This service was a direct-dial telephone information and advice service run by nurses, open from 9.00 am to 5.00 pm, Monday to Friday. It was funded by the Friends of Moorfields and served two main functions: to offer help with diagnosis and management of urgent problems and to advise callers about conditions of which the diagnosis was already known. Specialist ophthalmic guidelines were incorporated into the software package designed to assist the nurse-advisor, and the dialogue between nurse and caller was recorded. The service was advertised on the Trust's Internet website, as well as in booklets and on posters around the Hospital, and soon became a popular service, averaging around 40 calls per day. It was viewed with approval by the Commission for Health Improvement when they inspected the Trust and was a valuable addition to the Hospital's portfolio of services.

Nursing management

With the transformation of nursing practice in the last quarter of the 20th Century, a commensurate change in management was inevitable. The foundation for this was probably laid much earlier, with the change in culture induced by the nationalized health service, as a part of the transmogrification of the 'them and us', 'upstairs/downstairs' social structure swept away by the Second World War. Just as doctors no longer dispensed charity to the poor whilst they were rewarded by the rich, so nurses were no longer prepared to accept the archaic conditions of employment and rigid hierarchy of the past. No longer was nursing something that only the well-off (for charity) or the very poor (to keep body and soul together) could afford to do, and a new breed of well-educated, middle-class nurses emerged, with egalitarian views and the wit and power to express them. The old-fashioned matrons and sisters and downtrodden, subservient juniors gradually disappeared, to be replaced by more open-minded individuals, who envisaged a rewarding career, combined with a normal family life and expectations of reasonable pay and working conditions.

Nevertheless, well into the second half of the century, an ethos persisted that nurses were inferior to doctors and were their hand-maidens, there to do their bidding. Such a state of affairs was allowed to continue and was even encouraged by politicians, who saw a soft-hearted, willing workforce, prepared to work tirelessly for little financial reward, as an invaluable resource. Sadly for the NHS, however, this threadbare state of affairs could not last, and slowly it became apparent that, even with the influx of nurses from abroad, more prepared to suffer poor conditions, the nursing profession was desperately short of person-nel. Furthermore, the nurses were aware of their potential worth and struck out for decent conditions, training facilities and the pay and credit they deserved.

In ophthalmology, as is so often is the case, the situation was plain for all to see. Even at Moorfields, during the 1970s and 1980s, it became increasingly difficult to recruit nurses, and it was not until better pay and career opportunities were offered that the situation began to improve. The changes introduced by Roslyn Emblin, improving the range and scope of training, offering university qualifications and gain-ing recognition by the Nursing Council, were crucial to its survival and subsequent forward progress. Even with the greatly enhanced job satis-faction and range of opportunities, however, so much damage to the image and ethos of the nursing profession had already been done and the job opportunities for women were by now so diverse that recruit-ment was still a major problem. Emblin's efforts were aided and abetted by John Atwill and the Board of Governors, whose forward-looking approach, with the development of primary care and the community outreach eye services, together with the specialist service groups, demanded a different type of nurse, with new skills, to work alongside and gradually to replace the non-consultant career-grade doctors who had kept the service going for so long.

During the 1990s relentless pressure from above, first of all by the Conservatives with their Patients' Charter, and then by New Labour with its NHS Plan and determination to control every aspect of the Health Service, led to demands for a greater devolvement of power, and this was bound to extend to the running of nursing services. The House Governor, Ian Balmer, saw the need to spread the administrative burden more evenly and, in the first instance appointed a Director of Operations, a move that proved, like the curate's egg, to be good only in parts, for while she was extremely efficient, her efficiency was matched only by her ability to upset almost everyone on the staff. Subsequent to her departure, there were further calls for change, but the period of uncertainty that followed New Labour's changes to the structure and running of the NHS and the unhappy episode involving the resignation of the Chairman of the Board of Governors delayed their implementation. At last, after much discussion and debate, it was decided in 2001 to devolve management into three divisions, each having at its head a clinical director (a member of the consultant medical staff) supported by a nurse manager and a general manager. The nursing posts were filled by existing members of the senior nursing staff, Ann Hughes, Lyn Heywood and Kate Lowe, all of whom had managerial experience within the Trust.

The aim of the exercise was to spread decision making across a broader tier by introducing three clearly defined parallel lines of management, with greater opportunities for true devolvement of power downwards and across them, the nine divisional managers meeting regularly and having control over their own budgets. Nevertheless they were still only nominally in control of the latter, so their power was limited, overall control resting with the Treasurer and ultimately with the House Governor himself. Roslyn Emblin chose to remain in post and ensure that the situation was stable following this restructuring, before, in 2002, she stepped down from the post of Chief Nurse and Deputy Chief Executive and, after a period of nearly 20 years of dedicated service to the Trust, left Moorfields.

The new Director of Nursing and Development, Sarah Fisher, had much in common with her predecessor, coming as she did with the experience of more than two years as Assistant Director of Nursing at a large London teaching hospital (University College), but with an even wider range of experience. Starting out in the oil exploration industry, with a degree in environmental science, she had trained as a nurse at a District General Hospital before joining the cardiac team at St George's Hospital. She then worked as a specialist community nurse, before doing a Master's degree in health sciences and moving to King's College as a lecturer. Her move to Moorfields she regarded as a leap back into the 'rough and tumble of NHS life', contrasting as it did with a huge teaching hospital that 'changed shape every year'. She found Moorfields very tight-knit, a place where 'four or five people made all the decisions' and where 'everyone knew each other so well that there was no need to write anything down'. Corporate responsibility appeared to be weak and accountability implicit rather than explicit.

She wanted to see more explicit accountability amongst the nurses, with a greater emphasis on shared objectives and regular appraisals. Questioning and innovation were expected and senior nurses were required to manage and take decisions on their own initiative. She could see opportunities for redeveloping the roles of the existing work-force, whilst introducing opportunities for non-professionally qualified health-care assistants in a strategic, coordinated manner. Her door was always open and she was addressed as 'Sarah', rather than 'Matron' or 'Miss Fisher'. She alone attended meetings of the Management Executive, to avoid duplication of senior representation and to allow the divisional nursing directors to focus more on delivering their remit.

Sarah Fisher could see the difficulties of modernizing one part of the service without linking it to those supporting it. It was not long before she and the new Medical Director, Bill Aylward, were jointly presenting a paper to the Board of Directors on their shared vision of how, by modernizing services to match patient flows, the clinical agenda could be put more firmly back into the centre of the Trust's activities. It was evident too that, if she had her way, it would not be long before financial management was devolved to the divisions, a possible source of tension with the Director of Finance. Time alone would tell.

The introduction into the management of the Hospital of such a dynamic personality with modern ideas was sure to have far-reaching effects, especially on its corporate functions. Her new eyes could see flaws and weaknesses hitherto hidden to others from view. Private practice had been allowed to stay largely outside the remit of the Trust's corporate responsibility, a situation that she, in common with the Manager of Moorfields Private, Elizabeth Boultbee, perceived to carry a high risk, but one that had long been tacitly accepted. She perceived that nursing sisters were all too often not fulfilling a management role and were not familiar with how to manage budgets or recruit staff. Few but the most senior nurses were used to making strategic decisions or really 'punching their weight' with their medical colleagues. In spite of their numbers, the voices of the nursing staff at Moorfields were not being sufficiently well heard. The old model of nursing hierarchy frequently stifled innovation, and the skill-mix and deployment strategy needed to be improved. The academic association with Thames Valley University, based as it was at Ealing, was unsatisfactory, contact being difficult, and research as a consequence being hard to undertake. It was essential, as Roslyn Emblin had previously identified, for Moorfields to grow nurse consultants and thereby keep senior, innovative individuals in the clinical arena. In short, the time had come to transmute the management of nursing at Moorfields and ensure that it would continue to take its place at the forefront of ophthalmic care in the 21st century. Time alone would tell if these perceptions were valid and, if so, what effect a change of course would have on the Hospital's future direction.

Meanwhile, as the present account goes to press, it is well to recall the long service quietly and unassumingly provided over the past 40 years by many members of the nursing staff at all levels. Amongst these, the present author remembers especially Gina Smith, Sister on Top Corridor for several years, Janet Porter, Sister on Alexandra Ward until its closure (and then a stalwart in the Nursing Office), Sisters Janet Smith, Ann Thomas, John Berrino and Sue Evans, Nurse Mary Dowkes and many others who served the Hospital well and long ago moved on. Many others, like Irene Sze and Patti Evans, continued to serve in different roles. Meanwhile, it lost several of its most loyal and long-serving nurses recently, including Helen Gorman and Charles Ramsurran who retired in May 2003, and Margaret Flood in December (**Figure 35**). To them all the Hospital and its patients owe their thanks.

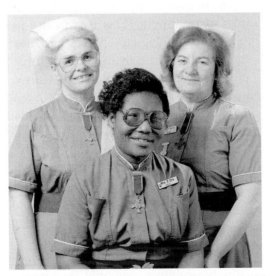

Figure 35   Three of the senior nurses whose dedicated service to Moorfields spanned several decades – *from left to right:* Sister Susan Stevens, Sister Omotayo Ero and Sister Helen Gorman.

CHAPTER 4

Clinical Support Services

Background

The Hospital's clinical activities are backed up by a number of support services that are fundamental to its performance as a centre of excellence, and essential if its ethos and standards are to be maintained. Most of these services have grown bigger, in parallel with their increasing sophistication and importance, as time has gone by, while in some instances their role has altered completely. They are all stand-alone departments meeting a broad spectrum of different clinical demands, although some of them necessarily subserve certain specialties more than others.

Electrophysiology

Amongst the scientific support services, probably none is more important today than the electrodiagnostic service, providing, as it does, information vital in making diagnoses, estimating prognoses and assessing the results of treatment. This was in the past by no means always the case, electrophysiological studies and investigations, until about 15 years ago, yielding little in the way of information that was really crucial to clinical management. Since that time, however, a sea-change has taken place. This is particularly true since the emergence of molecular biology, gene therapy and the role that this new technology is playing in the diagnosis and treatment of inherited conditions affecting the brain and central nervous system.

The Electrodiagnostic Department (EDD) first came into being in the late 1960s, when Geoffrey Arden, medically trained, but academically minded, joined the Institute of Ophthalmology's physiology department and began a lifelong interest in the electrophysiological responses of the human eye. Arden remained firmly within the academic milieu throughout his career (in the Department of Visual Science), eventually receiving a personal Academic Chair, but his research was clinically related and he therefore ran an investigative service at the Hospital. In this he was joined by John Kelsey, a consultant ophthalmologist at University College Hospital, with a keen interest in electrophysiology. Together, for many years they ran an electrodiagnostic clinic on the second floor of the Hospital at City Road, undertaking electroretinograms (ERGs), electro-oculograms (EOGs) and visually evoked responses (VERs), in response to requests from ophthalmologists at Moorfields and outside, and reporting the results of their findings. These were helpful in differentiating between grossly different conditions affecting the retina and optic nerve and between those with genuine neurophysiological disorders and those without, but were not initially of much use in the finer points of diagnosis. For this reason, the EDD was not, in its early days, always held in the highest esteem by busy clinicians wanting simple answers to baffling problems, although that did not deter some of them from making unreasonable demands of the electrodiagnosticians.

John Kelsey recalled receiving a referral request from a consultant at a London teaching hospital that simply said: 'Dear John, this lady is a complete mystery. Can you help?'

The inability of electrophysiological investigation in its early days to provide answers to complex clinical questions should not detract from the brilliance and inventiveness of both Arden and Kelsey, especially Arden, who carried out excellent research and developed methods of investigation that proved to be of seminal importance. In 1976 they were joined by a technician, Chris Hogg, with a passionate interest in all matters electronic, and the partnership between Hogg and Arden blossomed. Technical advances came steadily, with standardization of tests, including pattern ERGs, and tests of colour and of dark adaptation, and with gold-foil corneal electrodes replacing the cumbersome and uncomfortable contact lens electrodes, as a result of Arden's efforts and the grants and other funds solicited by him. From then on, the EDD grew steadily, both in stature and in physical size, the range and quality of tests and their applicability, especially to the differentiation of retinal dystrophies, becoming increasingly important in diagnosis. It also played a vital role in confirming the diagnosis of demyelinating disease in patients presenting with loss of vision from optic neuritis, with the demyelination causing delayed conduction in the optic nerve, and exhibiting delay in the VER.

In 1991, however, disaster struck. The review body set up by the Director of the BPMF reported unfavourably on Geoffrey Arden's research output, even going so far as to recommend his early retirement, a view supported by the new head of Visual Science, Adam

Sillito. Great bitterness ensued, until Arden reached retirement age and left to carry on his pioneering research at the City University, even at the time of writing, continuing to produce and publish new work.

With the loss of both Arden and Kelsey (who retired in 1995), and the increasing importance of the EDD's role in the diagnosis, prognosis and evaluation of results of gene therapies, the Hospital realized the need for a more structured and full-time clinical service. In 1995 Graham Holder was appointed as departmental head. A full-time NHS employee of Moorfields, he had previously acquired wide experience of running an electrophysiology service for the neurological and neurosurgical units in South East Thames Region and held higher degrees in neuropsychology and neurophysiology. He was nevertheless appointed with the express intention of running a clinical service and this he set out to do, with considerable success. He was well equipped to do so, his appointment in South Thames many years earlier having coincided with the demonstration by Halliday, just a year before, of the value of the VER in the diagnosis of demyelination of the optic nerve, thereby releasing a deluge of clinical referrals. His arrival at Moorfields was greeted with enthusiasm and relief, the department rapidly expanding from 6 to 12 staff, including 2 more scientists.

The service was required in particular to meet the demands of the Medical Retinal Service, which accounted for 40% of the internal referrals, as well as channelling many patients referred to Professor Bird for an opinion by outside consultants, and of John Sloper's paediatric practice, while the neurologist, Dr Gordon Plant, relied heavily on its services. Under Graham Holder's leadership it remained the busiest and most prestigious department of its kind in the country. This in itself was sufficient to attract students from all over the world, Holder becoming the Director of Education for the International Society for Clinical Electrophysiology and one of the very few British authors in his subject, writing for the American Academy of Ophthalmology.

Meanwhile, Chris Hogg, who had originally contributed hugely to the Hospital's early struggle to develop information technology (**Figure 36**, Plate 18), continued to pioneer advances in equipment, in particular the development of the Ganzfeld stimulator, a big project for which he received great credit and one leading to much improved methods of assessment. The battle to introduce computerization in the 1970s and 1980s had brought the Hospital to rely heavily on Hogg's expertise in this comparatively new field, and his unstinting efforts and unfailing good humour were instrumental in assisting many of the staff to master its fundamentals. Furthermore, advances in computer technology were to transform electrodiagnostic testing, Chris Hogg's skill and enthusiasm playing no small part in this quiet revolution.

Hogg recalled that the first computer acquired by the hospital, in 1976, had little more than the power of the pocket calculator of the year 2003, and cost £30 000, or about £200 000 at 2003 values.

Unlike Arden, whose brilliance was matched by a prodigious capacity for absent-mindedness and whose attention to teaching was somewhat limited, Holder was practical and down-to-earth and held weekly teaching sessions for Fellows and Residents from the Medical Retinal Service, which were well attended not only by the juniors but also by Professors Bird and Moore. He also contributed to the courses of instruction in macular disease and uveitis run by the Hospital's Education Department. The increasing involvement of the EDD in the work of the Medical Retinal, Paediatric and Genetic Services bore testament to the fruits of Arden's research and to the newfound ability of electrodiagnostic testing to differentiate between the numerous different causes of poor vision, not just between macular or optic nerve disease, but also between cone dystrophies, rod dystrophies and cone/rod dystrophies, and between congenital night-blindness and vitamin A deficiency or supracortical visual loss. The benefits of this were to be found not only in accurate diagnosis, but also in estimating prognosis and in the capacity to gauge the results of therapy, in the prevention and treatment of genetically determined disorders of the retina, and in the treatment of vitamin A deficiency in malabsorption syndromes such as Crohn's disease.

Although strictly a clinical service, the EDD managed to produce six or more scientific papers annually, many of them in association with Alan Bird, Andrew Webster and members of the Medical Retina team. Graham Holder and Chris Hogg, although not Institute employees, also worked in collaboration with workers there, both basic and clinical scientists, including Phil Luthert in Pathology, Shomi Bhattacharya in Genetics and Fred Fitzke in Psychophysics, while Hogg was also still involved with Geoffrey Arden, at City University, developing colour-sensitivity tests for glaucoma, diabetes and age-related macular degeneration. The Moorfields EDD soon became, without exception, the best clinical electrophysiological department in the UK, rivalled only by some centres in the USA, and, what is more, attracted a considerable income for the Trust from outside referrals. Furthermore, with the development of the International Children's Eye Centre, there was the likelihood of more laboratory space and clinical work becoming available in the future.

Imaging services

X-ray Department

The appointment of Glyn Lloyd as consultant radiologist in 1962 turned out to be an inspired choice. With a joint post at the Royal Throat, Nose and Ear Hospital in Gray's Inn Road, his special interest was in radiology of the head and neck, but he was also highly innovative and intent on developing new techniques at Moorfields. This soon led to a happy and fruitful collaboration with John Wright, who saw the opportunities presented by Lloyd's expertise, for radiology of the orbit. Wright had, while a Resident at City Road, tried injecting contrast medium into the orbit to outline tumours with hypocycloidal tomography, but with poor results. In 1968 he visited Milan and learned from Professor Passerini how to perform orbital venography, and between then and 1973 he and Lloyd used this technique extensively, Lloyd soon becoming the internationally acknowledged expert in the interpretation of its results. The method was, however, difficult and unpleasant for patients and investigators alike. When computed tomography (CT) came on the scene, Lloyd was quick to realize its potential, as early as 1973 sending patients to the Atkinson Morley Hospital for scans, a practice that continued until 1977, after which Moorfields shared the scanner at Queen Square. The close collaboration between Lloyd and Wright continued until the former's retirement, the weekly meeting to review and discuss cases becoming a formidable exercise in clinical teamwork and teaching.

When Dick Welham took over as lacrimal surgeon, he and Lloyd capitalized on the method pioneered by Barrie Jones, using a fine nylon catheter and an oily contrast medium with high viscosity to demonstrate abnormalities and obstructions of the lacrimal drainage system (the dacryocystogram, DCG), by combining this with an imaging technique that greatly magnified the field without loss of definition. Taking advantage of the enormous throughput at Moorfields, and consequently the unrivalled clinical experience available (300 DCGs per year compared with 20 in most other units), he made the very most of such opportunities to polish his technique in successful collaboration with the up-and-coming surgeons of the time. Lloyd was also responsible for the development of a greatly simplified method for detecting and localizing intraocular foreign bodies.

In the early days there were many plain films to be done, X-rays of chests prior to surgery, skulls on suspicion of intracranial disorders, and similarly, plain films of orbits. As time went on, however, these were superseded, first by CT and then, only 10 years later, by magnetic resonance imaging (MRI) (from one year to the next, the number of plain skull X-rays fell from 800 to 50). While CT remained the method of choice for demonstrating pathology in the orbit, MRI transformed the diagnosis and delineation of abnormalities of the intracranial pathways, such as chiasmal lesions. Advances in both surgical methods and anaesthetic techniques meant that routine chest X-rays were no longer necessary, while the different approach to 'blow-out' fractures of the orbital floor meant that emergency plain films of the orbit became obsolete, repair being carried out as a planned procedure, preceded by CT scanning.

The 1980s saw a change of emphasis in the imaging services. Derek Kingsley, a neuroradiologist at the London Hospital, was appointed and, before the retirement of Glyn Lloyd in 1987, Ivan Moseley, from the National Hospital for Neurology and Neurosurgery, Queen Square, took up his post. (**Figure 37**, Plate 19). The interests of the three radiologists overlapped considerably, and the emergence of a distinct subspecialty in its own right, head and neck radiology, was increasingly apparent. The unique experience offered by the interaction between Moorfields, Queen Square and the Royal Throat, Nose and Ear Hospital in neuroradiology and head and neck imaging was recognized as part of the radiology training programme in North Thames Region.

As soon as MRI came into being in 1983, Glyn Lloyd recognized its importance, referring patients to the Hammersmith Hospital, when necessary, until it was available four years later at Queen Square. Ivan Moseley had been a visiting professor in San Francisco when the first work was being done on MRI of the orbit, contributing thereby to the first paper to be published on the subject, in the *British Journal of Ophthalmology*. Its importance was plain, the low level of ionizing irradiation causing no risk to the crystalline lens or retina, while with later developments, even the levels of blood flow in the cerebral cortex and their variation with visual activity could be demonstrated.

Trained in head and neck and neuroradiology at Queen Square, Kathryn Miszkiel arrived in 2001 to take over from Ivan Moseley, having had a very different training and coming to a very different place from that which Glyn Lloyd had entered in the 1960s. Computerization of the reporting system had transformed the running of the department, while modern techniques greatly reduced the need for manpower, especially as the Hospital did not have its own CT or MRI scanners, patients being sent to Queen Square for these investigations. As a result, although imaging of the eye and its adjacent structures remained as important as ever, the department was smaller and quieter than of old and there were now one and a half whole-time equivalent radiographers instead of three, including Pat Skelley, mainstay of the department for more than 30 years.

Diagnostic ultrasound

As well as the huge differences in X-ray techniques that have evolved during the past 40 years, an entirely new technology grew up in the late 1960s, largely as a result of its usefulness as an industrial tool. The use of high-frequency sound waves as a means of detecting solid objects and indicating their position had long been recognized, both in the animal world as a means of navigation by bats and in war and peace by surface vessels to detect underwater hazards. Its use as a tool for detecting fine cracks and irregularities in aircraft components and in pipes was exploited by the aircraft and allied industries, while at the Harwell Atomic Research Establishment it was used to identify metal fatigue.

The pioneer in ophthalmic ultrasound was Douglas Gordon, radiologist at the High Holborn branch of Moorfields, who used an A-scan technique in the late 1960s. He and Lloyd tried scanning some patients with orbital pathology, but the technique was limited by the quality of the apparatus. In 1969, however, Lloyd was sent a leaflet advertising a lecture on the use of holographic ultrasound in industry. He went to the lecture and spoke afterwards to the lecturer, an engineer from Harwell, and he and John Wright subsequently paid a visit there, when they were greatly impressed by some scans of a bull's eye. The engineers at Harwell were sympathetic to the concept of establishing the use of ultrasound in helping to solve the problems of eye disease, but they needed money to build a prototype machine. Wright applied for and was awarded a large grant by the Medical Research Council, and two years later the first ophthalmic ultrasonic holography machine was built and installed at Moorfields. Thus was the Ultrasound Department at the Hospital founded.

Initially, the equipment designed by the Harwell engineers, although superbly designed and ahead of its time, depended on a large, oscillating transducer, which could not therefore be applied directly to the eye. Nor could it be satisfactorily used through the eyelids, so it had to be applied to the cornea through a water-bath, an effective but cumbersome arrangement, which could sometimes produce unanticipated complications, not least when used, as was occasionally the case, in an anaesthetized patient. It was not long, however, before the equipment became more sophisticated. Improvements in the image grey-scale capabilities helped to increase diagnostic accuracy. Solid array probes, which could be applied directly to the closed eye via a coupling gel, also became available. These probes comprised multiple transducer elements that were fired electronically, in sequence, to simulate a single moving transducer.

A hospital physicist was initially assigned to the task of operating and looking after the equipment, but it was not long before Marie Restori, a young physicist with a Master's degree in radiobiology, was appointed to the post of ultrasound physicist (**Figure 38**, Plate 19). It was due to her expertise and enthusiasm that the Ultrasound Department developed as it did, standard A- and B-scan apparatus being purchased to provide a fully comprehensive service for clinicians. It soon became apparent, however, that its value as a diagnostic tool for orbital disorders was limited. The CT scanner had just been introduced, and it was obvious that CT was far superior to ultrasound for demonstrating orbital pathology. Coincidentally, however, in that same year, closed vitrectomy was started at Moorfields and it seemed possible that ultrasound could be ideally suited to the demonstration of intra-ocular abnormalities, where there were no dense tissue structures to distort and deflect the sound pulses.

John Wright continued to have responsibility for the Ultrasound Department, but was keen to transfer it to the care of one of the vitreo-retinal surgeons. A brilliant young ophthalmologist, David McLeod, freshly off the residency programme at Moorfields with an expressed interest in vitreoretinal surgery, was deputed to work with Marie Restori to develop the new diagnostic method. The partnership between them turned out to be a highly successful one, the combination of a pure scientist with a well-trained and intellectually gifted clinician conspiring to produce a welter of new findings and understanding. Diagnostic ophthalmic ultrasound had come to stay.

The rapidly developing specialty of vitreous surgery launched a raft of diagnostic dilemmas, while the demonstration of surgical pathology enabled by ultrasound was impressive. Growing clinical experience made it possible not only to differentiate between the different intra-ocular tissues and identify pathological changes in them, but also to demonstrate dynamic changes accompanying eye movements. Even retinal tears could be identified and located, when the ocular fundus was totally obscured by blood or other debris. The introduction of intra-ocular lens implantation in the latter half of the 1970s meant that A-scanning of the globe became an integral part of ocular biometry and threatened to overwhelm the service until cataract surgeons were encouraged to perform their own scans and train others to do so.

Ironically, the Iran/Iraq war during the 1980s had a powerfully positive effect on the Ultrasound Department at Moorfields. Huge numbers of Iranian soldiers with serious eye injuries (sometimes as many as 15 or more at a time) would be sent over, following land-mine explosions. In many of these cases the intra-ocular contents were so badly disrupted that it was difficult to make out the internal topography. One way of doing so was to identify the direction and velocity of flow along blood vessels in the disorganized tissues, for example, in the retina, and this could be done using colour flow mapping and spectral Doppler techniques. Not only did the department gain unique experience from this tragic state of affairs, but it also brought in large amounts of money for the research fund. It was not until the publication of the 'Satanic Verses', and the resulting fatwah issued by Iranian Muslim clerics against its author Salman Rushdie, calling for his punishment by death, that the ensuing security clampdown caused the flow of these unfortunate patients to cease.

In later years the use of ultrasound became increasingly wide-ranging. In the 1990s B-mode resolution improved further and improvements in both the resolution and sensitivity of colour flow mapping increased diagnostic reliability. Although the majority of referrals still came from the Vitreoretinal Service, an increasing number were sent by a broad spectrum of consultants, including babies with congenital glaucoma from Peng Tee Khaw and patients with tumours from John Hungerford. The type of pathology included children with suspected retinoblastoma and adults with vascular anomalies in the orbit, such as carotico-cavernous fistulae, suprachoroidal haemorrhages and a wide range of other disorders. In some instances these cases could be scanned quickly, while in others the intra-ocular pathology was complex. Unlike other specialties, where biopsies were commonplace, in ophthalmology, the eye being a superficial organ, ultrasound often became the investigation of first choice. The vast throughput and clinical experience soon made the department at Moorfields, and Marie Restori in particular, a world leader in the field.

Although much of the original equipment was funded by the Medical Research Council, and Harwell were generous, from the time of its inception the Ultrasound Department used private patient fees, routed through the Special Trustees, not only to sponsor research but also to buy new equipment. While the hospital management were not completely deaf to entreaties for new and better equipment, they were far from magnanimous. A share in a generous donation from a wealthy benefactor helped and the Hospital came to the rescue when its arm was twisted. The active support of the Surgical Vitreoretinal Service, including the advocacy of Bob Cooling and provision of emergency cover by the Fellows, was also much appreciated.

Medical Illustration and the Retinal Diagnostic Department
Founded by Peter Hansell, when the Institute of Ophthalmology opened in November 1948, the Department of Medical Illustration has always played a vital part in the Hospital's activities. Hansell himself was an inspiring and authoritative figure. Medically qualified, he was a keen amateur photographer, who was awarded a Nuffield Scholarship to visit the USA to study medical illustration and returned to set up his own departments at both the Westminster Hospital, then one of the prestigious London medical schools, and at the new Institute of Ophthalmology. He founded the London School of Medical Photography and the Institute of Medical and Biological Illustration, wrote several books on medical photography, and went on to train a generation of medical photographers and illustrators who subsequently became heads of audio-visual departments throughout the UK.

The department at the Institute flourished, Hansell attracting some especially talented individuals, including Terry Tarrant, Kulwant Sehmi and Alan Lacey, who were to have a major impact on the development of the specialty at Moorfields. Tarrant was a draughtsman of outstanding ability, who developed a skill in painting the ocular fundus, unmatched either before or since. He learned to use the Fison binocular indirect ophthalmoscope and became as proficient in its use as most retinal surgeons. Because he was (as he explained to the present author) not an artist, he made no attempt to embellish or adapt what he saw (the main fault of most medical illustrators), producing as a result perfect reproductions of the fundus, equal to or better than any photograph. As it was several years before fundus photography developed sufficiently to enable wide-angle views of the fundus that were of equivalent quality, and because all his work was outstanding, he became indispensable, producing exquisite drawings and diagrams to illustrate every aspect of the human eye, healthy or diseased, and contributing to vast numbers of scientific publications.

Kulwant Sehmi completed his training at the London School of Medical Photography in 1968, and planned to return home to India. The course at the school included field visits to a number of different working departments, including the Institute of Ophthalmology. Dr Hansell, spotting Sehmi's obvious talent, suggested that he might apply for a vacancy at Moorfields, where the newly formed Retinal Diagnostic Department (RDD) was looking for a photographer. Sehmi rang his father, who agreed that this experience would be useful in his future career back home, and felt that a few more months away would do no harm. So began the career of one of the world's most distinguished ophthalmic photographers and the loyal and dedicated head of the Department of Medical Illustration at Moorfields. Sehmi's appointment was aimed at developing the new science of fluorescein fundus angiography (FFA) (**Figure 39**, Plate 20), which had been started at Moorfields not long before, by Sohan Singh Hayreh and David Hill. This soon set off a chain of events that was to have a major impact on the practice of medical retina in the UK (see Part 2).

Fluorescein angiography had already been used in the USA for some time, especially in Miami, where Alan Bird was doing his Fellowship, and the medical photographer there, Johnny Justice Jr, was already the unchallenged expert. On Bird's return, therefore, the scene was already set for him, Rolf Blach, recently appointed consultant at City Road, and Sehmi to set up a combined retinal diagnostic service and research team. Sehmi rapidly gained unique experience and, like Justice in the USA, became the doyen of retinal photographers in the UK. The department at Moorfields, from a shoestring affair in a corner of the Professorial Unit, with Sehmi going to the Institute to do his processing, soon moved to customized premises on the second floor, with its own dark-room, Peter Hamilton joining in 1971, and the weekly number of FFAs rapidly growing from 50 to 250, as more and more patients were referred.

A photographer came over from the Institute to undertake other types of photography, Sehmi remaining exclusively devoted to fundus photography. He developed his own films and a weekly fluorescein conference was started, Sehmi choosing the most interesting cases he had photographed and submitting them to Alan Bird for his selection. As the team of doctors in the RDD led by Alan Bird grew, and the number of FFAs increased, a formal weekly reporting session was held, which not only provided valuable experience and teaching for the Fellows and others in reading angiograms, but also ensured that referring doctors received reports promptly. By the end of the 1970s the RDD had outgrown its premises and it was rehoused in the area previously occupied by Edward Ward, until in 1985, with the refurbishment of the lower ground floor, it moved to a purpose-built clinical area there, including examination rooms, offices and laser suite.

The Department of Medical Illustration was until 1981 part of the Institute and it was there in 1970 that Alan Lacey joined its staff as a scientific and technical photographer. He found it a busy and friendly place and was soon absorbed in routine work, including the preparation of diazo slides and other teaching material. It was not long, however, before he became involved in movie-making, at first on 16 mm celluloid film, producing in 1975 the first films of 'live' vitreoretinal surgery. He rapidly became more and more involved with Alan Lane and Walter ('Buck') Buchanan, the technical staff in the television studio above the operating theatres at the Hospital, and when they retired, took over the running of the television studio and all aspects of film and video-making work. His aptitude for, and skills in, electronic audio-visual techniques developed steadily during the 1980s and 1990s, as he moved seamlessly from U-matic to VHS recording and, by the turn of the century, to digital imaging, acquiring on the way a unique position in the pantheon of ophthalmic illustrators.

In 1981 the financial plight of the Institute forced it to close the Department of Medical Illustration. The Board of Governors, deciding that the service it provided could not be foregone without serious detriment to the Hospital, made provision to take it over, albeit not without considerable rationalization, including the retirement of Terry Tarrant, and a considerable reduction in other staff. Sehmi was, by this time, firmly established at the Hospital, as was Alan Lacey, and they were joined there by Tony Sullivan. Sehmi was the obvious choice to head the newly restructured department. That he was not made head did those involved in the appointment little credit, nor was it in retrospect a sensible decision to bring in as director an inexperienced if well-meaning journeyman from outside. Within three years they were to realize their mistake and make amends, Sehmi duly taking over as head of the department, the number of commissions rising to 18 000 per year and the staff increasing over the next 20 years, from 3 to 10.

Meanwhile, at the High Holborn branch, Tim Ffytche had initiated an FFA service in 1969, and was joined, on the closure of the Royal Eye Hospital in 1973, by Professor David Hill. A photographer from City Road was seconded there, on a rotating basis, a system that worked well and offered a different brand of experience. Although it was by all accounts less highly pressured than the service at City Road, it provided opportunities for independent thinking and individual expression not so readily available at the latter, and so was, for all that, enjoyed and appreciated. Because of the strength of the all-round training provided by the Moorfields' Department of Medical Illustration, and although there were strong departments elsewhere, notably in Manchester and Dundee, the majority of ophthalmic medical photographers in the UK received at least some of their training at Moorfields.

The pattern of work at Moorfields changed over the years. Perhaps surprisingly, the number of FFAs dropped, from around 250 to 150 per week, as ophthalmologists became more discriminating, while the development of oculoplastic surgery and later the proliferation of outreach centres altered the pattern of demand for photographic records. The change from Kodachrome to Ektachrome film enabled all processing to be done 'in house', and the department achieved such high standards that it received quality recognition by Eastman Kodak, alongside that of commercial units, until in the 1990s the emergence of digital imaging rendered the use of film virtually obsolete. The resulting desuetude of expensive processing equipment and the purchase of two new digital processors, costing £70 000 each, was balanced by savings in running costs.

In 1998, in a bid to keep down capital costs and at the same time make the best use of expensive equipment, a Mobile Unit (a large articulated lorry) fully equipped to carry out FFA and laser treatment at the different outreach sites, was purchased by the Hospital, with the help of donations from members of the consultant staff (see **Figure 28**, Plate 15). This facility, although appealing and imaginative in design, was only partially successful, problems with parking such a large vehicle sufficiently close to where it was needed limiting its usefulness. Sad to say, the new Director of Operations, Christine Miles, whose brain-child it was and whose energy and determination brought the project to fruition, caused much distress and lowering of morale in the department of medical illustration by her insensitive attempts at micro-management and conflict with Sehmi – an unfortunate effect that was to last until 1999, when she left the Trust.

Meanwhile, in the TV studio, Alan Lacey was producing an ever-increasing range of high-quality movies and other real-time images, on video-cassette and later with digital software. In contrast to what happened in the department downstairs, he fared well at the hands of Christine Miles, her efficient business style, coupled with the obvious attraction of producing high-quality movie presentations of the Trust's work, leading to a transformation in the audio-visual equipment in the operating theatres, at a cost to the Special Trustees of more than £100 000. The increasing ability of the new-style ophthalmologists to use audio-visual technology themselves also meant that Alan Lacey was free to spend more of his time on designing and developing pro-grammes and producing top-quality presentations for the Hospital. As the new century began, the Department of Medical Illustration looked to be in as healthy and progressive a state as it had ever been.

Medical social workers

The emphasis on progress and improvements in treatment, in all aspects of eye disease, can easily obscure the sad reality that, in spite of best efforts, loss of sight is sometimes inevitable. A small number of patients with intractable conditions ranging from dry eyes (Stevens–Johnson disease), corneal ulceration, glaucoma and uveitis, through to diabetic retinopathy, complicated retinal detachments and retinitis pigmentosa, pass tragically along a remorseless path to blindness, in spite of all that modern medicine has to offer. Sometimes such individuals belong to families in which hereditary disorders leading to loss of vision are understood and accepted, and in which family support is strong, but in others there is no supportive home environment and visual incapacity leads to loneliness and despair. It is in such cases that the medical social workers play a vital role, offering comfort and compassion and helpful advice and directing those with severe visual impairment towards the facilities and benefits offered by the State and by voluntary organizations.

Originally, in the days when Moorfields was a charitable institution, lady almoners were employed to assess patients' needs and ability to pay for medical services and to help them access whatever benefits were available. With the coming of the NHS, this role became a more far-reaching one, almoners becoming medical social workers (MSWs), and at Moorfields there was a strong and effective department, headed from the 1960s through to the early 1980s by Mary Howarth. They did a great deal of invaluable work, counselling, advising, supporting and rehabilitating patients in whom treatment could not preserve sight. In 1974, however, a major change in the provision of social work took place, responsibility for MSW departments being transferred to Local Authorities, in Moorfields' case the London Borough of Islington. While for large district general hospitals this arrangement was sensible, patients being rehabilitated in their own locality by their local social services, thus guaranteeing continuity of care, for a single-specialty hospital like Moorfields it was plainly the reverse. Patients came to the Hospital from all over London and further afield (only about 3% from Islington), and to maintain continuity of care was nigh on impossible. Furthermore, during the ensuing decade, Islington not unnaturally sought to reduce its funding, and without the intervention of the House Governor, John Atwill, staffing of the MSW Department would have fallen to levels at which it was no longer possible to provide an adequate service.

In 1977 Jackie Howe, a medical social worker from Somerset, arrived on the scene. Invited by Dr Barry Jones, the consultant paediatrician, to join the Childrens' Department as a Family Support Service counsellor, she worked for eight years with only a small emolument provided by the Friends of Moorfields, until in 1986 she joined the substantive staff of the MSW Department. In 1988, on the retirement of Mary Howarth, she took over as its Head, but moved back to the Family Support Service in 1992 when funding became available from the Royal London Society for the Blind, and Chris Poole took over the MSW Department. The 1990s were turbulent and difficult years, as funding was cut and support from the Hospital limited. It was a bleak episode in the life of the MSW Department and in the lives of its staff and patients alike, and when Poole left in 1998, it reached its nadir.

In 2001 Islington finally withdrew all support and, however reluctantly, the Hospital again assumed responsibility for the department. Mandy O'Keefe, who had joined in 1992, became its senior practitioner. There was never again to be an MSW Department employing four full-time MSWs, as had been the case in its heyday. In truth, because of the huge changes in every aspect of healthcare, including better treatments, rapid discharge and speedy return to activity after surgery, this was not as serious as it sounds. Further, the Hospital now employed a Patient Support Sister to meet some of the patients' emotional needs, and the MSW department no longer took responsibility for children. The department was further strengthened by the addition of Barbara Norton, a qualified social worker, herself blind, who had worked since 1992 with Professor Alan Bird's team counselling those with inherited retinal dystrophies.

Many of the improvements in public services were, however, of only the most meagre kind. The MSW would often only see a patient once, for the purpose of blind or partially sighted registration, with very little follow-through in the community, while although jobs for the visually handicapped were quite plentiful for those who were literate (especially computer-literate), and the Disability Discrimination Act of 1994 obliged employers with more than 15 employees to take on disabled staff, they were scarce otherwise, and only 25% of those registered were able to find employment.

Nevertheless, changes in attitude throughout the Hospital and the introduction of multidisciplinary policies and thinking, with increasing cooperation between groups of staff, led to some fundamental improvements. Surprisingly, until the arrival of Sarah Fisher as their Head in 2002, collaboration with the Nursing Services seems to have been less than one might have expected, Mandy O'Keefe and her colleagues feeling that they received little support and encouragement from that direction. Under the new Director of Nursing, more and better cooperation with the nursing services seemed to be a realistic possibility. Furthermore, a more open and frank relationship between surgeons and patients, the former being more prepared to discuss the possibility of failure of treatment and consequent visual deterioration with their patients and to confront with them the practical prospects for rehabilitation, led to a closer working relationship with the MSWs.

Children's Services

In 1969 Mary Digby, a Norland-trained children's nurse, was appointed to the post of play leader in the Children's Ward. This was an informal arrangement and not one approved wholeheartedly by everyone, although the then Matron, Margaret Mackellar, and the House Governor, John Atwill, were enthusiastic, and the medical staff were in favour. Mary was paid by the Save the Children Fund and her acquisition was a great success. She worked tirelessly to provide comfort and emotional support to the children and their families, as well as establishing 'Play in Hospital' courses and lecturing to students from many countries, in the process earning an international reputation. When Dr Barry Jones arrived, and in 1977 invited Jackie Howe to join the department as Family Support Counsellor, they together formed a strong team, greatly aided by the Friends of Moorfields, who were always supportive and paid Jackie's expenses, as well as providing for equipment and numerous other amenities in the Children's Ward.

Between them, they founded the Retinoblastoma Society, which soon became a recognized organization nationwide, and they also managed to persuade the Sick Children's Trust to fund the purchase of a house nearby, in which parents of children needing to remain in the hospital overnight could stay. Sadly, however, this closed a few years later, due to lack of funding. In 1989 Mary Digby retired, leaving behind her a greatly changed culture and a huge legacy of experience and improvement in facilities, as well as a remarkable archive of diaries, drawings and other memorabilia from her 20 years of devoted service to the children of Moorfields. Jackie Howe (now Martin) restored the Family Support Service in 1992, and continued to give devoted service to the children and their families until 2003, when she too retired.

Optometry, contact lenses and ocular prosthetics

Contact Lens Department

The first foray into the field of contact lenses at Moorfields was conducted by Ida Mann, who set up a Contact Lens Clinic in 1937. After the Second World War, Frederick Ridley joined her in running the clinic, and in 1951 he was appointed director of the first Moorfields Contact Lens Department (CLD), premises being acquired adjacent to the Hospital at No. 177 High Holborn. The lenses were initially for therapeutic purposes only, and although Ridley became a renowned authority on contact lens technology, his contribution was entirely restricted to therapeutic scleral lenses. He was joined by Charles Trodd SRN, who had been working in the Casualty Department at Holborn and who went on to become an expert in manufacturing scleral lenses and shells. Much later, Monty Ruben, who had originally set out studying ophthalmic optics, but subsequently trained in medicine and went on to become a Fellow of the Royal College of Surgeons, joined the department.

Ruben was both clever and ambitious. He saw the future for corneal and soft contact lenses and when, on Ridley's retirement in 1968, he assumed the Directorship of the CLD, he was quick to introduce this new technology. He was made a consultant at Moorfields, with operating rights, although in spite of this was never fully accepted by the other members of the consultant staff. Nevertheless, he was a highly effective director and carried out a great deal of excellent research in the field and in 1970 was made Professor. Ruben attracted staff of the highest calibre. Among these was Geoff Woodward, an outstanding individual of great charm and integrity as well as academic flare who in 1976 joined the department as senior optometrist. Together, he and Ruben wrote a textbook on clinical optics. They also collaborated with Tony Bron, later Professor of Ophthalmology in Oxford, setting up a keratoconus clinic, the first of its kind in the world. Woodward went on to gain his PhD degree with a thesis on the progression of keratoconus, before he too was made a professor and left Moorfields to be Head of Optometry and Visual Science at the City University.

Such was the demand for contact lenses as the years went by that eventually there was insufficient space at the premises in Holborn, and in 1977 the CLD moved to new and bigger quarters in Cayton Street, adjacent to the Hospital in City Road. Occupying the ground and lower ground floors of the building, it provided lens and prosthetics manufacturing facilities and a lecture theatre, as well as the Consulting and Dispensing Department. In 1981 Roger Buckley, who had completed his training as a Resident at City Road, before going on to work with Peter Wright and Emil Sherrard on specular microscopy of the cornea, joined Ruben as consultant and assistant director in the CLD, and three years later, on the latter's retirement, he took over as its director. The CLD remained in its Cayton Street premises until 1996, when it moved across to the Red Clinic in the main hospital building, to share activities and space there with the External Diseases Clinic.

Optometry

From its earliest days, Moorfields, like all eye units, was involved in the assessment of vision, provision of spectacles and other visual aids. Initially, refraction was provided, at both branches of the Hospital, by a mixture of optometrists (ophthalmic opticians, as they were then called) and ophthalmologists, working under the supervision of a senior optometrist, Norman Hudson. In 1969, when the latter left, his place as Senior (later Principal) Optometrist at the City Road branch was taken by Janet Silver, an energetic and dynamic individual with a special interest in low vision (see **Figure 33**, Plate 17), who recognized that its assessment and treatment at Moorfields, hitherto limited to the provision of the odd magnifier, was inadequate. She soon started a Low Vision Aid (LVA) Clinic at City Road, which flourished and grew steadily year-by-year, under her direction. As time went on, more and more preregistration optometry students were taken on, several when fully trained joining the departmental staff. Others went on to head departments elsewhere in the Hospital Eye Service, and several were appointed to professorial chairs.

In 1978 the department at City Road, up to that time called the Department of Ophthalmic Optics and represented by a consultant (in turn Alex Cross and Desmond Greaves) at the Medical Committee, was put in overall charge of a consultant ophthalmologist, Arthur Steele, and renamed the Visual Assessment Department. It assumed a wider role, taking in visual field testing as well as refraction and low-vision clinics, and continued to prosper, moving premises several times within the hospital building. Janet Silver collaborated with Elizabeth Gould, the first of many pre-registration students, and other colleagues in important clinical research into low vision, and successfully completed her Master's degree. She also collaborated with Rolf Blach and Alan Bird, and with members of the staff at the Institute of Ophthalmology, and studied for and obtained her Fellowship of the British Institute of Managers, the department achieving a high profile both in the UK and abroad.

Thus it was that, by the mid-1970s, there were two quite separate departments at Moorfields specializing in the assessment and improvement of visual function, both of them comprising optometrists of the highest calibre, with one specializing in contact lenses and prosthetics and the other in refraction and low-vision aids. While both the Contact Lens and Visual Assessment Departments were acknowledged as prestigious units, under the direction of world leaders in their own special fields, it was inevitable that the Trust should wish ultimately to merge them and rationalize the situation.

When Janet Silver retired in 1995 (honoured with the award of an OBE), the Visual Assessment Department employed some 40 staff, albeit most of them part-time, and was responsible for teaching Residents, other doctors and optometrists at both the Institute and

Hospital. In Cayton Street the Contact Lens Department was similarly active and involved. Both John Dart and Steve Tuft were lecturers there, prior to their appointments to the consultant staff. Ken Pullum was a world leader in scleral lenses, Nigel Sapp had taken over from Charles Trodd in the manufacture of ocular prostheses, and Geoff Woodward was soon to leave to become head of Optometry and Visual Science at City University (his place to be taken by Christine Astin). It was decided that the time had come to merge the two departments with the Corneal and External Disease Service, and in 1996 Louise Culham took over as head of the new combined Department of Optometry, the Prosthetics Department moving to its own premises on the first floor of the Hospital. Meanwhile, in 1997 Roger Buckley was appointed to a Professorial Chair in Ocular Medicine in the Department of Optometry and Visual Science at City University, the first and only ophthalmologist to hold such a position in an academic department of optometry.

Louise Culham brought to the new department not only a different style of management but also a fine intellect and strong academic back-ground. Qualifying in 1987, she had done a Master's degree with Alan Bird and Janet Silver, before going on to undertake a PhD with John Marshall and Fred Fitzke at the Institute of Opthalmology, using the scanning laser ophthalmoscope to study eccentric viewing. Like her predecessor, her special interest was in low vision, but, in contrast, she was strongly committed to basic science research and continued, throughout her time as head of the department, to share responsibility for PhD students, both ophthalmologists and optometrists, with Professor Gary Rubin in the Department of Visual Rehabilitation Research at the Institute.

She was active in promoting shared working with the ophthalmologists, recognizing that the retirement of many of the clinical assistants, who had previously fulfilled such an important role in the out-patient clinics, left a potentially serious gap in the service. An optometrist, Michael Banes, had set the pattern, working in glaucoma clinics as part of the clinical team, rather than as simply a refractionist, and on Louise Culham's arrival she saw the wisdom of his example and started to reward him for this work. She worked hard to introduce other optometrists into the clinics as full members of the clinical team, working to strict proto-cols with, amongst others, Steve Tuft in the Cataract Service, Keith Barton, Ian Murdoch and Ted Garway-Heath in Glaucoma, and Phil Hykin and Jonathan Dowler in Medical Retina. Not only was this good for the Hospital, but as Moorfields optometrists demonstrated their con-fidence and expertise, the word spread outside. While earnings at the

Trust could never fully match those in the high street, senior optometrists were well rewarded for work that was both challenging and exciting. In fact, Janet Silver had initiated the process of hospital optometrists working closely with clinicians in outreach clinics in the late 1980s, as a result of her acquaintance with a paediatrician in a nearby Health Centre, children as a consequence being referred to Moorfields for further investigation and treatment. Furthermore, a study conducted with Rhodri Daniel in the Primary Care Clinic at about that time had showed that optometrists working there were as reliable in their diagnostic assessments as were the doctors.

The department continued to be a leader in both contact lens work and visual assessment, Roger Buckley, Geoff Woodward, Ken Pullum and Dan Ehrlich continuing to work there. Meanwhile, Andrew Milliken led the Visual Assessment Service with unfailing commitment, skill and good humour, the introduction of four metre bays and LogMar charts for the assessment of visual acuity providing evidence of a more modern approach to clinical assessment (see **Figure 30**, Plate 16). Nor was the commercial side neglected, a strong commitment to the dispensing service, particularly the budget range of spectacle frames, with its own contact lens manufacturing and glazing laboratories, earning the Trust upwards of £350 000 per annum. By the time Louise Culham left the Trust, for personal reasons, in 2003, and Dan Ehrlich took over as its Head, the Optometry Department comprised 85 members of staff and was in as healthy a state as it had ever been.

Ocular prosthetics
From its earliest days, the CLD made artificial eyes as well as scleral lenses. In the late 1950s and early 1960s, following the discovery that they were well tolerated in human tissues, thermoplastic materials were developed that were ideal for making contact lenses and prostheses. One of the technicians in the CLD took to making artificial eyes, and it was not long before Charles Trodd, who had been nursing in the Casualty Department, became interested in this field. He soon developed an expertise all of his own and started making artificial eyes in conjunction with the National Artificial Eye Service (NAES), working from the CLD, free of charge. The then Southern Area manager of the NAES, Nigel Sapp, later joined the Moorfields staff and began to manufacture and paint artificial eyes on site. When Trodd finally retired in 1986, Sapp took over as head of the Prosthetics Department, and in 1995 it moved to its own premises on the first floor of the City Road building, all prostheses being made and fitted at the Hospital, in a free-standing unit having no connection with the NAES.

Pharmacy

It is difficult to imagine a world more changed and changing, during the past four decades, than that of the pharmaceutical industry. When Jill Bloom arrived at Moorfields in 1977 as a freshly minted young pharmacist, there were still a number of Winchester jars containing strange mixtures, tablets came loose and were put into bottles, and leeches had only recently been discarded. Nevertheless, much had already changed since the 1960s, when preparations were still made up in large drums and stirred on the bench top, and by the time she came, sterility and quality control were the order of the day. She found a friendly and happy department, under the direction of Bob Watkins, the Chief Pharmacist, who had replaced Alan Baker in 1973 on the latter's retirement. She also found herself the proud possessor of a Cardex formulary dating back to the 1940s.

The advances in ocular pharmaceuticals since the 1960s have been enormous, as has been the change in both the role and quality standards of the pharmacy. Timolol maleate, for the treatment of chronic simple glaucoma, came on the scene in the late 1970s, a battle ensuing between the Hospital and its manufacturers, Merck, Sharp and Dohme, over production costs and patents. Similar problems arose with other drugs and the companies that patented them, such as the antiviral trifluorothymidine (F3T), and later with Pharmacia (now Pfizer Ltd) over the manufacture of hydroxypropylmethylcellulose (HPMC) and healonid (Healon) for cataract surgery. In the 1970s and 1980s it was permissible to test a new drug in the clinical setting to see if it was effective, and consultants like Professor Barrie Jones, Peter Wright, Roger Hitchings, John Dart and others would work with the chief pharmacist to develop new drugs for ocular use. In this way Moorfields was at the forefront of pharmaceutical research, pioneering the use of artificial tears BJ6 (Barrie Jones' formula number six) for dry eyes, sodium cromoglycate for the treatment of allergic conjunctivitis, acetylcysteine 5% for mucoid keratitis, retinoic acid for hyper-keratinization of the cornea, and guanethidine and adrenaline (Ganda) for glaucoma. Much of the early work on antiviral agents, such as idoxuridine (IDU) and F3T, culminating in the development of acyclovir, a drug non-toxic to the host tissues, was also done at Moor-fields, before the days of strict (some might say restrictive) regulation.

By the 1990s, increasingly stringent regulations laid down by the Medicines Control Agency (MCA) made it difficult, if not impossible, to do such ad hoc clinical research. Nevertheless, Peng Tee Khaw introduced mitomycin C and instigated a national multicentre trial of 5-fluorouracil in the outcome of filtering surgery, Susan Lightman

pioneered the widespread use of immunosuppressants in the management of ocular inflammatory disease, and John Dart the biguanides for
Acanthamoeba keratitis. In 1983 John Lee introduced the hospital to
botulinum toxin for the management of squints and essential blepharospasm. In cataract surgery, changing methods demanded the production of increasing quantities of balanced salt irrigating solutions, to
save buying-in commercially available alternatives. Because of their
volume and methods of delivery in the operating theatres, these
demanded the most stringent quality control, both to ensure that they
were sterile and to eliminate toxic by-products. Likewise, in vitreoretinal surgery, complex retinal detachments often needed silicone
fluid, a material that had acquired a bad name as a result of its use by
plastic surgeons for cosmetic surgery, and the pharmacy was forced to
go to great lengths to avoid using expensive alternatives. In the 1980s
the cost of perfluorocarbon liquids (PFCLs) caused a similar headache
for the chief pharmacist, lengthy negotiations with their manufacturer
only finally being rewarded with a satisfactory compromise.

The increasing demands of what was now called Quality Assurance
meant that the days of the pharmacy continuing to manufacture and
deliver its own preparations were numbered. Indeed, the MCA had, as
long before as 1992, declared it unfit to do so. Although sales of ocular
preparations had steadily increased during the 1970s and 1980s, forming a significant component of the Hospital's income, as the 1990s progressed it was clear that if this was to continue, it would be necessary to
revamp the Hospital's facilities for manufacturing pharmaceuticals.
The arrival of Christine Miles, herself formerly a chief pharmacist, as
the new Director of Operations in 1996 signalled a major review of the
pharmacy. Sadly, her review of the department exposed irregularities
that led ultimately to the resignation of Victor Andrews, the bright,
energetic and popular chief pharmacist, who had been instrumental
theretofore in much of the pharmacy's commercial success.

After an inspection by the MCA that highlighted the inadequacies of
the pharmacy's manufacturing capabilities, Miles and the House
Governor, Ian Balmer, set about exploring the possibility of developing
a purpose-built Pharmacy Manufacturing Unit (PMU), on a separate
site, to both continue and expand this commercial activity. Their drive
and vision led to the eventual construction, at a cost of £11m, of a
PMU on land opposite the Hospital, with the capacity to produce
10 000 bottles of drops and countless single-dose vials daily, instead of
the maximum of 1500 bottles per week previously possible (**Figure 40**,
Plate 21). This facility was under the direction of Alan Krol and opened
in 2003. It was quite separate from the Clinical Services Department,

which remained within the Hospital building under the direction of Elaine Ioannou, the Chief Pharmacist, promoted to that position in 2001, purchasing its own supplies from the PMU or elsewhere, according to cost and availability.

Not only was the range of pharmaceuticals continuing to expand rapidly but there were also enormous changes for the staff themselves. Just as the role of medications had changed completely, with alpha-2 agonists, beta-blockers and prostaglandin analogues replacing anticholinesterase agents for glaucoma, and the introduction of antiproliferative agents and the development of photodynamic therapy changing the face of ophthalmology, so too had the roles of the pharmacists at the Hospital. The hospital-based pharmacy was now responsible for medicines information and management, covering all pharmaceutical issues, including advice to patients and health-care professionals both within and outside the Trust, as well as for clinical pharmacy services. Technicians like Ali Safiee (**Figure 41**, Plate 21), who had been at Moorfields for more than 14 years, in that time rising from pharmacy assistant to be Chief Pharmacy Technician, now did the dispensing and found themselves more and more on the wards and in the day-case units, giving advice to patients, medical and nursing staff and seeing that drugs were prescribed and used with accuracy and safety. Gillian Oldham, Quality Assurance Officer, was in her new place at the PMU, while Jill Bloom now ran the Specialist Ophthalmic Medicines Information Department for the whole of the UK, bridging the gap between the consumer and the commercial market place.

Her role exposed her to new challenges and interesting observations, as when she attended a market-research seminar, where patient satisfaction and compliance with the new plastic single-dose vials was being assessed. The vials can be difficult for older people to use, so she was amazed to find that, of the 60 volunteers trying out the single-dose drop vials, only two were over the age of 60!

With the opening of the PMU in February 2003, and the continuing development of new drugs, there was no sign that the rapidity and extent of change in pharmacy practice at Moorfields was likely to abate. Furthermore, the greatly enhanced commercial possibilities made possible by the new PMU were of vital importance to the Trust's future survival and independence.

PART 3

Academe

CHAPTER 5

Medical Education

Background

Until the 1990s, postgraduate medical education in the UK was based on an old-fashioned apprenticeship model. As recently as the 1960s, following qualification (which simply meant obtaining a diploma from one of the bodies recognized by the General Medical Council (GMC) for training purposes), an aspiring doctor needed only to spend one further year of training, as a junior house officer in clinical posts recognized by the GMC, before being granted full registration as an accredited medical practitioner. He or she could then practise independently, in any branch of the profession they chose. In hospital medicine and in surgery, as in other specialist branches, the Medical Royal Colleges of England, Scotland and Ireland had instigated higher examinations of knowledge and expertise, with higher diplomas to match, but remarkably, until the 1970s, it was not mandatory to be in possession of one of these in order to be appointed to a consultant post. Indeed, there were many instances of consultant general surgeons who did not possess the Fellowship of the Royal College of Surgeons and of ophthalmic surgeons holding no more than a diploma in ophthalmology. Nor were they necessarily in any way inferior to their better qualified counterparts, so much of clinical medicine, especially surgery, depending as it did more on practical skills than on theoretical knowledge. Nevertheless, the chances of being appointed to a consultant post at the more prestigious institutions, like Moorfields, without the Fellowship of one of the Royal Colleges of Surgeons were small.

Because of its exclusively specialist nature and the enormous number of patients attending it, Moorfields had, from very early on, gained an unparalleled reputation, not only as a centre of therapeutic excellence but also for the quality of training it offered. From the time it moved to City Road in 1899, a medical school had been established there, with its own pathology department, and it was for its time a thriving seat of learning. Following the creation of the Institute of Ophthalmology in 1948, this school transferred to the new Institute. Even then, training at

Moorfields remained, for the most part, a one-to-one apprenticeship process, skills and knowledge being passed down from seniors to juniors, with comparatively little formal teaching. Academic distinction was not considered important and few Residents wrote scientific papers while 'on the House'.

The beginnings of a new era

During the 1960s and early 1970s, the emphasis on formal teaching at Moorfields increased. Barrie Jones, Dermot Pierse, Noel Rice and Peter Watson instigated microsurgical teaching workshops. Disorders of ocular motility were addressed in the Motility Clinic and their surgical management in the Squint Pool, by Peter Fells. Alan Bird, on his return from the USA, undertook early-morning teaching for the Fellowship examination (so-called 'early bird' sessions), and a weekly programme of visiting lecturers, interspersed with monthly clinicopathological conferences, was held in the Palmer Lecture Room at the City Road branch. There was also a very valuable six-month period of their training during which the Residents spent time at the Institute, their time being divided equally between the Pathology and Physiology Departments.

Barrie Jones well understood the difficulties encountered in learning a new and complicated subject and so was a brilliant teacher. He held weekly teaching sessions in external disease, which were keenly attended by Residents and Fellows alike, not without some frisson of fear and trepidation, for his penetrating questions could be discomfiting. Residents who had failed to come to a just and logical conclusion as to diagnosis and management could find themselves in hot water.

A lady from abroad had presented to the Casualty Department with a sore eye and the casualty officer had prescribed antibiotic drops for a non-specific superficial infection. Five days later she again presented, this time with a corneal abscess, and was speedily referred to the Professorial Unit. Intensive investigation revealed the source of infection and it was soon brought under control. The patient became the centre-point of the Professor's teaching round, however, and the hapless casualty officer was called and asked to account for himself. 'Was he not aware, when he first saw the lady, that the infection was on the very brink of an exponential growth phase in its development?' 'No, he was sorry, but this was not something which had occurred to him' (during the hurly-burly of a busy session in Casualty), he was forced to confess, much to the vicarious sense of self-satisfaction and amusement of all those present.

Lest it be thought that the Professor was being unfairly critical, another anecdote serves to put matters in perspective:

It is said that when he himself was a casualty officer, he saw a patient with an unusual and interesting condition, the cause of which had recently been elucidated by a doctor at the Royal Postgraduate Medical School, Hammersmith. Leaving his desk, Barrie Jones collected specimens and took a bus to the Hammersmith, returning some hours later, to a cool reception from his colleagues and a somewhat bored and puzzled patient, but with the correct diagnosis firmly established.

Because of its influence on the career path of aspiring ophthalmologists in the UK, the Fellowship Diploma of one of the Royal Colleges of Surgeons played a central role in the teaching and training ethos, its possession being the hallmark of excellence, and thereby the key to ultimate success, fame and fortune. It became customary for would-be Residents to pass the primary part of the examination before being awarded a place 'on the House' at Moorfields, and to take the final part during their three-year tenure there. The acquisition of both a place 'on the House' and the Fellowship of one of the Surgical Royal Colleges was usually enough to guarantee a successful, if not always glittering, career in the specialty. Indeed one can do no better than to quote from Professor Douglas Coster's account of his experiences on arriving in London from Australia as a junior doctor:

'...Had I known how much competition there was to get appointed to Moorfields, and how tortuous the process could be, I may have stayed at home...As it was I blundered on and had three unsuccessful attempts at getting on to the house. The manoeuvring to get appointed to a house job was something quite foreign to me and something I was not very good at. I had graduated from Melbourne University five years previously and had held posts at the Royal Melbourne Hospital and the Royal Victoria Eye and Ear Hospital, but had never been interviewed for any of the positions. Royal Melbourne was an absolute meritocracy and took notice only of the graduating class list and the results of postgraduate exams. It was not influenced by any factor other than academic achievement, not even bad behaviour, which some people thought was fortunate for my career prospects. Getting appointed to Moorfields was a more complicated process.

'What I didn't realize and what explained the seriousness with which the locals took getting appointed to Moorfields, was that being appointed to the house was the most important step in an ophthalmologist's career, more important than graduation, passing the Fellowship examinations, or marrying the boss's daughter. Once on the house at Moorfields, professional success was inevitable.'

At the Institute, there was a course devoted to teaching refraction and also a thriving course aimed at the Diploma of Ophthalmology, especially popular among foreign students, groups of whom were a regular sight during the 1960s and 1970s, clustered eagerly around consultants, in the out-patient clinics (see **Figure 19**, p. 65) and on ward rounds. Mostly, however, those studying for the Fellowship did so off their own bat, reading and studying for the first part (basic sciences), and then, when that had been passed, learning the clinical knowledge for the second, clinical part, by working as an ophthalmic registrar and by teaching one another. So prestigious and autonomous was Moorfields at this period that, once appointed to a registrar post, promotion to senior registrar was automatic after two years, even if the Fellowship had not been successfully passed.

The Dean of the Institute had little contact with those in training, except to offer advice and guidance, when asked to do so, and to preside over the running of the courses. The post of Dean was a prestigious one, however, always being occupied by a senior member of the Moorfields consultant staff, on a part-time basis, and was supported by both an academic and a clinical Sub-Dean, the former a member of the academic Institute staff, and the latter a more junior consultant from the Hospital, who together took responsibility for the day-to-day running of the educational programme. So far as the quality of the programme and its relevance to the needs of ophthalmology services nationwide were concerned, this would today be considered a somewhat loose arrangement, there being no formal links with the Faculty of Ophthalmologists, nor with the Regional Postgraduate Dean. By the standards of the age, however, this comparatively unstructured model of postgraduate training worked well, having stood the test of time and having been the accepted norm for as long as anyone could remember. Both Peter Wright and John Lee, clinical Sub-Deans during the period of this account (**Figure 42**), prior to the appointment of a Clinical Tutor in 1992, worked hard to ensure the high quality of the teaching programme, and did an excellent job.

In the 1950s there were 12 resident surgical officers at the City Road branch of Moorfields. By the late 1960s this number had risen to 24, both the amount and intensity of work and the demands for well-trained ophthalmologists throughout the country having increased proportionately. At the High Holborn branch there were six, and the appointment process was slightly different to that at City Road, as was the attitude to formal teaching, but the role of apprenticeship in the delivery of training was, if anything, even stronger. Senior Residents, as well as their chiefs, taught the more junior Residents, those who had

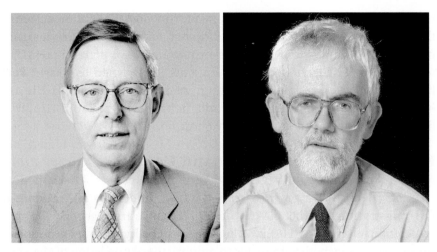

Figure 42   Clinical Sub-Deans, Mr Peter Wright (*left*) and Mr John Lee (*right*) who, with Mr (later Professor) Barrie Jay before them, were responsible for medical education, under the aegis of the Dean, prior to the appointment of a Clinical Tutor in 1992.

already taken and passed the Fellowship examination passing on their knowledge and skills. There were also a number of joint senior registrar posts between Moorfields and other hospitals. From the mid-1960s, there were in addition a number of lecturers and senior lecturers on the Professorial Unit at City Road, most of whom had been through the residency programme, who willingly gave instruction to the Residents and tutored them for the Fellowship examinations. These comprised, from the mid-1970s onwards, a particularly strong and enthusiastic group, including Douglas Coster, John Lee, Richard Collin and Tony Moore, and an increasing number of Fellows, to help with teaching. Both the Retinal (surgical) Unit, under Lorimer Fison and Alan Bird's newly formed Retinal Diagnostic Department (in which Peter Hamilton became an inspirational and charismatic teacher of fluorescein angiography and laser treatment in retinal vascular disease) also offered up-to-the-minute teaching of the highest quality, including a weekly Fluorescein Conference. For those who were post-Fellowship, including consultants, advanced specialist courses like the one on retinal detachments organized by Lorimer Fison, Rolf Blach and Michael Bedford at the Highgate Annexe, over a long week-end, sprang up in a range of different subjects.

The enlargement and extensive refurbishment of the Professorial Unit in 1973, to include the provision of a small lecture room and seminar rooms, made a big difference to the clinical teaching facilities. Furthermore, the move of the Dean's Department to Cayton Place, on the island site next to the City Road branch of the Hospital, in 1978 facilitated closer supervision and coordination of teaching and training by the Dean and his Sub-Deans, while the installation of a lecture theatre there greatly improved the quality and scope of the teaching programme. Similar, but less high-profile, improvements in teaching took place at High Holborn, Tim Ffytche, later joined by David Hill, running the medical retina teaching, and refurbishment of the old operating theatre area on the second floor yielding a well-equipped library and fluorescein angiography clinic.

Expanding role of Faculty and College

Medical training could be divided into three phases: basic medical training (BMT), as a pre-registration house officer, up to the point of full registration by the GMC, basic specialist training (BST), as a senior house officer (SHO) working in a specialty or, over a period of time, several specialties, in order to gain further knowledge of the skills required in various specialties, and higher specialist training (HST), as a registrar and senior registrar (SR), gaining training and experience, in a chosen specialty, (usually with the intention of making a career in that specialty). In ophthalmology, it became requisite during the 1980s for all trainees to have undergone two years' training in recognized SHO posts in ophthalmology, before entering HST.

During the late 1970s and throughout the 1980s, a radical change in attitude towards medical education and its delivery gradually took place. A number of different factors contributed to this: first the huge explosion of knowledge and technological advance rendering the simple apprenticeship model unequal to the task, secondly the new culture of understanding and awareness of doctors' competence growing amongst the public at large, and thirdly the Conservative government's increasingly strong political influence on the conduct of medicine. As a consequence, the methods and structures that had previously sustained professional performance were no longer sufficiently robust to withstand scrutiny. The bodies in charge of supervising medical training and standards of care came under enormous pressure to put their houses in better order, and to show that they were monitoring both the content and conduct of their teaching and training schemes, as well as ensuring satisfactory outcomes of understanding and proficiency.

As in so many matters, the Americans were the first to recognize that the evolution of modern medicine, and its consequent subdivision into distinct specialties, demanded specialist certification, and had therefore long since introduced a system of specialist boards, each demanding its own level of expertise, before offering accreditation in the specialty. In the UK it was not until the mid-1970s that the Royal College of Surgeons decided to introduce a form of self-regulation. The Faculty of

Plate 17

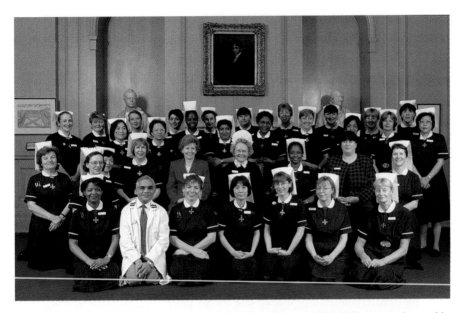

Figure 32   Miss Roslyn Emblin, Chief Nurse and Deputy Chief Manager, pictured in 2001 with senior members of the nursing staff.

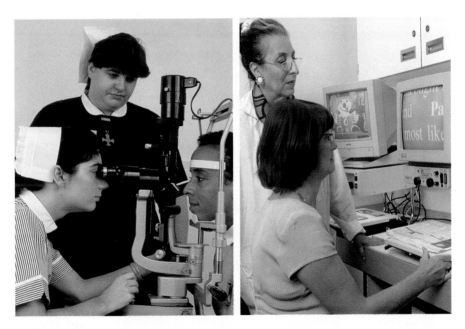

Figure 33   *Left:* The introduction of modern teaching methods led to the development of nurses with much broader clinical skills than ever before. *Right:* Janet Silver's pioneering work on the development of Low Vision Aids (see p. 191.) and her teaching had a profound influence on the development of the Hospital's optometry services.

Plate 18

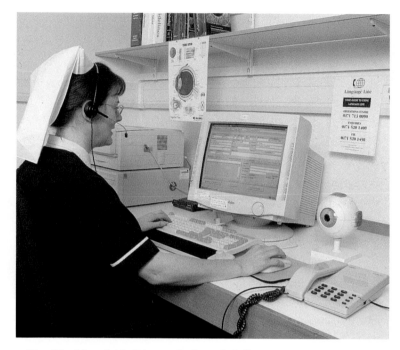

Figure 34 The Moorfields Direct telephone helpline, operated by experienced nursing staff, was instantly popular with the public. (See p. 169.)

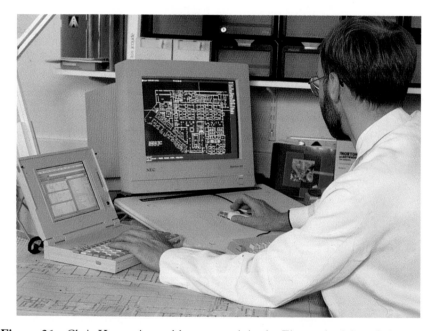

Figure 36 Chris Hogg, pictured here at work in the Electrophysiology Laboratory, was, inter alia, a central figure in the introduction and development of the Hospital's computer technology.

Plate 19

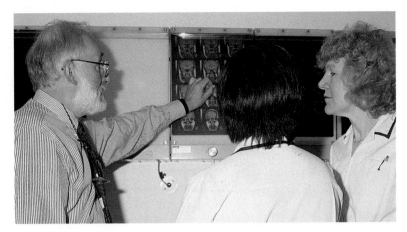

Figure 37 Dr Ivan Moseley, pictured in the X-ray department, reviewing CT scans with the Hospital's radiographers.

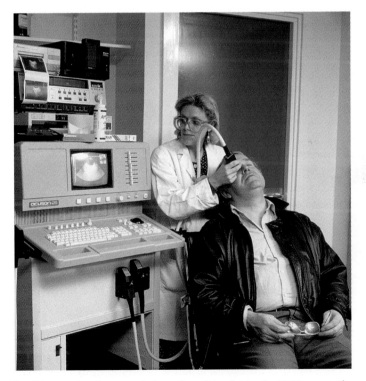

Figure 38 Diagnostic ultrasound, introduced in the early 1970s, soon became the province of Dr Marie Restori (*pictured*), ultrasound physicist.

Plate 20

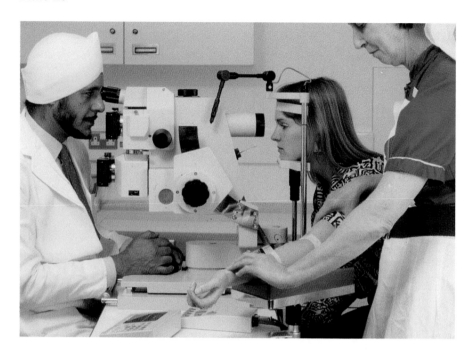

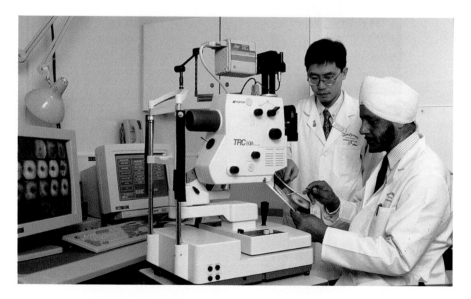

Figure 39 Fluorescein fundus angiography (FFA), started at Moorfields in the late 1960s, soon became, with the clinical expertise of Professor Alan Bird and the technical skill of Kulwant Sehmi and his staff (*pictured top and bottom*), an indispensable diagnostic service.

Plate 21

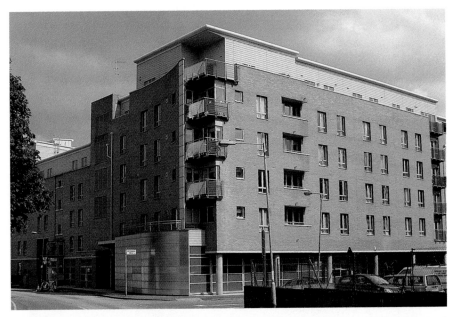

Figure 40   The new building opposite the Hospital, at the junction of Nile Street and Britannia Walk, housing the Pharmacy Manufacturing Unit on the ground and two lower ground floors, with accommodation for key members of hospital staff on the floors above.

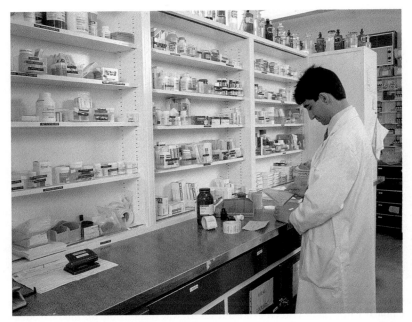

Figure 41   The nature of the hospital pharmacy changed with the course of time, as did the roles of its staff, many of whom began to play a greater advisory role. Ali Safiee, pictured here, became one of the new governors of Moorfields in 2004 when it became a Foundation Hospital.

Plate 22

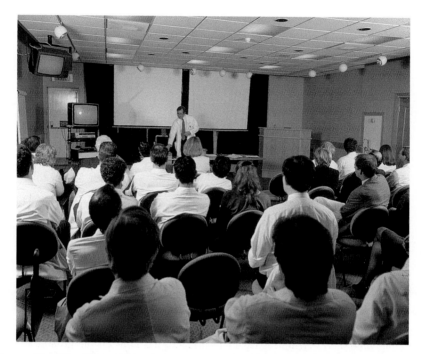

Figure 43 The Clinical Tutorial Complex was built in 1991, with the financial support of the Special Trustees and Friends of Moorfields, to provide modern teaching facilities. (See p. 205.)

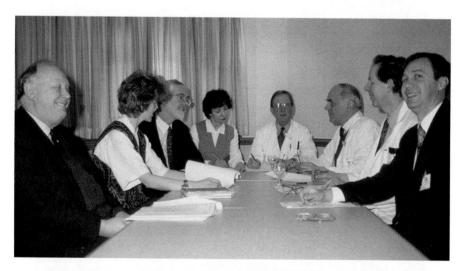

Figure 44 The original (1994) Postgraduate Medical Education Board, chaired by the Clinical Tutor (later Director of Education), was responsible for medical education in the Trust. *Pictured, from left to right*: Mr David Rhys-Tyler (Director of Finance), the Senior Resident Miss Genevieve Larkin, Mr John Lee (College Tutor), Mrs Brenda Aveyard (PA to the Clinical Tutor), Mr Peter Leaver (Clinical Tutor), Professor Alan Bird, Professor Roger Hitchings and Mr Ken Gold (Director of Human Resources).

Plate 23

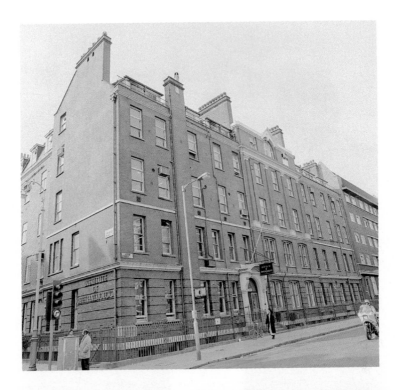

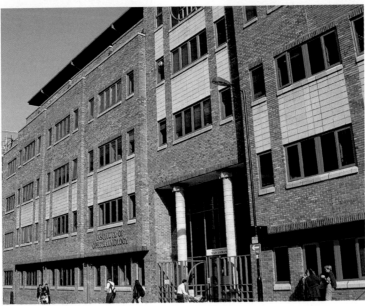

Figure 46 The Institute of Ophthalmology building in Judd Street (formerly the Central London Ophthalmic Hospital) (*top*). It closed in 1991, when the Institute moved to its new premises in Bath Street, on the island site adjacent to the Hospital (*bottom*).

Plate 24

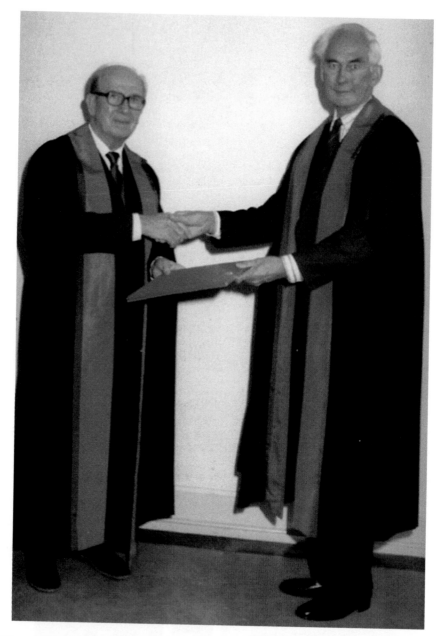

Figure 47 Professor Norman Ashton (*left*) presenting the award of Fellowship of the Institute of Ophthalmology to Mr Francis Cumberlege, Chairman of the Committee of Management.

Plate 25

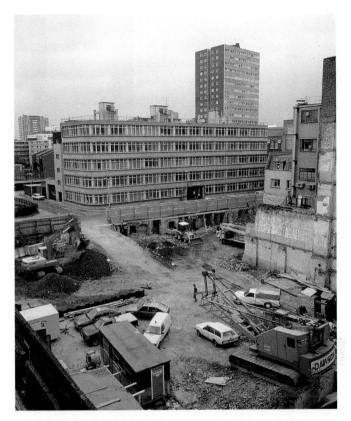

Figure 49 The new Institute of Ophthalmology building under construction on the island site in Bath Street in 1989.

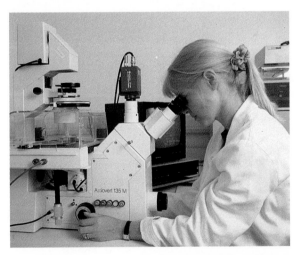

Figure 50 Research work in progress in the laboratories of the new Institute of Ophthalmology. The new buildings in Bath Street provided first class facilities for research and thereby enabled the Institute to reach and maintain a 5★ (top) rating.

Plate 26

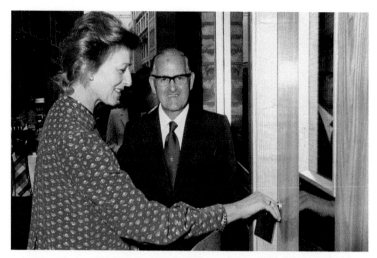

Figure 51 The opening of the International Centre for Eye Health, Department of Preventive Ophthalmology, Institute of Ophthalmology, in 1981 by HRH Princess Alexandra, who is pictured here with its founder and first director, Professor Barrie Jones.

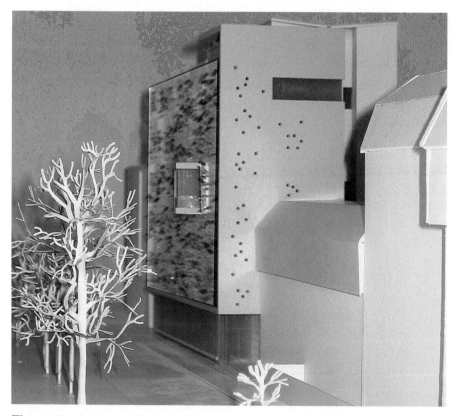

Figure 52 Architects' design for the proposed International Children's Eye Centre, to be constructed on the site of Fryer House, in Peerless Street (CAD drawing dated 2004). (See p. 256.)

Plate 27

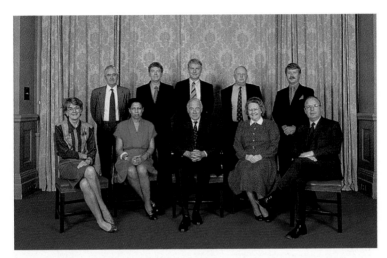

Figure 54 The first Board of Directors of Moorfields Eye Hospital NHS Trust (April 1994). *Seated, left to right*: Mrs Rosalind Gilmore, Ms Jude Goffe, Mr Hugh Peppiatt (Chairman), Miss Roslyn Emblin (Matron), Mr John Bach; *Standing, left to right*: Mr Noel Rice (Director of Research and Teaching) Mr Bob Cooling (Medical Director), Professor Adam Sillito (Director, Institute of Ophthalmology), Mr David Rhys-Tyler (Director of Finance) and Mr Ian Balmer (House Governor and Chief Executive). (The remaining non-executive member of the Board, Mr Clive Nickolds, was absent on the occasion this photograph was taken.)

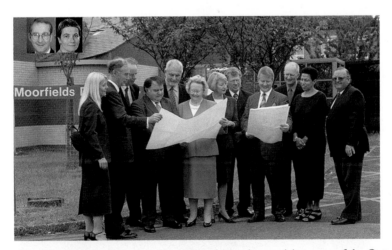

Figure 55 The Board of Directors in 2001, pictured on a visit to one of the Outreach Units. *Left to right*: Miss Anna Wigstrom (PA), Sir Thomas Boyd-Carpenter (Chairman), Professor Roger Hitchings (Director of Research and Development), Mr Ian Knott (Director of Finance), Professor Adam Sillito (Director, Institute of Ophthalmology), Miss Roslyn Emblin (Chief Nurse and Deputy CEO), Mrs Maggie van Reenen, Mr Bob Cooling (Medical Director until 2002), Mr Ian Balmer (House Governor), Mr Clive Nickolds, Ms Jude Goffe and Mr Elkan Levy. (Mr Bill Aylward and Miss Sarah Fisher (*inset*) took over from Mr Cooling and Miss Emblin as Medical Director and Director of Nursing and Development respectively in 2002.)

Plate 28

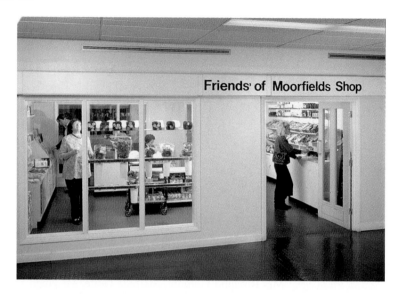

Figure 58 The Friends of Moorfields run a very successful and much appreciated shop in the ground floor waiting area of the Hospital.

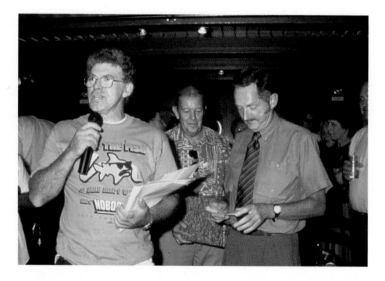

Figure 59 The Moorfields Surgeons Association provides funding for the benefit of Moorfields staff, which includes support for recreational 'days out'. Pictured here announcing the results of the raffle on such an occasion are consultant surgeons Mr Bob Cooling (*left*) and Mr Arthur Steele (*right*) and (in the background), Clinical Risk Manager Mr Cyril Peskett. (See p. 292.)

Plate 29

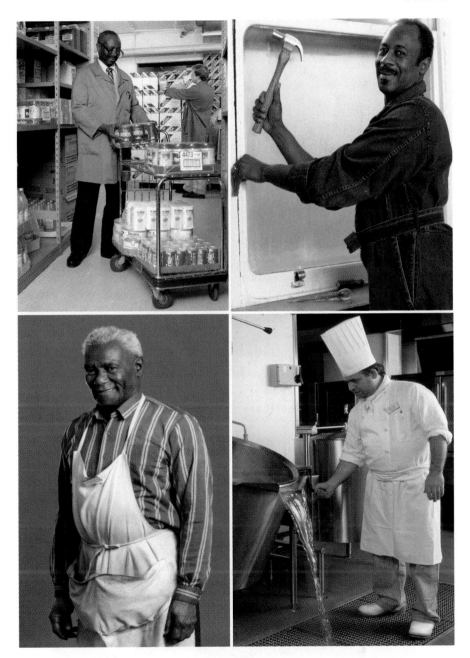

Figure 60   Some long-serving members of the support staff: (*top left*) Stanley Gallimore (Stores); (*top right*) Ron Green (Maintenance); (*bottom right*) Alex Olala (Chef); (*bottom left*) Rupert Bristol.

Plate 30

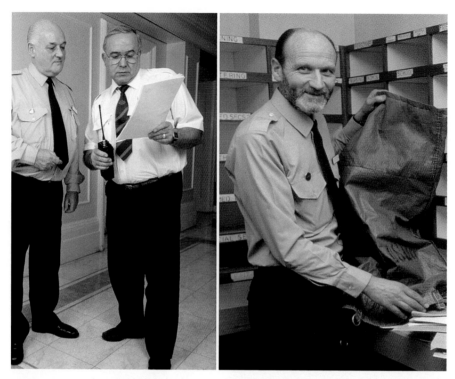

Figure 61 The high standards of portering and security services current today were largely established by the efforts of the Head Porter from 1974 to 1997, Tony Beltrami MBE (on the right in the left-hand photgraph, with Harry Walker) and his staff. George Horton, pictured right in the post-room, for many years sorted and distributed the Hospital's mail with charm and efficiency.

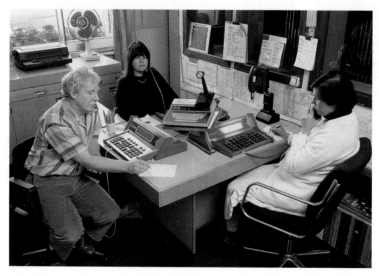

Figure 62 Several of the telephone switchboard staff stayed at Moorfields for many years, including Maureen and Ron Coggin and (*seated, right*) Pat Layzelle.

Plate 31

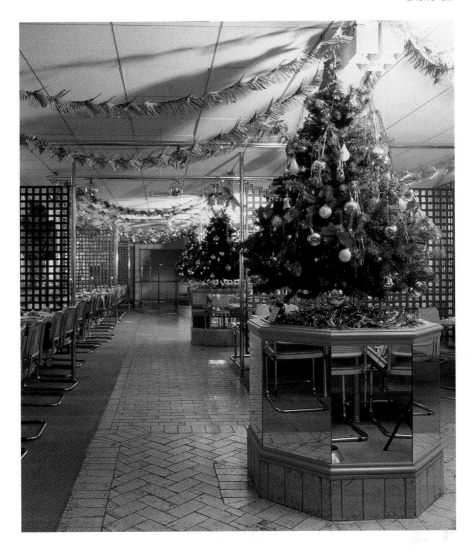

Figure 63 The new dining rooms (seen here decorated for Christmas) were completely redesigned and refurbished in 1987. They were an instant success, and have remained a popular and pleasant environment, shared by all members of staff, ever since.

Plate 32

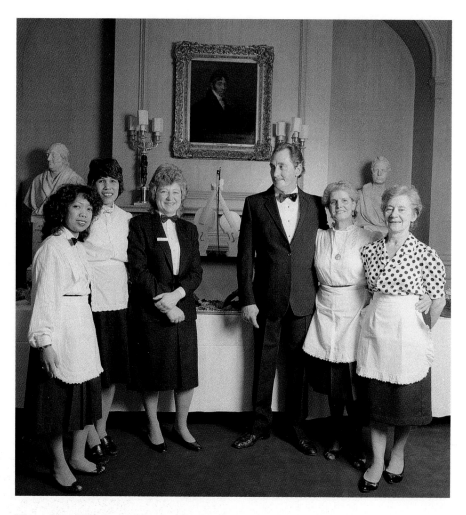

Figure 64 Members of the catering staff pictured above include Dominga Xavier (*second left*, still in Moorfields' service) and Diana Rowe (*third left*) and Ricky Lee (*third right*), both formerly Catering Managers.

Ophthalmologists decreed that all ophthalmic trainees should undertake a minimum period of three years' clinical training in ophthalmology, after passing the Fellowship examination, at least two years of which must be as an SR. Provided these conditions had been met and they were supported by a letter from their trainers, would-be consultants were considered to be accredited. The Surgical Royal Colleges set up Specialty Advisory Committees (SACs), independent of the Faculties, for all the subspecialties in surgery, including ophthalmology, to monitor and advise on teaching and training of Higher Specialist Trainees (registrars and SRs) within their specialties, and these became powerful adjudicators of teaching and training standards. It was also specified that promotion from registrar to senior registrar could only be undertaken on the recommendation of a statutorily constituted Advisory Appointments Committee. At Moorfields the days of promotion on little more than a nod and a wink were over.

In order to assess the standards not only of the trainers but also of the units in which they operated, a system of inspections was instituted, small teams, recruited from the membership of the SAC, travelling to each of the training units throughout the UK in turn. Where practice, fabric or equipment was found to be wanting, this was reported back to the SAC and the institution concerned was given reasonable time to put things in order before re-inspection. If conditions did not improve, training recognition could be restricted or withdrawn completely, providing a powerful incentive not only to the consultants but also to managers, to maintain high standards, as junior staff were unwilling to work in a department that did not offer approved training towards accreditation in the specialty. Trainees were expected to keep logbooks in which were recorded all the surgical procedures undertaken and the degree of supervision. In due course of time these were to become electronic records, and the amount of detailed information increased accordingly.

The role of the SAC and the process of accreditation grew steadily more influential during the 1980s, as the need for the profession to regulate itself and set high standards became increasingly pressing. At Moorfields the demand for improved teaching facilities within the Hospital itself, in addition to the small lecture theatre in the Institute building in Cayton Place, grew steadily, and in 1991 a brand new educational complex, comprising lecture theatre and seminar rooms, was opened (**Figure 43**, Plate 22). Titled the Clinical Tutorial Complex (CTC) and funded jointly by the Friends of Moorfields and the Special Trustees, this development became an integral part of the Hospital's educational activities, later being further developed to house the teaching office of the Department of Education.

Radical changes in the way in which teaching and training were undertaken, stemming from the report of the Chief Medical Officer as detailed below, led to the appointment of a Director of Education for the Trust, the first (appointed in 1996) being the present author and after him John Lee. In fact the Trust had taken steps to address the changes in educational leadership well before, when in 1993, on relinquishing the post of Dean of the Institute, Noel Rice became the Hospital's first Director of Research and Teaching. Traditionally, the formal teaching programme of courses, attended by ophthalmologists in training, from all over the country, had been the prerogative of the Institute of Ophthalmology. In spite of the fact that most of the teaching on these courses was clinical and was therefore carried out by Moorfields staff, the Institute enjoyed most of the financial reward. In 1996 it became clear that the additional funding previously provided by the Department of Health to support the Hospital's teaching activities was no longer forthcoming. The new Director of Education was charged with making good at least some of this shortfall. This he did, by transferring the management of the teaching programme of short courses from the Institute to the Hospital, setting up an office in the Clinical Tutorial Complex and appointing a manager there, Susan McKeever, who proved to be dynamic and resourceful, as were her successors in the post, first Maggie Maher and then Louise Halfhide. This action initially engendered considerable ill-feeling at the Institute, but was a necessary and successful change of direction, the short courses generating a considerable income, which was deployed amongst the clinical services to purchase teaching aids, the teachers themselves, mostly Moorfields consultants, in this way seeing for the first time some tangible rewards for their efforts.

The rise of the Postgraduate Deans and 'Calmanization'

In 1992 the Secretary of State for Health was made aware that the certification process for independent medical practice in the UK did not comply with a resolution of the European Parliament dictating that every member state must recognize the certificate of specialist competence of every other member state in the European Union. The Chief Medical Officer, Kenneth Calman, was therefore instructed to look into ways in which the UK could change its practices to comply with the directive. A man of considerable imagination and vision, Calman elected to re-examine the whole panoply of HST, and use the directive to bring about changes on a huge scale. He set up a working group, comprising a wide range of senior doctors and others concerned with higher medical education (including Presidents of Medical Royal Colleges, Postgraduate Deans, representatives of the GMC and the British Medical Association, and Chief Executives of Health Authorities), to explore the problem, and subgroups to meet with the Colleges, Faculties and others concerned with specialist medical training.

There were a number of training issues over which the profession was divided, probably the most contentious of which related, in all specialties, to the length of training required before accreditation as an independent specialist. It was not uncommon at this time for SRs, already fully trained, highly experienced individuals, capable of undertaking the entire spectrum of surgical work of their consultants (as they were not infrequently called upon to do), to remain as SRs for as long as five years or more, because there were insufficient consultant posts and little incentive to create more. Another concern was the great variability in training, not only from one part of the country to another but even within the same geographical region. There was no absolute requirement to ensure that trainees received instruction from a wide spectrum of trainers, and curricula were often vague. Because SRs depended on good references from their chiefs to help them to gain consultant posts themselves, and they often had only one or two trainers to provide them with these, there was considerable scope for oligarchy and patronage. Poor practice and outdated methods could therefore be easily perpetuated. Furthermore, the public were becoming increasingly unhappy, perceiving it as their lot under the NHS (albeit, in most cases, unfairly) to be cannon-fodder for trainees to practise their skills, while the consultants concentrated on their private patients. While some of these criticisms of the higher surgical training structure were undoubtedly exaggerated, they did nonetheless contain more than a grain of truth.

The Calman Report of 1993 set out a wide-ranging and groundbreaking series of measures, which had a profound effect on the whole of HST throughout the country, and which were to alter for ever the pattern of training at Moorfields. The most fundamental of these was the introduction of structured training programmes, whereby a number of specific training opportunities, in defined placements, were offered to each trainee, the trainee rotating to each unit for a year or more before moving on to the next placement. Of most concern to the existing consultant body, however, was the reduction in length of training (no more than seven years, in any specialty, from qualification to consultant appointment), which they considered detrimental to the production of well-trained specialists. This criticism, aimed squarely at Calman, was not entirely fair, for three reasons: first, because it had been argued by all and sundry, for a long time before the Calman Enquiry, that the length of training before appointment to a consultant post in the UK was too long; second, because it was the Medical Royal Colleges and Faculties, not the CMO, that proposed the durations of training, deeming these to be adequate for HST in their specialties; third, the detrimental effect on service provision, brought about by the reduction in training time recommended in the Calman Report, was compounded by the near simultaneous reduction in doctors' working hours demanded by the European Parliament.

The report set out to define with great clarity at whose door the responsibility for each aspect of HST lay: the Royal Colleges for setting the standards and curricula and the Regional Postgraduate Deans (with the aid of the Trusts to provide exposure to clinical practice) for their implementation. To facilitate this process, Clinical Tutors were appointed, jointly by the Deans and Trust Chief Executives, to take responsibility for the Higher Specialist Trainees in the Trusts and to administer the study-leave budget and other statutory obligations on their behalf. HST was simplified to some degree, by making it a continuum, there being only one grade, the specialist registrar (SpR), instead of two (registrar and senior registrar), but made more difficult to monitor, because of the removal of the well-defined hurdles placed in their path that had previously checked the progress of unsatisfactory trainees. Entry was competitive, with the lowest common denominator for entry to the SpR grade in ophthalmology being the possession of the MRCOphth, and exit by success in an assessment process, leading to the award of the FRCOphth. On the award of the FRCOphth, the Royal College would recommend to the UK competent authority, the Specialist Training Authority (STA), that the doctor be awarded a Certificate of Completion of Specialist Training (CCST) and the ophthalmologist's name placed on the Specialist Register (Ophthalmology) of the GMC. Only then would such an individual be eligible for consideration by an appointments committee for a consultant post in the UK. Provision was made for those (usually married women) who wished to work part-time whilst training, so-called 'flexible' SpRs, permitting them to train for a longer period, pro rata, in posts the same in every other respect as full-time ones.

The minimum length of the training period leading to the award of the CCST in ophthalmology, designated by the College, was four and a half years, one year of which had to be spent at a district general hospital. SpRs could be allotted a maximum of seven clinical sessions per week, two sessions being reserved for research and a further one for formal (bleep-free) teaching. The curriculum, developed by the RCOphth (largely the work of Professor David McLeod), was detailed and comprehensive, covering every aspect of the specialty, and the new electronic logbook (developed by David Wong) set out to encompass it. The ad hoc, poorly structured training of yesteryear was finally a thing of the past. The Postgraduate Deans in each Region were charged with implementing the training programmes devised by the Medical Royal Colleges in each specialty. At Moorfields a Postgraduate Medical Education Board was set up, and met bimonthly, chaired by the Clinical Tutor, to oversee teaching and training in the Trust (**Figure 44**, Plate 22). The Postgraduate Dean in North Thames looked favourably on Moorfields, having as it did such a concentration of teaching material, facilities and expertise, while the appointment in 1997 of a Moorfields consultant (the present author) to the post of Associate Postgraduate Dean for the surgical specialties won an extra point in its favour.

During the transition from the old system to the new 'calmanized' one, a major shift occurred in the power-base underpinning the education of doctors. Where formerly it had been down to individual units, directed by the Colleges and Faculties, to implement training, the Calman Report recommended that the Postgraduate Deans should in future be responsible for implementing it, and that to enable them to do so, they should have control over the budget. This meant that, from the time of commissioning the new process (in the case of ophthalmology, July 1995), the Regional Postgraduate Deans took over from the Trusts half of the SpR's basic salaries, as well as responsibility for the whole of their study-leave and removal expenses. Not only did the Medical Royal Colleges now carry out inspections of training units, the Postgraduate Deans also did so. Each Region became a separate teaching and training circuit, its trainees (SpRs) each being allotted a personal National Training Number (NTN) on appointment to the grade.

The NTNs were of crucial significance, the allotted quantity depending on the number of suitable training posts in the Region and hence the number of SpRs it could train. There was a national quota of NTNs for each specialty, carefully monitored, to balance the number of trainees and the number of consultant posts in that specialty. As can be imagined, there was intense competition for appointment to an SpR post and getting a NTN, the latter only being relinquished when the holder was deemed to have satisfactorily completed the period of training and been awarded his or her CCST. NTNs belonged to the Deanery, so appointments to SpR posts were in the Dean's hands, as was the assessment process (see below). Once HST was completed to the Dean's satisfaction, however, it was up to the RCOphth to recommend the award of the CCST, the NTN returning to the Dean's pool of numbers for redistribution. As noted above, the actual award of the CCST was the prerogative of the STA (later to be given even wider powers and renamed the Postgraduate Medical Education and Training Board), who then informed the GMC that the individual's name could be placed on the Specialist Register. This somewhat complicated arrangement was designed to distinguish the separate responsibilities of the different bodies involved in HST, the Medical Royal College (standards and curriculum), the Postgraduate Dean (implementation of training), and the STA and GMC (award of specialist recognition). Not only did this bring the UK into line with the rest of the European Union, it also established, for the first time, clear-cut lines of account-ability for achieving clinical competence.

Changes at Moorfields

Moorfields lay, by virtue of its geographical location, in North Thames Region (NTR). Where, immediately prior to 'calmanization', there had been 18 SRs and 6 registrars, spread over a three-year period of train-ing, 34 SpR posts were now identified at Moorfields, spread over five years, as part of the North Thames training programme, the latter comprising a total of 65 SpR posts in all. In practice this meant that each NTR SpR spent a minimum of two years at Moorfields, during the five-year period, and often longer. The appointment process for HST in ophthalmology in North Thames was carried out by the Moorfields Medical Staffing Department led by Jane Taylor, and later by Sarah Hollingshead and Kelly Burdekin, all of whom worked hard to ensure that it worked well. This was done in collaboration with the Postgraduate Deanery, on an annual basis, 12 applicants being appointed to 12 training rotations, each comprising five periods of one year in different units throughout the Region. During the six months leading up to the award of the CCST, and the six months following that, SpRs in each of the 12 rotations in North Thames were able to spend the year in an Advanced Specialty Training Opportunity in their chosen subspecialty (the equivalent of a clinical Fellowship), while still in HST, under the auspices of the Regional Postgraduate Deanery. After giving up his or her NTN, as required, within six months of the award of the CCST, the Dean was no longer strictly responsible for the individual's training and did not have a duty to find him or her employ-ment.

The numbers of trainees entering and leaving training programmes throughout the country could in this way (in theory) be kept in balance, while the numbers of consultant posts could also be kept under control. In fact (not surprisingly, but for reasons beyond the scope of this short account), this did not always prove to be the case, and serious imbalances between the numbers of accredited trainees and the numbers of available consultant posts frequently ensued. Nevertheless, the Calman scheme had some important intrinsic merits and advantages. First, it stimulated the Medical Royal Colleges, including the Royal College of Ophthalmologists, to produce carefully designed curricula, covering all aspects of current knowledge in the specialty. Secondly, it drove the introduction of broader-based training programmes, involving several different types of hospital, with different priorities and case-mixes, and it ensured that no trainee could be trained by only one unit, with a narrow course of instruction and heavy accent on patronage. Thirdly, because appointments to the training programmes became the responsibility of the Deans, these were carried out centrally, and impartiality could more easily be assured. Lastly, as the Deans paid half of the trainees' salaries, it was difficult for hospitals to exploit trainees by demanding service from them at the expense of training, without the risk of facing financial penalties and the removal of their junior staff.

On the other hand, there were a number of conspicuous disadvantages of the new system. The apprenticeship model, although it had inherent weaknesses, was beloved of many because it forged a close bond between trainer and trainee, to the benefit of both surgical teaching and job satisfaction. In the new order there was little opportunity for such bonds to develop, and this could foster a sense of frustration and apathy, on the part of both trainer and trainee. Because the training period was now a continuum, with no examination to pass or promotion to gain on the way to a more senior grade, trainees sometimes lost their driving ambition to do well and failed to attend teaching sessions or operating lists wherein they did not see any personal advantage. On the other hand, such was the intensity of competition for SpR posts that the academic standards of applicants rose to heights never before seen, many of the candidates already having higher degrees and impressive numbers of scientific publications to their credit. At Moorfields itself, the most notable difference from the previous situation was the change from a closely knit band of elite trainees (**Figure 45**), specially selected by the Moorfields consultants, to a shifting cohort, selected by a wider range of consultants from around the Region, spending one or more periods of their training at Moorfields, as part of the wider North Thames training programme. Whereas, formerly, Residents spent three years entirely at Moorfields, they were now able to spend only two years there, the rest of their time being spent at other hospitals in the Region. For some this was seen as a serious privation, although for others it seemed to offer a better balance.

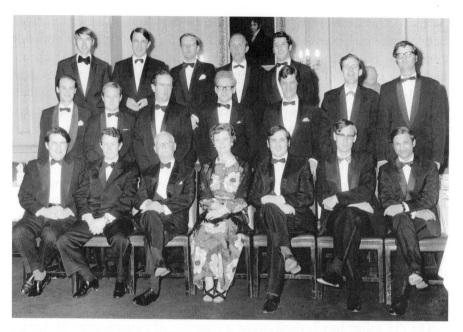

Figure 45 As this photograph, taken on the occasion of Harold Ridley's retirement in 1971, indicates, the Resident Surgical Officers ('Residents') were a closely knit body before the introduction of the Calman reforms. The latter had the effect of opening up the residency training period to all North Thames trainees, thereby bringing to an end the elitist nature of the old Moorfields Residency training programme. Pictured sitting beside Mr Ridley is the former Operating Theatre Nursing Superintendent, Miss Watkins, and on the far right her second-in-command, Mr Ryan.

Perhaps more serious than any other consideration arising from the implementation of the Calman recommendations, however, was the quandary in which they put the profession with regard to assessment of competence. Formerly, there had been a number of well-tried and established hurdles placed in the path of would-be consultants on the way to being fully trained, over which they were required to jump before they could proceed further. First amongst these was the Fellowship examination and second (and most important) was the ability to convince a statutorily convened appointments panel that they were competent to progress from the grade of registrar to senior registrar. Under the new regulations, there was a seamless progression through HST from the point of entry to the point of exit, halted only by failure to satisfy an annual assessment process (the Record of In-Training Assessment, RITA). True, it was still necessary to pass an examination to enter the training scheme, but this was (of necessity considering the relative inexperience of the examinees) less clinically searching than the previous Fellowship examination had been, and after that, whatever the opinions of their trainers, they were virtually guaranteed a consultant post at the end of the training period. The RITA process, a review of a mixture of documentation, including the trainee's logbook and written assessments from trainers, therefore assumed enormous significance. Because the trainers initially had little or no previous experience of the process, it got off to a somewhat indifferent start and, what is more, the final RITAs sometimes failed to indicate clearly whether or not trainees were fully prepared for independent practice as consultants, or had simply jumped through the hoops to the best of their abilities.

Other factors contributed to the difficulties experienced during the early days of the new regime, one of these being the reluctance of trainers to give honest references for their trainees, in an increasingly pejorative and litigious climate, even though, in view of the crucial importance of honest assessments of their competence, these had assumed greater significance than ever before. Moreover, the shortened period of training meant that some weaker trainees, who might otherwise have had the benefit of an extended period of time as a senior registrar, gaining experience under supervision, were now launched into the maelstrom of NHS consultant practice at a time when, as never before, political and managerial pressure to give value for money, as well as the spotlight of accountability, were at their most intense. It was therefore perhaps unsurprising that a number of supposedly fully trained specialists should, after appointment to consultant posts, be found wanting, the Trusts to which they were appointed expecting them to be as well trained and experienced as was formerly the case. Although this unhappy state of affairs was due as much to the outdated culture within the Trusts as to the inadequacy of the tyro consultants, it too was blamed on Calman.

Administration of the training programme in each Region was handed over to a Specialist Training Committee (STC), responsible to the Postgraduate Dean and composed of consultant trainers from Trusts around the Region. In ophthalmology, in North Thames, the first of these was chaired by Ron Marsh, senior consultant at the Western Ophthalmic Hospital, and comprised, as well as consultants representing the teaching hospitals, including Moorfields, and district general hospitals in the Region, individuals with specific remits, such as one to represent flexible trainees, a representative for academe and one for the Royal College of Ophthalmologists. It met every six months at the North Thames Deanery and was attended by Deanery representatives, as well as the ophthalmologists. In addition to the day-to-day administrative issues arising from a training programme for 65 ophthalmology SpRs, it was responsible for the appointments process and for deputing consultants to sit on the annual RITA panel and undertake the crucial task of annual assessments.

Together with the attentions of the SAC (later the Training Committee of the Royal College of Ophthalmologists), demanding better use of study time and formal lectures, and the changes to the training programme engendered by 'calmanization', Moorfields found itself greatly under the cosh during this period in its history, its cosy elitism no longer there to protect it from the ravages of national accountability. In 1992, with the declining influence of the Dean of the Institute, a Surgical Tutor was appointed, to take over the duties previously carried out by the Clinical Sub-Dean, and in 1994, when the Hospital became a NHS Trust (and Moorfields thereby came under regional control), he was formally appointed Clinical Tutor, the post officially recognized and supported by the Postgraduate Dean, to supervise training on his behalf. The present author was the first Clinical Tutor to be appointed at Moorfields, a post that, in common with many other Trusts, was in 1996 restyled Director of Education. Because the Moorfields programme formed its hub, it also fell to him to run the training programme throughout the North Thames Region. In 1997, however, on Leaver's appointment to the post of Associate Postgraduate Dean for the Surgical Specialties in North Thames, John Lee took over as Director of Education at Moorfields and James Acheson assumed the mantle of Training Programme Director.

As noted, 12 HST rotations in ophthalmology were established in North Thames, SpRs joining each of the six core subspecialty services at Moorfields for a period of four months during their two years at the Hospital, thereby gaining exposure to all aspects of the training programme. This was very different from the old-style arrangement, where Moorfields trainees spent the whole of their three-year period of HST at the Hospital, and at least six months with each consultant, but it did provide exposure for a far greater number of trainees to a greater range of consultants throughout the Region, with different knowledge, skills and ways of working. At Moorfields itself the new Clinical Tutor produced a comprehensive teaching prospectus for the Trust detailing all the educational opportunities available, and this was revised and updated in 1998. The teaching and training of medical staff was under the direction of the Postgraduate Medical Education Board, chaired by the Clinical Tutor (later Director of Education) and comprised a wide range of other senior personnel in both teaching and management roles, including the directors of Finance and Human Resources (see **Figure 44**, Plate 22).

Because BST encompassed a wide range of skills, across different specialties, and many SHOs were still undecided about their future careers, it was difficult to bring it into line with HST and incorporate it into the continuum of specialist training. BST therefore remained outside the Deans' purview, until much later, SHOs being appointed by the individual Trusts and not by the Deanery, the implementation of their training, as well as its content, ultimately being the responsibility of the Medical Royal Colleges. Moorfields took the step in 1993 of establishing six SHO posts of one to two years' duration. These posts were keenly sought and offered good training, several of their holders going on to become SpRs in North Thames and others obtaining research posts. The first appointees were Celia Hicks, Alex Ionides, Ordan Lehmann, Diana Mather, Adnan Tufail and Irene Whelehan, two of whom had done no ophthalmology prior to their appointments, but coped very well nonetheless. All six were a credit to the Hospital, going on to forge successful careers in a wide variety of different expertise, two of them (Ionides and Tufail) becoming consultants at Moorfields. The Trust also provided a surgical skills laboratory to encourage the development of manual skills, which was later incorporated into a multidisciplinary teaching facility for both junior doctors and nurses.

In 2002, however, a government white paper 'Unfinished Business: Reform of the Senior House Officer Grade' was published, suggesting the establishment of a two-year foundation programme of BST, one year pre and one year post registration, before SHOs were able to specialize. This seemed set to throw a very large spanner into the works for ophthalmology SHOs, committed as they were to a two-year period in the specialty before being able to take the entry examination for HST in ophthalmology. SHO posts at Moorfields were now deemed inappropriate, and in 2003, ten years after they were introduced, they were abandoned in favour of an increased number of SpR posts.

The effect on Moorfields of these fundamental changes in the conduct of medical education was considerable, and opinions about their influence for good and bad varied widely. There was a near-unanimous feeling, amongst juniors as well as seniors, that although the regional scheme of training, rather than bringing it to an end entirely, merely reduced its intensity, the loss of the apprenticeship model was a step backwards. So far as the reduction in time spent at Moorfields was concerned, it could be argued that the old system was unhealthily elitist and that time spent in other environments, with a wider range of colleagues (a cynic might say 'in the real world'), was time well spent. The latter was, in any event, bound to happen to some extent, with the spread of the outreach programme. Moreover, while the exposure to lower standards of practice in some weaker units in NTR could be said to be detrimental to their training, it could equally be argued that such experience was valuable, and furthermore that the presence of top quality SpRs in such units would encourage better standards there. Perhaps more worrying was the effect that clinical-risk management might have on the ability to offer trainees the opportunity to practice independently, before they became consultants and were forced to do so. Already, the RCOphth no longer approved unsupervised operating lists for senior SpRs, as it had stipulated previously for SRs. Trainee ophthalmologists were in danger of becoming better taught, but less well trained, under the new governance.

The introduction of well-defined curricula and structured programmes was seen as both desirable and inevitable, in the light of the specialty's increasing sophistication and complexity, and the relentless demands of accountability and evidence-based medicine. In truth, it is probable that the change in culture was simply hastened by the Calman Report, and that it would in any case have evolved in the course of time. Probably the most controversial aspect was the loss of the Registrar/SR barrier, in favour of a continuum, and the problems it engendered in ensuring competence. Even this, however, is open to question, history reminding us that, long before Calman, instances of incompetence were not unknown, while the capacity to perpetuate outdated treatments was legendary.

Continuing medical education, continuing professional development and revalidation

The unremitting drive, from the beginning of the 1990s, to modernize the medical profession and deter doctors from resting on their laurels, continued without pause into the new millennium, reaching its peak in 2001 with the publication by the Department of Health, of the NHS Plan. This set out a number of organizational objectives, including the introduction of formal Continuing Medical Education (CME) programmes for those who had completed their training, and the award of CME points for educational activities. The Royal College of Ophthalmologists had in 1996 introduced a logbook for its Members and Fellows to record their accredited CME activities and keep score of the points gained thereby. In due course of time, the minimum annual or triennial score required was published, points being awarded for different types of educational activities, including attendance at scientific meetings, giving lectures, and many others. Failure to reach the minimum laid down by the College could result in action being taken to penalize the individual concerned, or even an adverse report being sent to the GMC. While the conduct of CME could be criticized for its reliance on personal integrity and the temptation to contrive activities to gain points, while gaining little educational benefit from them, its value as a signal of the profession's commitment to keeping its members up to date was difficult to gainsay. Standards of teaching and training had indeed come a long way during the last 40 years.

Similarly, the establishment of the Cochrane Library, enabling members of the profession to access up-to-the-minute data, based on large-scale reviews of available scientific evidence from clinical trials, was a fundamental step forward. No longer could doctors easily hide behind curtains of doubt, while avoiding the charge of falling behind the times and prescribing treatments for which there was little scientific justification. On the other hand, there was less encouragement to explore new methods for which there was no conclusive evidence of efficacy, so that, especially in the case of rarer conditions, the opportunities for progress could be reduced. It had been argued for a long time by some that professionalism represented a dangerous threat to patient safety, when doctors were encouraged to act solely on their own initiative and decide for themselves, regardless of scientific evidence, what was best for their patients. Now, with the boot firmly on the other foot, it remained to be seen if the craving for evidence-based medicine would ring the death-knell for surgical initiative and innovation.

In addition to CME, the introduction of clinical governance and risk management, embodied in the NHS Plan, demanded far more than just the assurance that consultants would keep themselves up to date. It was also decreed that they should undergo regular appraisal and assessment of their performance, part of so-called Continuing Professional Development (CPD). Not only did the GMC demand that there should be a formal personal assessment process for consultants, comprising review of a portfolio of clinical and academic activities, leading to regular revalidation, but managers were also expected to carry out regular appraisals. Whereas assessment implied an open, objective, judgemental process, appraisal was, in contrast, confidential and non-judgemental, focusing on career development and allowing two-way discussion of aims and objectives and the best way of achieving these. Again, the medical profession was ill-prepared for such measures, relying as it always had on professional pride and independence to see it through. Furthermore, it was announced that fresh legislation would underpin the new measures, with an over-arching competent authority, the Postgraduate Medical Education Standards Board, replacing the STA.

There was a predictable outcry, so many and so great were the combined pressures placed upon doctors, especially hospital consultants, in such a short space of time. Nevertheless, there was little doubt that, in the climate of public opinion fuelled by medical disasters highlighted in the popular press, political correctness would win the day and that the measures taken by the Royal College of Ophthalmologists and the Postgraduate Deans to strengthen training standards would be seen eventually to be of great importance for the future of ophthalmology. So important an issue did Moorfields consider clinical risk management to be that it took the step of appointing a broadly trained ophthalmologist (FRCOphth), epidemiologist (PhD) and public health doctor (MSc), Parul Desai, to spearhead clinical governance in the Trust. This she accomplished, in collaboration with the Clinical Governance Committee (headed by Clive Nickolds, a member of the Board of Directors), with great efficiency.

Library services

The main hospital library, previously housed in the City Road building, moved to the Institute when it opened in 1948. From that time on, until the move to the new building in 1991, the fabric changed but little, rows of sturdy wooden shelves and glass-fronted cabinets in fine weathered oak lining its walls, with desks and chairs to match. The quality and range of journals, textbooks and archive material was, however, unrivalled, as were the qualifications and knowledge of Sarah Lawrence, Librarian from 1977 until 1997, who was their conscientious, helpful and efficient custodian, as well as that of the small museum. At the High Holborn branch there was also a small library, the contents of which were offered to the main library in Judd Street in 1988, when the branches were merged.

In 1992, with the completion of the Phase IV building of the Institute in Bath Street, the library moved across to a space in the lower ground floor of the new building, so small and cramped that it was almost impossible to negotiate a path between the shelves without occasioning unacceptable intimacy with and disturbing the concentration of other users. Meanwhile, the museum was moved to the Royal College of Ophthalmologists. In November 1988, prior to the library's relocation on the island site, the Hospital, largely at the instigation of the nursing body, opened its own Joint Study Facility (JSF) on the fourth floor, housing what was previously the Residents' Library and the collections of textbooks and journals from the School of Nursing, Pharmacy and Orthoptic Department. This facility was well equipped, well designed and extremely accessible and was staffed by two part-time librarians appointed by the Hospital, but under Sarah Lawrence's supervision. It functioned well and was used by a wide range of hospital staff, particularly nurses and Residents. There was also a separate reading room stocked with current journals. With the advance of computerization, the latter was provided with computer terminals and converted into a reading and searching facility.

When Phase VIA of the new Institute was opened in 1999, the library found itself with much improved accommodation, the new area quadrupling its space and allowing the provision of desks, computers and extended shelving, so transforming the facilities and enabling the Hospital to close the JSF and transfer its contents to the new Joint Library in Bath Street. This move, providing as it did much needed office space at the Hospital, for the Education Department, was a mixed blessing, for, while the Joint Library was well able to provide space, it was, unlike the JSF, geographically separated from the hospital building, and difficult to access at week-ends or 'after hours'. Nevertheless, the rapid development and availability of 'on-line' search and reference facilities largely offset this perceived disadvantage, while the impending imposition of a statutory working time limit for all members of staff in any case made its use out of hours technically illegal.

Sarah Lawrence retired in 1997, and her place was taken by Debbie Heatlie, another highly qualified librarian who had previously been at University College Library and who therefore understood the workings of the Institute and of the North London Libraries well. She did much to cement the relationship between the Hospital and Institute, providing advice and help to both scientists and clinicians with equal charm and kindness, and imbuing her staff with similar qualities.

The Joint Library remained a valuable resource, the integrated collection of journals running back to the mid-1800s and books from as long before as 1585. It had a collection of over 23 000 books, many of them donated by eminent alumni such as Edward Nettleship, Herbert Parsons and Stewart Duke-Elder, and it subscribed to 119 current journals. It was soon evident, however, that the scientists at the Institute preferred on-line facilities to books and journals, while the clinicians were more conservative in their approach. Nevertheless, with the colossal proliferation of electronic journals and similar, though less dramatic, advances in textbooks, as well as the increasing use of Medline (by doctors) and Cinahl (by nurses) to search literature, it was evident that paper would gradually be supplanted by the computer screen and that the role of the librarian, like everyone else's, would soon change completely. Debbie Heatlie remained contracted with both the Hospital and Institute, her remuneration being shared equally between the two, but it was not long before the new North Central Workforce Development Confederation took over responsibility for NHS library policy and direction. This fitted in well with the Joint Library's commitment to a multidisciplinary role, all the hospital departments using it in some measure, while it provided the scientists at the Institute with an invaluable resource. The Library, jointly owned and managed by Moorfields and the Institute and affiliated with University College, gave all library members access to a wide range of (on-line) resources, while a Joint Library Committee, jointly chaired by the Hospital's Director of Education and the Institute's Senior Researcher, was responsible for its overall direction.

CHAPTER 6

Research

The Institute of Ophthalmology

Background
Many years prior to the Second World War, there were proposals to establish an institution for the purpose of encouraging research and teaching in ophthalmology, under the auspices of London University (see Volume II of this *History*, pp. 83–84). In 1948, following amalgamation of the Royal London, Royal Westminster and Central London Ophthalmic Hospitals, and the inauguration of the National Health Service, the Institute of Ophthalmology was founded, under the aegis of the British Postgraduate Medical Federation (BPMF), a school of London University. The building that had previously housed the Central London Ophthalmic Hospital was converted for this purpose, an arrangement that had been proposed and accepted, in principle, some years before (**Figure 46**, Plate 23).

Sir Stewart Duke-Elder, whose brainchild the Institute was, became the first Director of Research and the Earl of Rothes the first Chairman of its Committee of Management. There were four departments, including Pathology under Norman Ashton and Medical Illustration under Peter Hansell. Transfer of the laboratories, library and museum from what had been the Royal London Ophthalmic Hospital created much needed space at City Road, while teaching activities, previously undertaken in the Medical School, were also transferred to the new Institute. Many of the scientists who were to translate understanding of ocular function into the modern era worked there during the first three decades of its existence, including Hugh Davson, the father of ocular physiology, and David Maurice, Geoffrey Arden and Robert Weale, who did much to elucidate the mysteries of corneal endothelial function, of the electrophysiological responses of the retina, and of physiological optics respectively. To compensate for the reduction in their direct influence and clinical input to teaching, the Moorfields surgeons were invited to provide the holder of the post of Dean of the Institute, a position that in

Duke-Elder's day had more prestige than power, and one that was usually awarded to a senior member of the consultant staff who would not 'rock the boat'. Clinical research was partly financed by endowment funds, with the understanding and acquiescence of the Hospital.

In 1954 two additional departments were set up: one for the study of intra-ocular inflammation headed by Terry Perkins, the University's new Reader in Ophthalmology, and one for research into the causes and treatment of trachoma, the latter a step that would doubtless have pleased John Cunningham Saunders, and one that would later turn out to be a platform for the advances in ophthalmology inspired by Barrie Jones.

Meanwhile, as Duke-Elder pressed on with his work on the *Textbook of Ophthalmology* and the direction of the new Institute, Norman Ashton was busy establishing his place in the pantheon of fame, with his seminal work on retinal vascular pathology. Barrie Jones was at this time still a resident surgical officer at the City Road branch of Moorfields, but had already made a strong impression with his extraordinary ability to identify the crux of a problem and apply his energy and skill to solve it. After leaving 'the House' in 1956, he joined the staff of the Institute as a part-time lecturer, and began to pursue his studies in the field of clinical microbiology, with particular reference to viral infections and trachoma, while maintaining his surgical interests and skills, with appointments as a senior registrar at the London Hospital and as a clinical assistant at Moorfields. Soon after this, he was made a senior lecturer with honorary consultant status, in which position he continued until the creation of the Professorial Chair of Clinical Ophthalmology in 1963, to which he was finally appointed.

It is evident from even the most cursory review of historical accounts and reminiscences that Duke-Elder 'ruled the roost', in the academic and socio-political world of ophthalmology from before the Second World War until the early 1960s. A colossus in terms of academic ability and productivity, and with political and social skills of the highest calibre, he bestrode the national and world ophthalmic stage as no single figure had done since Bowman. As Director of Research at the new Institute, he continued to do so, until the emergence of two major figures on the academic scene, first Norman Ashton and shortly afterwards Barrie Jones.

The Chair of Clinical Ophthalmology

To understand the dynamics at work within the academic world of ophthalmology in this period, it is helpful to recall something of the personalities involved. Duke-Elder, already firmly established as the doyen of the ophthalmic world, was by all accounts polished, urbane and outgoing. Ashton (**Figure 47**, Plate 24), holder of a personal Chair in Ophthalmic Pathology since 1959, was equally polished and brilliant, an outstanding public speaker with a keen sense of humour and razor wit, but vain and easily offended, while Jones was charming, unpretentious, equally capable, and fired by relentless determination and ambition. Alongside the latter stood Terry Perkins, a delightful, unassuming, pipe-smoking, clinical academic of more modest ambitions, who had nevertheless made a considerable impact on academic ophthalmology and who, having already served as Reader since 1954, rightly commanded the respect and support of Sir Stewart and his colleagues.

When in 1963 the University finally agreed to fund the first substantive Chair of Ophthalmology, Barrie Jones' standing amongst his clinical academic colleagues, after six years of clinical research at both Hospital and Institute, was unchallenged, and he was, without any doubt, the Hospital's preferred candidate. Duke-Elder, however, as Director of the Institute, was duty-bound to support his incumbent Reader. The appointments panel was therefore placed in an invidious position and was unable to come to a decision between the two candidates for the post. In the event, such was Duke-Elder's position and influence that he was able to persuade an independent funding organization, The Sembal Trust, to finance an additional Chair, of Experimental Ophthalmology, so that the claims of both Jones and Perkins could be appropriately recognized. Thus did Barrie Jones became Professor of Clinical Ophthalmology and Terry Perkins Professor of Experimental Ophthalmology, a compromise solution that spared the blushes of all concerned.

Hospital and Institute united

Ashton had already established an unrivalled position of supremacy worldwide in the field of ocular pathology, and was shortly (1965) given a substantive University Chair. Nevertheless, he was not by any means a team player, preferring to appoint staff who would not present any threat to his standing, and would promote his own position and that of his department, rather than that of the Institute as a whole. His relationships with the Hospital were, likewise, not especially easy, the consultant staff standing somewhat in awe of his reputation and sharp intellect, while he, in his turn, despite his honorary consultant status, felt excluded from the clinical world.

Indeed, the story goes that on one occasion, arriving at the Hospital for a meeting and entering the consultants' cloakroom, he was informed by a member of the consultant staff that this was for the sole use of consultant surgeons and that he should hang up his coat elsewhere. (If this was indeed the case, then his reticence in dealing with the Hospital is scarcely surprising.)

Consequently, although he and the new Professor of Clinical Ophthalmology had the greatest respect for one another's academic abilities, they were not destined to become close colleagues. Indeed, it is fair to say that while Barrie Jones, recognizing Ashton's genius for pathological observation and interpretation, tried very hard to cultivate his friendship and cooperation, his efforts in this respect were not fully reciprocated. Ashton too must have found it difficult to cope with Barrie Jones' relentless enthusiasm and determination. In fact he is said to have described him as *'like an oak tree growing up through concrete'*.

The pathology department was, by all accounts, extremely busy, providing a vital service, not only to Moorfields but also to many other hospital eye departments throughout the land. While Ashton pursued his research interests, his staff undertook a heavy clinical load, as well as teaching the Moorfields resident staff and the students on the Diploma of Ophthalmology course. Specimens would arrive from far and wide, including a delivery service to and from Moorfields, by van. Ashton's juniors were therefore kept busily occupied in the laboratory, examining histopathological and other specimens, and in the lecture theatre, with little time to conduct research themselves or to make contact with their colleagues at the Hospital. It was, in the words of one, *'like being on an island, or in a watertight compartment'*. It was understandable, therefore, that with the exception of the professor's own contribution, less original research came from the department than might otherwise have been expected, and that a service-orientated culture tended to prevail amongst the junior staff.

Barrie Jones himself recalled that when he was a junior in Ashton's department, no one was allowed to visit a laboratory in another institution without the professor's express permission and personal intervention. Finding that he got on well with other workers in his field, he ignored this edict, much to Ashton's displeasure and opprobrium.

Nevertheless, in the words of Professor Douglas Coster, who worked with both Ashton and Barrie Jones for some years before returning to Australia, and knew them both well, Norman Ashton was a far warmer and more charismatic character than he might at first have appeared:

'Ashton ruled the department in the manner of a 19th Century German Professor. He was able to get away with this for two reasons. First, he was a towering figure in his profession and he was always prepared to be judged

alongside his colleagues in the regular public and competitive examinations of masked pathology slides held in the department. Secondly, he had a sophisticated and disarming sense of humour. He was fun to be with. On one occasion he hosted a party at the Institute, which was attended by a large number of friends and supporters. He introduced me to a group of guests, telling them that I was doing a good job bringing together the laboratory microbiology and the clinical management of ocular infections. Inappropriately keen to take advantage of the situation, I remarked that I could do better if given access to a modern microscope, rather than the brass monocular microscope he had provided me with – the one Louis Pasteur had once used and discarded. Ashton quickly retorted "My boy, at least he did some good with it", turned on his heel and left me to contemplate my out-of-place remark, much to the mirth of those with whom I was standing.'

On Sir Stewart Duke-Elder's retirement from the post of Director of Research in 1965, it is hardly surprising that this position was not perpetuated. Sir Stewart became President of the Institute, while its direction was left in the hands of a Committee of Management, headed by a non-academic, and an Academic Board whose chairman was elected by its members, thereby obviating the need to identify an all-powerful director amongst the senior academic staff. Meanwhile, until the 1980s, apart from the spell between 1976 and 1980 when it was occupied by Professor John Gloster, the post of Dean continued to be held by hospital clinicians with only a passing interest in research, and little direct influence on the Institute's future destiny.

This notwithstanding, Barrie Jones's ability to combine academic flair with clinical understanding and bring together academics and clinicians paid dividends. Never, in its entire history, has the Institute shared with the Hospital such a close and fruitful relationship as it did during the period when he was Professor of Clinical Ophthalmology. Such was his standing at the Hospital and the strength of his department at the Institute that he was able to bring his influence to bear on almost every activity at both. At the former he championed the use of microsurgical techniques and promoted specialization in many areas of eye disease, while at the latter the Department of Virology investigated the causes of and possible treatments for a wide range of conditions caused by bacterial, fungal, viral and chlamydial infections, as well as those associated with inflammation and disorders of the immunological system.

A man apart: Barrie Jones
The twists and turns of fate, conspiring, as they so often do, to rearrange the best laid plans of mice and men, played no small part in

shaping the career of Barrie Jones, one of the most remarkable in the history of modern medicine. To sum up the character and portray the profile of such a giant figure would present a challenge even to someone who had known and worked with him for a lifetime, let alone the present author, whose knowledge was limited to brief periods of his career. It has been the present author's good fortune, however, to have the opinions and advice of others who knew him much better, including Professor Coster, who worked closely with Barrie Jones for several years and whose searching wit and insight have been invaluable, and one can do no better than to again quote verbatim from his account:

'...I was fortunate to be given a position with Professor Barrie Jones in the Cornea and External Disease Service. This involved working on a number of clinical research projects and spending a little time in the Pocklington Eye Transplantation Laboratory at the Institute of Ophthalmology. The attachment altered the course of my life. It was at this time that I decided to pursue a career in academic medicine. During the year I learned how to plan and conduct trials, how to read and write papers, and had my first experience of presenting material at meetings. The Cornea and External Disease Clinics were very strong at that time. Barrie Jones had established several groups that were international leaders in fungal, viral and chlamydial eye disease and were also amongst the leaders in corneal transplantation. The standing of the group attracted Fellows from all around the world and many of them went on to establish major reputations in ophthalmology...

'...Although I worked with Professor Jones for a number of years and was privileged to spend quite a lot of time with him, I could never claim to know what made him tick. He had a drive which set him apart from anyone else I have ever met in the field. Certainly he had a remarkable intelligence and he worked very hard. But he had more than this. He was able to identify the areas of ophthalmology where advances needed to be made and where advances were feasible. Often he was working in a number of disparate fields at once, assembling willing collaborators around London and the rest of the UK and indeed the world. Each of his pursuits was attacked with extraordinary enthusiasm and effectiveness. Often the time from identification of the problem to a rounded symposium at the Oxford Congress or the OSUK would be as short as a few months, but nothing was ever half done. The ability to focus intently on important and emerging issues and to get to a point of tangible contribution quickly was one of Professor Jones' attributes.

'There was another aspect of his character that contributed to his success. He was a shy man, but a showman, nevertheless. His showmanship had an

unusual configuration. Never a self-promoter in the manner of so many latter-day rock-star eye doctors, he was a most energetic promoter of his cause, which was the eradication of avoidable blindness. He had a remarkable facility with language. He had natural talent in this regard, but he also worked on it. Every paper was carefully crafted and worked through various drafts. Nothing went out until it was word perfect. He once told me that when writing you have to 'think until it hurts'. When writing or preparing for an oral presentation, he gave great importance to finding the perfect words and considered carefully not only the meaning of the words he used, but their weight and rhythm, much as an orator like Churchill must have done. He would toss over phrases until the correct phrase popped out. Many of his terms and expressions quickly found their way into the ophthalmic vernacular. Phrases such as the 'burden of avoidable blindness' are constantly repeated and have been for 30 years. Such expressions were generated by someone who understood the power of language.

He was also capable of seriously understated showmanship. He was into the mega-lecture before the multimedia presentations of today were dreamt of. His three-screen, fade-in, fade-out, presentations were spellbinding and out of character with his shy personality or any other aspect of his life or work. He believed in what he was doing and presented his findings accordingly and with maximum impact.'

It had been Barrie Jones' original intention to take advantage of the educational opportunities that London had to offer, prepare a PhD thesis in microbiology and, after getting his higher degree, return to the Antipodes, most probably to take over Rowland Wilson's Chair at his alma mater, the University of Otago. He also felt bound to repay a debt of some £600, borrowed from his grandfather's estate, to enable him to come to the UK in the first place. All thought of the former disappeared in a whirlwind of research and clinical activity, his unquenchable enthusiasm and boundless capacity for hard work taking him relentlessly along paths he had not sought or been prepared to tread. Duke-Elder, in particular, encouraged him to set up his own laboratory, with funds from an oil company, which he had at his disposal. An invitation to apply for the newly created professorial chair in Melbourne, which could well have derailed him, seemed attractive, until the job specification of the post changed at the last minute, when unacceptable conditions were imposed. So it was that Barrie Jones remained in London, was appointed Professor of Clinical Ophthalmology in 1963 and went on to change, for ever, the face of British ophthalmology.

Large numbers of young ophthalmologists from all over the UK and abroad were attracted to the Hospital and Institute, in addition to a strong core of home-based, Moorfield-trained individuals, who saw the opportunities created by working jointly with clinicians and academics. Would-be ophthalmologists, who had trusted formerly in honing their clinical skills alone, now took advantage of the opportunities provided by the proliferation of joint clinical research studies and controlled trials to improve their knowledge and understanding of ophthalmology, and thereby improve their chances of gaining appointment to the Moorfields training programme. At the other end of the training pathway, those who had completed their formal training and could thereby have realistically applied for consultant posts were persuaded to enhance their skills further by undertaking research projects as lecturers or senior lecturers in the Professorial Unit.

The effect of this explosion of learning and research on the development of modern ophthalmology in the UK (and further afield) is difficult to quantify, but it was undoubtedly hugely influential, leading as it did to widespread changes in surgical technique, improved methods of treating corneal and external diseases, and a far-reaching improvement in all aspects of ophthalmic care. It is, perhaps, a reflection on the weakness as well as the strength of the NHS, in its symbiotic relationship with private practice, that the majority of those whom Barrie Jones inspired to take up the new subspecialty interests eventually left the Clinical Academic Department in favour of independent practice. This was, however, not invariably the case. When Alan Bird returned to the UK after completing his residency at the High Holborn branch of the Hospital and spending a year as a Fellow in the USA, he joined the Academic Department and went on to found the Retinal Diagnostic Department, remaining in full-time academic practice throughout his career. Others, such as Noel Rice, Peter Watson and Peter Wright, remained in the department as senior lecturers, in a part-time capacity, sometimes, as in Watson's case, travelling to London from considerable distances to do so.

Barrie Jones himself pioneered many of the advances made in the diagnosis and management of ocular infections, in particular those strongly resistant to treatment, caused by viruses, *Chlamydia* and fungi. Not only was the Department of Clinical Ophthalmology influential in the Professor's own spheres of special interest, but it also promoted and encouraged developments in other fields. As well as Bird's early work in the use of fluorescein angiography to elucidate medical retinal disorders, the first clinical trials in ophthalmology, studying the effect of photocoagulation in the treatment of diabetic retinopathy, were initiated by Barrie Jones in collaboration with the Royal Postgraduate Medical School. These were undertaken by Rolf Blach, Hung Cheng,

Peter Hamilton and Eva Kohner. In other fields, there were major advances too: John Wright soon became a world authority on orbital tumours, Peter Wright and Tony Bron on lacrimal disorders and Peter Watson on inflammatory diseases of the sclera. Indeed, the close cooperation between the Hospital and the Institute during this period spawned what was perhaps the most exciting and productive era that British ophthalmology has ever known. Even in cataract surgery, in which field, since the ill-starred pioneering efforts of Harold Ridley 20 years before, Moorfields had lagged seriously behind the rest of the UK, Barrie Jones was influential, encouraging Arthur Steele to initiate a controlled clinical trial and thereby promoting the development of lens-implant surgery at the Hospital.

Sadly, this golden age was not to last. Soon after Norman Ashton reached retiring age in 1978, Barrie Jones became seriously ill, and was forced to spend three months away on sick-leave. Although he made a full recovery from what was a life-threatening condition, it proved to be a turning point, not only in what was already a remarkable career but also in the relationship between the Hospital and Institute. On his return to work, it quickly dawned on him that things had already moved on, and that rather than fall back into the familiar pattern of his previous role, he would do better to steer his energies in the direction of preventive ophthalmology, the cause that had always been his top priority. To this end, he set about raising funds and canvassing support for the establishment of an International Centre for Eye Health. Owing to his standing and reputation, he achieved his aim with remarkable speed, so that the new department, accommodated in the Institute's Cayton Street premises, was formally opened in September 1981 (see **Figure 51**, Plate 26), and he was able to resign from the Chair of Clinical Ophthalmology to become its director (see below).

The 1980s, a decade of academic turmoil

The replacement of two such critically important figures as Ashton and Jones with individuals of comparable stature and abilities proved, perhaps unsurprisingly, to be beyond the compass of either institution. In truth, this was partly circumstantial. In the first instance, there simply were no candidates for the post of Professor of Ophthalmic Pathology of such enormous intellectual capacity and forceful personality as Norman Ashton. In the event the position went, with Ashton's wholehearted approbation, to one of the two existing Readers in the department, Alec Garner, thereby precipitating, soon afterwards, the other's resignation. Shortly after the new Professor's appointment, there began a series of financial cuts, imposed (indirectly) by the new

Tory government, which further weakened the Department of Pathology and entailed rationalization and redundancies, causing even more concern. Indeed so serious was the financial crisis that the Institute decided that it could no longer support the Department of Medical Illustration, forcing the Hospital to take it over.

In the second instance, when Barrie Jones relinquished the Chair of Clinical Ophthalmology, in spite of all efforts by the new Dean, Barrie Jay (who even travelled to the Antipodes in the course of his search), all efforts to find a replacement for him also failed. Out of numerous candidates for the post, some of them more suitable than others, only two appeared to be seriously interested. One of these was finally offered the job, accepted the appointment and then turned it down after a lapse of six months, while the other, after thinking things over for a short period, also withdrew. The reasons for their withdrawal are not entirely clear. Indeed in the case of the first it is hard to understand his reasons for accepting the appointment and then withdrawing 6 months later. In the second instance the appointee made it plain that he would expect the Hospital to offer realistic financial support for the Professorial Unit and this assurance was not forthcoming. It seems that Moorfields, although it was a Special Health Authority, did not see the need to devote any of the extra funding that it received from the Department of Health (up to 40% more, pro rata, than that granted to a district general hospital) to the support of its research activities. Failure to appreciate that its special status and exalted position made it duty bound to provide high-quality research would, 10 years later, rebound badly, when the government and its advisers sought to account for the extra funding given to the SHAs (see below). The once most prestigious academic post in ophthalmology in the UK thus remained vacant and unwanted for almost four years, until in 1985 the then Dean of the Institute, Barrie Jay, was persuaded to take it on.

Although there were many academics of considerable stature working at the Institute during the first half of the 1980s, some of them internationally acknowledged experts in their chosen fields, the lack of clear direction and strong leadership became steadily more corrosive as the decade wore on. The sudden and totally unexpected death in December 1986 of one of its brightest stars, Chris Ernst, did nothing to lighten the gloom. This was not helped by the attitude of the Hospital administration, nor by the apparent lack of a clear vision for the future on the part of the Dean. In spite (or perhaps because) of the fact that the Chairmen of the Committee of Management of the Institute and of the Board of Governors of the Hospital were one and the same person (Francis Cumberlege), the two institutions were at variance with one another, and the House Governor, in particular, was unsympathetic to the Institute's plight. The Institute's financial position became steadily more parlous and, as the most senior academics appeared unable to resolve the situation, the Dean was forced to take firm control, which he did, with considerable effect, by balancing the books. So serious did the situation at one time become, however, that without the financial assistance of Norman Ashton's Fight for Sight charity, it is unlikely that the Institute would have survived this period in its history.

It is one thing to put the books in order, and quite another to inject enthusiasm and a sense of direction into an academic institution in which disorder and disenchantment have taken root. In this respect the exercise was clearly a failure, and when the government ordered all research institutes to undergo Research Assessment Exercises (RAEs) on a triennial basis, the Institute of Ophthalmology scored very badly. At the second RAE, it fared little better than it had at the first, resulting in a warning from the Chairman of the University Grants Committee that if things did not improve dramatically then funding would be withdrawn altogether, in effect threatening its closure. Drastic action was consequently required.

A new broom

As a consequence of Barrie Jay's appointment to the Chair of Clinical Ophthalmology in 1985, the Dean's post at the Institute fell vacant, prompting an upsurge of support for a different style of candidate. This emerged in the shape of Rolf Blach, a man with a strong track record of vision and imagination, albeit as a clinician rather than a scientist (**Figure 48**). He was duly elected. Blach's appointment coincided with the retirement of the most senior professor at the Institute, the head of the Department of Visual Science, giving him the opportunity to take the initiative and introduce new blood. In this endeavour he had, not surprisingly, the strong support of (indeed a mandate from) an advisory panel, headed by the Director of the British Postgraduate Medical Federation (BPMF), Professor Michael Peckham.

In casting around for a suitably high-quality candidate to take over the Department of Visual Science, it was soon clear to Blach that Peckham had ideas of his own, and he was intrigued to receive an enquiry from a very senior professor, then Head of Physiology at the University of Wales in Cardiff, a position he had held since 1982. With a background in the neurophysiology of vision and considerable experience of and success in running university departments (having already done so in Birmingham, before moving to Cardiff), there was no question that Adam Sillito had impeccable credentials. As a result of efforts to down-

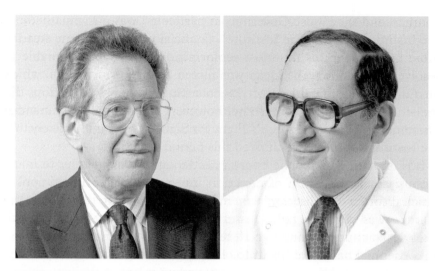

Figure 48　Professor Barrie Jay (*left*), Dean of the Medical School from 1980 to 1985 and Mr Rolf K Blach (*right*), Dean from 1985 to 1989.

size his department in Wales (allegedly due to poor financial management on the part of the University), he was looking to move elsewhere and had already been viewing the possibility of a post in the USA.

When he first came to see the Institute, then still housed in the original building in Judd Street, Sillito recalls that he simply spoke to one or two people there, took one look at the gloomy and archaic premises and promptly fled back to Wales. Further discussion with Michael Peckham, however, and his reluctance to go abroad, convinced him that the prospect of rescuing the Institute (assisted by the University's apparent willingness to fund its relocation alongside the Hospital) could be rewarding and, so in 1987 he applied for and accepted the post of Director of the Department of Visual Science, charged with building up that department before going on to rejuvenate the organization as a whole.

Adam Sillito brought with him several of his team from Cardiff, effecting an immediate and dramatic improvement in the Department of Visual Science. Meanwhile, the other departments continued in much the same way as before, individuals pursuing their own agendas, more or less effectively, but with little teamwork or clearly defined research strategy. Several departments had over the years become more and more focused on their service roles, to the exclusion of, or with a serious reduction in, basic research, so that such research as was being done was of insufficient weight to pass muster in a stringent examination of scientific quality.

In 1990 Michael Peckham instituted a programme of peer review, to assess the research programmes of all the postgraduate institutes and see for himself how they were performing. A review group was convened, consisting of distinguished academics in a wide range of fields, including ophthalmology, which visited the Institute of Ophthalmology in February of that year to listen to submissions by representatives of all the departments, outlining their previous work, ongoing activities and future plans. While some individuals came out of this exercise with credit, few departments performed well overall, especially when the review group considered the potential for productive basic and applied research, in an organization closely allied to a centre of excellence of the calibre of Moorfields, with its enormous amount of clinical material.

Perhaps unsurprisingly, Visual Science was the only department that earned unstinting praise. Whatever the case – and there were many different views – the report was very damaging to the established staff. It was clearly evident that the writing was on the wall and that drastic changes were inevitable. There were calls for the resignation of the Dean, and several of the more senior staff were called upon to take early retirement, while the Hospital faced the prospect of losing the services of the Department of Pathology altogether if the quality of its research did not improve. There were bitter recriminations, not only amongst the Institute and Hospital staff, but more widely. An editorial in the *Lancet*, highly critical of the report, drew angry denials and expressions of outrage from Peckham and Blach, and further correspondence of a critical nature from others.

It was soon obvious that Rolf Blach's position was becoming untenable and that relations between him and Adam Sillito were strained. The Dean found a powerful lobby ranged against him, including the Chairman of the BPMF, the Chairman of the Academic Board, the House Governor of the Hospital and the Professor of Clinical Ophthalmology, as well as Sillito himself. As a result, in spite of strong protestations from the Chairman of the Hospital's Medical Committee and others, it was not long before he resigned, in favour of Noel Rice, whose appointment was strongly supported by both Peckham and Sillito. In fact, Peckham, who was all powerful, felt (perhaps with some justification) that clinical deans, without strong academic records, were not the best people to run research institutes and that their replacement by scientists was to be commended. Rice, who had long made it plain that he concurred with this view, thought it right for Adam Sillito to be the Research Director of the Institute, with full authority to undertake the role. In 1993, therefore, when the former finally relinquished the post of Dean to become the Hospital's first Director of Research and

Teaching, Adam Sillito became the unchallenged custodian of the Institute's fortunes.

In line with proposals going back as far as Todd's in 1969, the report of Sir Bernard Tomlinson's 'Inquiry into London's Health Service, Medical Education and Research', published in October 1992, contained a strong recommendation that the postgraduate medical institutes should be closely linked with multifaculty schools. In contrast with previous advice, suggesting that it should go to the medical school at Barts, however, it was now recommended that the Institute of Ophthalmology should be subsumed into University College London (UCL). This arrangement was endorsed by Peckham's research review of 1993, and implemented shortly thereafter, thereby dissociating the Institute still further from the Hospital and consolidating the autonomy of its director.

Meanwhile, over at Bath Street, on the island site adjacent to the Hospital, the major redevelopment of the Institute had at last begun (**Figure 49**, Plate 25). It will be recalled that Phases I–III, comprising the conversion and renovation of the old Metal Box Company building in Cayton Place, to house the Department of Pathology, the Dean's offices and later the Department of Preventive Ophthalmology, had taken place many years earlier. Phase IV, started in 1989, consisted of a brand new, purpose-built establishment, on five floors, housing, amongst other things, state-of-the-art laboratories and a new library (**Figure 50**, Plate 25). It was completed with the help of a £1.1m donation from the Fight for Sight charity and opened in 1991.

> *Its completion was, according to Sillito, not entirely without incident, the previous planning team comprising a group of academics who, to use his own words, 'could not have pitched a tent', the consequence being that little attention had been paid to practical details, such as the provision of window blinds or air-conditioning for the laboratories.*

The start of Phase V, an ambitious project (some would say over-ambitious), comprising laboratories, a lecture theatre and accommodation for clinical research, to interface with the Hospital, was postponed indefinitely. In the first instance this was because costs per unit of floor space were seen to be vastly higher than those of the other phases (more than four times so, pro rata); in the second, it might be surmised, it was as a result of scepticism on the part of both Institute and Hospital concerning the feasibility of creating a workable interface between the two institutions.

> *Indeed, it is alleged that when the Wellcome Trust was approached with regard to the funding of Phase V, the then Chairman of the Wellcome,*

Professor Stan Peart, retorted: 'Now they want us to pay the Institute of Ophthalmology to speak to Moorfields'.

Phases VIa and VIb went ahead, as planned, however, in 1998 and 2002 respectively, VIa incorporating a shared facility, supported by a £2 million contribution from the Special Trustees to encourage and enable joint research work between Hospital and Institute. Phase VIb, the Joint Infrastructure Fund (JIF) building, was an equally exciting new development. Enabled by a £9.2 million grant from the Wellcome Trust it created a centre for 'the development of novel strategies for the treatment of ocular disease', sending out a strong signal that there was real determination, as the 21st Century began, to translate basic science into clinical practice (in perfect harmony with the title of the Institute/Hospital's new joint research strategy, 'From Basic Science to Better Sight').

A *clean sweep*

Once in a position of absolute power at the Institute, the new director set about purging it of its weaker elements, a task rendered easier for him by the voluntary resignations of most of the established academics with solid reputations, who left to take up posts they were offered in university departments in London, Birmingham, Manchester, Liverpool and elsewhere. In some instances these departures were to be expected and some had indeed been recommended in the peer review report of 1990. In others the baby might be said to have been thrown out with the bathwater, the Institute losing the services of excellent clinician scientists, such as Alison McCartney, and researchers with a keen clinical research interest, such as John Marshall and Ian Grierson, all of whom were able to bridge the gap between basic science and clinical ophthalmology. This was a loss keenly felt by the Hospital too, as these workers had provided relevance to the collaborative efforts of those keen to maintain clinical research.

Whatever the whys and wherefores relating to this period in the history of the Institute – and there are widely differing views, not only about the wisdom of the changes that took place but also about the methods of achieving them – it is certain that there was an overriding need for radical change, if the institution was to survive. So low had its research rating fallen and so poor was morale when Adam Sillito arrived that a total overhaul was inevitable, if only to restore credibility. This he achieved with extraordinary success, albeit with brutal severity, dismissing those who were unable to score highly in the UGC ratings exercise and virtually emptying the Institute of clinical academics, most of whom were unable to spare the time for, and were ill-equipped to undertake, high-grade basic research in the course of their clinical duties.

In all fairness, there were very great pressures on Adam Sillito and the Institute that forced such drastic measures upon them. The government's squeeze on research funding was universal (Oxford University reacted by going so far as to refuse an Honorary Degree to its exalted alumna, the Prime Minister – an unprecedented snub), every research institute and medical school across the country being affected. There simply was no room any more for the weaker elements of clinical academe. To make matters worse, Malcolm Green, who took over from Michael Peckham as Director of the BPMF, declined to honour the latter's commitments to the Institute. In Sillito's own words, *'we struggled forward despite, rather than with, BPMF support at that time'*. Only the intervention of the Fight for Sight charity and its Chairman Ian Steers, redirecting funding to the support of core posts, enabled the Institute's survival, and led in the course of time to the successful revival of its fortunes. Nevertheless there was great bitterness and ill-feeling.

In Pathology there were especially serious tensions. Alec Garner, who succeeded Norman Ashton as Professor in 1978, had made every effort to improve the relations between his department and the Hospital, encouraging collaboration and involving himself in Hospital activities as much as he could. His research performance, however, was said by the new director to be weak, and he soon found himself marginalized and under-funded. *Indeed, a senior member of Garner's department described Sillito's modus operandi in graphically pathological terms as 'metastasizing to all departments (throughout the Institute) and infiltrating pathology'.* Tensions increased, between him, Sillito and Susan Lightman, after her appointment to the Duke-Elder Chair, and between her and Alison McCartney, who had seemed likely to be Garner's successor, but who now departed to St Thomas' Hospital, as did John Marshall. To his everlasting credit, Garner, who was strongly supported by the Hospital, stayed on until his retirement was due, even 'shadowing' his successor, Phil Luthert, who, having no experience of ocular pathology, went off to the USA for three months to learn about it prior to taking up his appointment.

Luthert was one of a new breed of clinician scientist. Coming from a background of neurosciences, he had intended to be a neurologist, until (as he alleges) he found he 'couldn't stand out-patient clinics'. He switched to neuroscience and was head-hunted from the Institute of Psychiatry in 1994. Unlike the traditional model of pathologist, he was interested in exploring the mechanisms of diseases, using as his tools knowledge of cell biology and immunology, as well as pathology, and an understanding of how they could be modified to effect cures. After this, there were numerous appointments to the Institute staff of scientists without ophthalmic backgrounds, or understanding of clinical practice, who nevertheless seemed to assimilate the ophthalmic ideal quickly, as well as a few clinicians like Peng Tee Khaw, able to bridge the gap between pure science, clinical medicine and surgery. Indeed, Khaw was one of the very few of these new appointees to whom the opening words of Barrie Jones' Bowman Lecture of 1975 could be truthfully said to apply:

'He who seeks to become an excellent clinician should, like Bowman, devote himself effectively and totally, to the disciplines he encounters in preparation for medicine; but, like Bowman, must never lose sight of the objective of applying these disciplines to solving the problems that patients present.'

In all truth, however, it was clear that the 'Clinical Interface' (see below) could only make headway if it was supported and nourished by a strong base of knowledge provided by top-quality basic scientists. Nowhere was this more true than in the fields of molecular genetics and cell transplantation, where the arrival of Shomi Bhattacharya, and later of Ray Lund (already a researcher of huge distinction and a Fellow of The Royal Society), underpinned the work of the clinical academics. When, in the latter days of this account, the tide of clinically directed research really turned, the bank of knowledge provided by these outstanding scientists (in Lund's case a legacy, for he soon moved on) was to prove crucial, not only to Alan Bird's work on retinal dystrophies and Peng Tee Khaw's on wound healing, but also to the work of Tony Moore, John Greenwood, Andrew Webster, David Charteris, Lyndon da Cruz and other clinical academics working in related fields.

Alan Bird in particular enjoyed a unique position. His ability to see the wider picture, interpret the relevance of scientific advances to clinical problems and bring these together was fundamental to the development of many of the multidisciplinary initiatives underpinning the future of the Hospital and Institute. This was particularly true where progress in molecular genetics was concerned, a field in which the Institute of Ophthalmology excelled. Bird's international reputation and standing amongst both clinicians and visual scientists was without precedent. The Department of Molecular Genetics, inaugurated in 1992, with Bhattacharya the new Sembal Professor at its head, was largely established as a result of his efforts, producing many high-impact publications and attracting huge amounts of grant income, both of which were key factors in raising the Institute's profile and in its achieving 5* status.

Khaw too was fast becoming a powerful force. A clinical scientist, with initially just two fixed clinical sessions (though he worked many more), and with a sufficiently high rating from the Higher Education Funding Council for England (HEFCE) and a personal Chair to justify his position on the Institute payroll, he yet remained free from the direction of the Clinical Academic Department, preferring to work instead with Luthert in Pathology. So outstanding was his contribution to clinical research, both at the Institute and at the Hospital, not only in wound healing and stem cell research, but also in the field of paediatric glaucoma and new surgical techniques, that he had already at the time of writing, begun to establish a special position amongst the clinical academics.

The new-found reputation of the revitalized Institute, in its brand new buildings on the island site close to Moorfields, swiftly attracted a host of younger academics with excellent credentials, as well as more senior scientists able to attract grant monies and satisfy the periodic attentions of the Research Assessment Boards, although few, were involved directly in clinical work. The new staff were grouped into multidisciplinary divisions, working in different areas of research: molecular genetics, cell biology, pathology, psychophysics, neurophysiology and visual rehabilitation. Both the quality and amount of research increased exponentially, with the result that HEFCE awarded it a grading of 5 in 1993, and subsequently a further rise, to the highest possible level, 5*, which was maintained throughout the remaining 1990s and into the 21st Century.

Meanwhile, the merger with UCL brought its problems, as well as its advantages. Tensions arose, because the Institute was deemed by UCL to be effectively one of its departments and UCL was inclined to think that any spare capacity in the Institute's funds was rightfully its own and could be appropriated accordingly, when the need arose. Even given that grant monies and UGC funding awarded to their employees could be construed as the property of UCL, considerable sums, donated by both the Fight for Sight charity and by Moorfields Special Trustees, were clearly intended for the use of the Institute of Ophthalmology alone. Nor did the aims and objectives of UCL and the Institute always coincide.

On the other hand, as the dust settled and time healed the wounds incurred during the cathartic upheaval of the late 1980s and early 1990s, there were signs that the Hospital and Institute were coming closer together and that shared perspectives were re-emerging. Changes in government policy, with a greater emphasis on research as a tool to improve patient-care, began to have their effect, with shared objectives and common goals enshrined in a Joint Research Strategy. The Research Directors of the Institute and Hospital began to work more closely together, while Adam Sillito supported Hitchings's appointment to a personal academic Chair. Liaison Meetings between the two institutions, comprising Sillito and Phil Luthert, respectively Director and Deputy Director of the Institute, and Sir Thomas Boyd-Carpenter, Ian Balmer and Bill Aylward, respectively Chairman, Chief Executive and Medical Director of the Hospital, began to take on a new dimension.

The Department of Preventive Ophthalmology

The foundation of the International Centre for Eye Health in 1981 was the culminating event of Barrie Jones' lifelong aspiration to demonstrate the importance of prevention rather than cure (**Figure 51**, Plate 26). From his earliest, formative years in medical training, he had been imbued with the desire to translate knowledge and understanding of microbiology and pharmacology into the practical prevention and cure of infectious diseases, especially in the developing world. Success and recognition in the developed world had done nothing to dampen his ardour or lessen this ambition. As early as 1961, he had visited the MRC Research Unit in West Africa, and throughout the 1960s and 1970s had conducted trachoma surveys in the Middle East, including Iran, where demographical data were especially accurate and easy to collate. He was accompanied on these many field trips by a number of ophthalmologists from the UK, including Peter Watson and Arnold Freedman, and also by his wife Pauline and by Zorab Darougar, the latter himself an Iranian citizen with wide connections there. In the late 1970s and early 1980s these expeditions extended to fieldwork on filariasis (onchocerciasis) in Cameroon, and to both trachoma and onchocerciasis in the Sudan.

In 1979 Barrie Jones became the Senior Vice-President of the International Agency for the Prevention of Blindness and he represented that organization on the International Council of Ophthalmology, subsequently (1985) becoming its European Regional Chairman. The titles of many of his lectures and publications, including the 1975 Bowman Lecture, provide supporting evidence (if such be needed) of this passion to seek ways of preventing blinding eye diseases. It was hardly surprising, therefore, that when fate forced on him the opportunity to re-order his life, he should have chosen to make the most of it by founding an institution linking Moorfields and the Institute of Ophthalmology with epidemiology and preventive medicine.

A more prosaic (but charming and entirely believable) explanation for his decision, given to me by Barrie Jones' successor as Professor of Preventive Ophthalmology, Gordon Johnson, is that Pauline Jones said to him one day, during a break in activities on one of the many field-trips: 'when are you going to stop all this research and do something for these people?'

It was not immediately obvious, however, whether such an institution should be based at the Institute of Ophthalmology or at the London School of Hygiene and Tropical Medicine (LSH&TM), where there was already an established infrastructure. In the event, the matter was decided when the latter declined to provide accommodation for the new department and happily the Institute of Ophthalmology was prepared to do so.

The International Centre for Eye Health (ICEH), as it was officially known, and Department of Preventive Ophthalmology, as it was called at the Institute, had the seal of approval of the World Health Organization (WHO) from the outset, and was set up with funding from a number of different sources. With the support of Barrie Jay (a trustee), the Wolfson Foundation financed the refurbishment of premises in Cayton Street, within the building already occupied by the Dean's Department and the Department of Pathology. The Rothes Foundation, via the Fight for Sight charity, provided for the professor's salary. Other salaries were sponsored by the Royal Commonwealth Society for the Blind, later renamed Sight-Savers International (whose director Sir John Wilson was a strong supporter), and the Coca Cola company, whose European director was equally so.

In the mid 1970s Barrie Jones had been joined by a young Iranian-born ophthalmologist, Darwin Minassian, who, imbued with the desire to do serious research and inspired by his example, soon became his right-hand man. Sadly, however, as that decade drew to a close, Zorab Darougar, who had taken charge of the *Chlamydia* microbiological service for the Hospital and who had trained Minassian, became disaffected, falling out with Barrie Jones, Minassian and Moorfields, and playing no further part in the work of the Department of Preventive Ophthalmology. So it was that, until the arrival of Jock Anderson as a lecturer, there were only Barrie Jones and Darwin Minassian in the new department. The Hospital was supportive, however, seeing the need for involving itself in epidemiology and agreeing to provide excellent ophthalmology teaching for the students. The latter came from all over the world, often sponsored by their governments or by non-governmental organizations, such as Sight-Savers, the Christoffel-Blindenmission and the British Council.

A fully integrated teaching programme was designed, with Barrie Jones, Minassian and Anderson all playing equal parts, to instruct students in the skills required to enable them to return to their countries and set up ophthalmic care programmes of their own. The course led to a Diploma in Community Eye Health (DCEH), which was recognized by the WHO, providing the returning doctors with the authority to lead preventive programmes in their own communities.

There was close cooperation with the School of Hygiene, especially with Professor Geoffrey Rose, an eminent epidemiologist and inspiring teacher there, in the training of aspiring preventive ophthalmologists, notably by Darwin Minassian and Jock Anderson, who formed the nucleus of the new teaching department, and, later on, Allen Foster, Gordon Johnson, Clare Gilbert, Richard Wormald, Ian Murdoch and Parul Desai. The standard of research was also high. Indeed, so good was the work of Minassian that he obtained a Wellcome Foundation Fellowship to undertake field studies in cataract in India, which were to form the basis of a case–control study, the first of its kind in the world, the results of which were published in the *Lancet*. The low impact factor of such journals was, however, to prove costly for the department when it came, later on, to the issue of the Institute's RAE ratings.

Barrie Jones himself was involved in every aspect of the new department and with the promotion of measures to prevent blinding eye diseases worldwide, travelling all over the globe on behalf of the WHO and the International Agency for the Prevention of Blindness, and lecturing at international ophthalmological conferences, as well as taking care of the teaching and administration in London. It was a punishing schedule, particularly for a man who had, not so long before, flirted so intimately with death. He nevertheless appeared to thrive on it, giving named lectures too many to recount and finally, in 1985 (and not before time), being made a Commander of the Order of the British Empire (CBE), an honour richly deserved.

As time went by, the DCEH programme was made into a course leading to a Master's degree of London University, and with the retirement of Barrie Jones in 1986, the pattern and ethos of the ICEH began to change. Minassian, Barrie Jones' natural successor, did not want the post of professor, with its administrative and sociopolitical burdens, and did not apply for it. The new Professor, Gordon Johnson, was, as was only to be expected, of a very different character from his predecessor. No less determined and equally unassuming, he had worked for many years in Canada and had been inspired by the ICEH and its founder during a sabbatical trip to the UK. He too had conducted population-based research in remote areas of the globe, but his presence was low-key rather than high-profile.

The new order at the ICEH coincided with the nadir of the Institute's fortunes, so that independent funding was essential for it to survive. The support of Sight-Savers and the Christoffel-Blindenmission was vital, Foster's position and influence with the latter underpinning its future. The teaching courses flourished and went from strength to strength, the ICEH remaining independent of University funding and thereby free from threat. The Dean, Rolf Blach, was strongly supportive of the department. Gordon Johnson, for his part, worked tirelessly to maintain its profile and joined in the clinical work of the Hospital, working in the Glaucoma Out-Patient Department and promoting good relations with the clinical staff.

During Adam Sillito's rise to power and the consequent upturn in the Institute's fortunes during the 1990s, after he became its director, he showed little interest in the Department of Preventive Ophthalmology, leaving it to run its own affairs, funded as it was by its teaching activities. It was clear that he had no personal interest in preventive ophthalmology, but was happy to tolerate the department, as a necessary and cost-free part of the Institute's armamentarium. Relations between him and Johnson were courteous, but cool. When in 1994 Moorfields decided to support epidemiology through the Glaxo donation, the ICEH's position was weakened by the creation of what was, in effect, a rival department of epidemiology at the Hospital. Similarly, five years later, when the Glaxo unit failed, partly for want of the Institute's support, no attempt was made to redirect those resources in the direction of the Preventive Department.

On Gordon Johnson's retirement in 2001 there was no immediate move to replace him, and Fight for Sight ended their support for the Rothes Professorial Chair. Allen Foster, supported by Johnson, seeing the writing on the wall, had already moved to the LSH&TM, in 1999, a venue probably better suited to the teaching programme and one that was only too pleased to take this on. Both Sight-Savers and the Christoffel-Blindenmission also demanded assurances from Adam Sillito that he was unable to give, so that finally Gilbert too decamped to the LSH&TM, leaving behind only Minassian, who had agreed to remain as acting head of the department, and Ian Murdoch, a consultant in the Glaucoma Service with a 50/50 clinical/research contract. Now called simply the Department of Epidemiology of the Institute, this was a sad fate to befall Barrie Jones' visionary concept, and, as its premises lay largely empty and vacant, occupied only by Minassian, it could only be hoped that a new leader would soon be found to rejuvenate it. Meanwhile, at the LSH&TM, Allen Foster was now a full professor and the unit thrived, with huge research grants, the largest trachoma research group in the world, and brand new premises in Bedford Square. Joined there by Clare Gilbert and most of the research fellows, he continued to run the teaching courses, the Resource Centre and the *Journal of Community Eye Health*.

Hospital-based research

The issues surrounding the conduct of clinical research are often controversial and tortuous, exciting, as they do, feelings ranging from indifference and apathy to those of injustice and outrage. From time immemorial, clinicians have attempted, with more or less scientific credibility, to report findings relating to the diagnosis, treatment and outcomes of conditions suffered by their patients. In so doing, they have often employed large amounts of their spare time, without tangible rewards other than the satisfaction afforded by a greater understanding of disease, the gratitude of their patients and the commendation of their peers. Evidence of the willingness to undertake such studies has always been a criterion in the selection process for appointment to a consultant post, particularly one at a teaching hospital. The extra effort expended by clinicians in carrying out clinical research has always been judged as a sign of dedication and commitment likely to enhance the future reputation of the institution to which they are appointed.

Throughout its history, most members of the consultant staff at Moorfields have contributed, more or less energetically, to the publication of clinical papers, originally in hospital reports and subsequently in the annals of national, and occasionally international, ophthalmological societies. Furthermore, they have always been expected to undertake the teaching and training of young ophthalmologists, and have, for the most part, fulfilled these duties well and with enthusiasm. The development first of a medical school, museum and library at the Hospital and, subsequently, at the inception of the NHS, of the Institute of Ophthalmology was an explicit avowal of these objectives. British ophthalmology was fortunate to have leaders in scientific endeavour, like Bowman, Doyne, Davson, Mann and Duke-Elder, who laid the foundations of clinical science, long before it came to assume the importance that it has today. Furthermore, Moorfields and its Institute were lucky, later on, to attract men of the calibre of Norman Ashton, Barrie Jones and Alan Bird, to usher in the new era of clinical science and research. As a result of this fruitful relationship, a spirit of uninhibited enthusiasm and progress reigned during the 1960s and

1970s, and joint activities between clinicians and scientists were commonplace and, for the most part, productive.

In the 1980s everything began to turn sour, partly as a result of the retirement of key figures, as already described, but also for reasons of sociopolitical change. The loss of two such patrician figures as Ashton and Jones could not be borne without detriment. Not only was there no one to replace them, but also the underlying infrastructure was weakened by the loss of Duke-Elder's leadership and of the firm hand of the Institute Secretary, Clifford Seath (who had left in 1976). This meant that many of the previously excellent relationships forged between clinicians at the Hospital and scientists at the Institute broke down, with the consequent demise of collaborative research. Furthermore, the laissez-faire attitudes and lack of accountability fostered by the socialist administrations of Harold Wilson and James Callaghan during the 1960s and 1970s had permeated all aspects of life throughout the UK, and led to the election of a Conservative regime that sought to restore the values of free enterprise and self-sufficiency. Academe was viewed with suspicion and, not without some justification, its value for money was questioned. The Institute of Ophthalmology had lost its way and its financial position was parlous.

The incoming Prime Minister in 1979 could not have been less in the mould of her predecessors, and her instincts favoured tight fiscal control and good housekeeping. After an initial period spent in overcoming some of the excesses of socialist dogma rife at the time of her election, she set about developing firmer management and financial accountability. While Moorfields was well able to respond to this new order, the Institute was poorly equipped to do so. As a result, during the 1980s, the Hospital forged ahead strongly, leaving the Institute to look to its own salvation, a course of action that proved, in the event, to be dangerously short-sighted.

The 1990s turned out to be as testing an era for the Hospital as the 1980s had been for the Institute. Just as the 1960s had been a decade of scientific awakening, the 1970s a period of clinical and technological progress, and the 1980s a time of rebuilding and consolidation, the 1990s were dominated by self-appraisal and introspection. From the time of the 1973 NHS Act, when the postgraduate teaching hospitals escaped the government's net and retained their special status, Moorfields had steered a careful and well-charted course through often-troubled waters. The forward-looking policies pursued by the Board of Governors and the leadership shown by Francis Cumberlege and John Atwill had ensured that it gained Special Health Authority status in 1982. The move towards primary care and the provision of community services driven by Atwill and Bob Cooling had maintained its viability in the face of the Griffiths Report and the creation of Clarke's Internal Market. Even Tomlinson was sufficiently impressed to leave the Hospital unscathed. In some ways, with the retirement of Cumberlege in 1991 and, little more than a year later, that of Atwill, the start of the last decade of the 20th Century marked a watershed in Moorfields' affairs.

Cumberlege's successor as Chairman of the Board of Governors, Hugh Peppiatt, had very different views concerning the respective roles played by the Hospital and the Institute, and was not prepared to take on the Chairmanship of the Institute's Board of Management as had his predecessor. It was Peppiatt's view (and one shared by some members of the consultant body) that having a foot in both the Institute and the Hospital camps posed a conflict of loyalties. He therefore declined to serve on the Institute's Board, feeling that it was his duty, as primarily an officer of the NHS, to defend the Hospital's interests, with particular respect to any financial demands that the Institute might make. Opinions differ with regard to the effect this policy may have had on Hospital/Institute relations throughout the 1990s. It is certainly true to say, however, that after the inception of the Hospital as a Trust in 1994 and the union of the Institute with University College shortly thereafter, the strategic thinking of the two organizations diverged further from one another than ever before, and that the prospect of joint working, far from becoming more of a reality, became for a time less so.

The Hospital/Institute relationship explored

In 1993, just as the Hospital was shaping up to apply for Trust status, attention once again turned towards the Special Health Authorities (SHA) and the justification for their existence. After the peer review of research activities of the seven London postgraduate research institutes instigated by the BPMF, the report of which in 1990 highlighted the plight of its Institute, the spotlight was once again focused on Moorfields itself, leading to embarrassing questions being asked about its extra funding for teaching and research, and the role it played in contributing to joint research output.

Margaret Thatcher's demise from the premiership in 1990 had made no difference to the mood and intention to impose self-governance on hospitals and turn them into self-financing Trusts. In March 1993, less than six months after the Tomlinson Enquiry into London's Medical Education and Research had reported its findings and recommendations (which approved Moorfields' *'imaginative proposal for the development of all ophthalmology services north of the River Thames'*), Michael Peckham, now Director of Research and Development at the

Department of Health, ordered a research review of the SHAs, to assess their ability to sustain their independence as centres of postgraduate excellence. The Review Advisory Committee was headed by Professor Sir Michael Thompson, Vice-Chancellor of Birmingham University, and the Expert Advisory Group delegated to investigate Moorfields contained five ophthalmologists, Professors Easty (Bristol), Fielder (Birmingham), Forrester (Aberdeen) and McLeod (Manchester) and Mr Brian Martin (Leeds).

Moorfields did not come out of this exercise with a great deal of credit. Much of the clinical research described in the Hospital's submission to the Expert Advisory Group was found to be contrived. Only two of its research teams attracted an A+ rating, and a lack of focused research strategy was identified, with poor links between the SHA and its Institute. A number of recommendations were made, including the demonstration of greater commitment to research by the consultant staff, the association of the Institute with a multifaculty school and a greater emphasis on research into conditions relevant to the NHS in general. While there was no immediate threat, implied or otherwise, to force the Hospital into partnership with an undergraduate teaching hospital, as had been mooted in the past, it was clear to all concerned that Moorfields would need to look to its research laurels as a matter of urgency if it was to survive for long as an independent, single-specialty hospital.

In the meantime, several important changes had taken place. As already noted, Noel Rice had taken over from Rolf Blach as Dean in 1991, a post that he was to hold for three years, before handing over the Directorship of the Institute to Adam Sillito. In the same year, Susan Lightman, who headed a very strong ocular immunology programme (graded A+), was appointed to the Professorial Chair founded on the death of Lady Duke-Elder, in Sir Stewart's memory. Lightman had become a vitally important contributor to the research activities of the Hospital. The importance of her work was recognized by both the Institute and the Hospital, although her personal reputation was somewhat marred by clashes of personality and undercurrents of mistrust. Two years later she was appointed to the substantive University Chair of Clinical Ophthalmology, on Barrie Jay's retirement, the Duke-Elder Chair being given to Ray Lund, a world-renowned expert in transplantation techniques, who, as previously noted, was invited to join the Institute's staff to raise its profile in the field of retinal transplantation. Both of these appointments were seen to strengthen the Hospital/Institute relationship, while Alan Bird's stature as Moorfields' and the Institute's ambassador on the world ophthalmic stage further enhanced it. Indeed, the Department of Clinical Ophthalmology was shortly to be restyled the 'Clinical Interface'.

Further apart than ever

Notwithstanding these attempts at joint working, it was apparent that the Institute and the Hospital continued to dance to different tunes and that the perceived inability of the new Trust to carry out research of high quality throughout all parts of the organization, non-medical as well as medical, was a threat to its continued independence. The government's insistence that only basic scientific research of the highest standard qualified for funding did little to improve the situation. With Professor Sillito now indisputably at the Institute's helm, Noel Rice assumed the role of Director of Research and Teaching at the Hospital, which set out to justify its application for Trust status by including in its prospectus a research strategy comprising cell biology, immunology, molecular biology, molecular genetics, neurobiology and pharmacology, visual psychophysics, and epidemiology. Fortified by the appointment of its own Director of Research and armed with this hastily assembled programme for future collaborative research with its academic partner, the Hospital was able to demonstrate that it had the capacity to remain (uniquely) an independent, single-specialty, postgraduate teaching hospital. Application to the Secretary of State was successful and in April 1994 the Hospital became a NHS Trust.

Moorfields now saw itself as a more independent organization, which indeed it was, and although it stood to benefit indirectly from collaborative research, it could not afford to be encumbered by dependence on the Institute or be beholden to UCL. There was a paramount need to develop and expand its own research strategy, in conformity with that outlined in its Trust application prospectus. Nor could it rely on the contribution of clinical academics developing collaborative projects, because the reborn Institute's recruitment policy, driven by the demands imposed on it by the Research Assessment Exercises, did not permit the employment of clinical lecturers. The only clinical academics on the Institute pay-roll were now Professors Bird, Lightman, Luthert and Khaw, all major figures on the national and international stages and each attracting large amounts of grant monies in their own right, but nonetheless under the direction of Adam Sillito, and subject to review by the HEFCE panel like everyone else in the Institute's employ. Even the Duke-Elder Chair was now occupied by a pure scientist under Professor Sillito's direction.

It may be pertinent here to outline, in the broadest terms, the funding policy of the University Grants Committee (UGC) towards the research institutes within its remit. The Research Assessment Exercises (RAEs), conducted at three- to five-year intervals, were designed to take into account the quality of publications and grant monies attracted by individual workers, the standard expected being extremely high, and consequently rarely achievable by clinical academics doing part-time research amongst their clinical commitments. All staff having a university title (e.g. Lecturer), whether paid by the University or by the Hospital, had to be included in the RAEs. This meant that only those producing research of sufficient quality, and in sufficient quantity, to satisfy the panel were able to contribute positively to the research assessment rating. In addition, the overall funding provided to an institution by the UGC depended on the total number of employees recognized by the HEFCE panel at the time of the assessment. It was therefore essential that any changes in the number of staff, whether by dint of retirements, resignations or appointments, were made well before the RAE took place, or the 'volume' of the workforce recognized by the UGC might not match the reality, and the institution might thereby risk being underfunded for up to five years.

In fact, an example of such a problem was to occur in the year 2000. The Director of the Institute, thinking well ahead and wishing to make an appointment to a clinical research post, shared between the Institute and the Hospital, to replace a high-profile clinical academic who was shortly due to retire, somewhat hastily invited two extremely distinguished and senior clinical academics to apply (thereby pre-empting the forthcoming RAE), in the belief that the Hospital would approve the appointment of either candidate. This was not the case, however, the Hospital having reservations about the clinical component of the joint post and its costs, both in terms of finance and of clinical risk. The Director's attempt to put pressure on the Board of Directors of the Trust, with the complicit involvement of its Chairman, Dr Leila Lessof, led eventually to Dr Lessof's resignation and to much confusion and embarrassment all round.

The employment of any but the most prestigious and well-established of scientists was discouraged, HEFCE demanding at least four publications in journals with an impact factor of four or higher, thereby excluding most papers published in clinical journals. For the Institute to maintain its 5★ ranking, therefore, Professor Sillito could only afford to engage top-grade scientists, so clinical academics all but disappeared from the academic departments. The work of outstanding scientists such as Shomi Bhattacharya in molecular genetics, Ray Lund in retinal transplantation and Fred Fitzke in psychophysical imaging was designed to back up that of the clinical academics and was a strategic direction of vital importance for the future of the Institute. Multidisciplinary teams of scientists to underpin core areas of ophthalmic research were an essential principle of the strategy drawn up by Michael Peckham, Noel Rice and Adam Sillito in the late 1980s. Nevertheless, this did not always seem to be helpful or relevant at a clinical level. Strictly patient-orientated clinical research could now only be undertaken by very exceptionally talented and committed people with relatively circumscribed clinical commitments, such as Bird, Lightman and Khaw. The result was that the Institute was no longer as clinically driven as many would have liked, 'blue-skies' research, often clinically related, but not strictly relevant to a specific disease, being the order of the day. Such criticism may later appear to have been misguided, if the pioneering work of Robin Ali in gene therapy, Steve Moss in cell biology and Santa Ono in immunology proves in the coming years to be successful in producing novel treatments. Indeed, the key to unlocking the store of talent, knowledge and expertise at the Institute, and allying it to the wealth of clinical acumen and spirit of enquiry amongst young consultant staff, might well rest in the Hospital's hands, and in the way it responds to the future demands of its political masters and their apparent obsession with service targets.

The quest for accountability

Following on from the development of stringent controls over money provided to the research institutes, which had its origins in the 1980s, a similar process developed with respect to their associated clinical partners. In the early 1990s, in a move towards greater accountability, all hospitals were required to undertake clinical audit. Furthermore, under the Patients' Charter introduced by John Major's government, waiting times, responses to GPs' letters and a host of other data were required to be collated and reviewed. This ponderous and time-consuming move towards a more 'hands-on' approach to the management of clinical resources was shortly to be mirrored by an equally bureaucratic oversight of clinical research.

Thus Moorfields was soon to find itself the subject of intense enquiry into the way in which money provided to it for research and teaching was utilized. It had emerged from the 1993 Research Review that there were fundamental weaknesses in the funding arrangements of the SHAs, whereby additional monies provided to them for research and teaching sometimes found their way instead into the general pool, to support cash-strapped patient services. This was perfectly understandable, given the consistent under-funding of the NHS over the previous two decades, but it was nevertheless clearly a misapplication of funds that could not be countenanced. One of the members of the Research Review's Advisory Committee, Professor Anthony Culyer, from the Department of Economics in York, was therefore asked to conduct a review of the way in which funding was distributed, throughout the NHS, and to come up with a mechanism for ensuring that it went where it was supposed to.

The Culyer Report, published in 1994, recommended that all hospitals (now NHS Trusts) should report on their research activities annually, and justify their research funding. The funding itself was to come from a levy on purchasers' allocations nationally and would be divided into three categories: (1) for direct and indirect costs of research and development (R&D) projects, (2) for associated service costs and (3) for maintenance of facilities and staff enabling such R&D programmes, but not specific to any single project. Initially, the 'Culyer' funding for each Trust was based on the previous annual allocation (so-called 'grandfather accounting'), but thereafter it was subject to stringent examination, and the Trust was required to demonstrate its ability to gain research grants equivalent to the sum allocated by the Department of Health (the levy) from other sources, such as the Medical Research Council or the Wellcome Foundation. Culyer made it clear that in order to be supported, NHS R&D must (a) be relevant to the aims of the NHS, (b) follow a clear protocol, (c) be subject to peer review, (d) be properly managed, (e) report its findings and (f) be generally applicable.

In common with so many initiatives set in motion as a result of political intervention, 'Culyer', as it became generally known, was changed, on the election of New Labour in 1997, to a somewhat different system of financial management, designated 'Support for Science, Priorities and Needs', a title impervious to the application of eponym or acronym alike. The importance of hospital research was now obvious and the need for skilful management of the Trust's resources paramount. Monies designated for Support for Science could be used only to fund supporting facilities, such as the remuneration of nurses taking blood samples for pure science research projects, while those for priorities and needs could be used to fund the infrastructure for clinically orientated research, but not for salaries. In each case, the use of the funds had to be precisely identified and a formula used to dictate how much was to be allocated.

Close monitoring of research activities within NHS Trusts, including Moorfields, with precise protocols and detailed audit trails for all projects, continued from the mid-1990s, openness and accountability being the watchwords of the day. Never again was there to be internal allocation of locally organized research funds or informal audits carried out 'on a whim', by clinical staff. From now on, specific questions were to be asked, such as: 'What is the need? What don't we know? What will be the improvement in clinical practice as a result?' and a clearly defined outcome reported, supplying the answers: the 'knowledge circle'. Such a change in the direction and performance of clinical research was deemed to be necessary, if improvements in patient care were to accrue as a result of government funding. Indeed, New Labour were to prove as determined as the Tories, if not more so, to obtain 'value for money'.

A major restructuring of the Hospital's research programme was undertaken in the wake of the Culyer report, to justify the existing level of funding and to create more opportunities for research that would attract further funding. In November 1994 the Glaxo Department of Epidemiology opened; this was a Hospital-based Institute facility, financed by a £1.45m donation to Fight for Sight from Glaxo Holdings, originally made four years earlier to finance an extension of the Department of Preventive Ophthalmology. A senior clinician with an epidemiological background was sought to head the new department, and Richard Wormald, a consultant ophthalmologist with a Master's degree in epidemiology, who had done several research studies in glaucoma and was already on the staff of the Western Eye Hospital, seemed to fit the bill. He was duly appointed, with a brief to study, under the general direction of Professor Sillito, the incidence, causes and prevention of eye diseases in specific groups of people in the UK, with the expectation that he would attract additional funding, as time went by, to build up the department and produce results in this area of epidemiological research. This did not happen, and after five years Sillito made it plain that he was no longer prepared to support the venture. The department therefore closed, its erstwhile director retaining his position as coordinating editor of the Cochrane Eyes and Vision Group and remaining on the consultant staff as a glaucoma specialist and cataract surgeon, while the Institute recaptured the Glaxo funding. The Department of Preventive Ophthalmology, already marginalized and keeping itself afloat by dint of fees charged to students from overseas, with little support from within the Institute, thus found itself also deprived of the funds that should have come its way from Glaxo's generous donation to promote preventive ophthalmology.

On the retirement of Noel Rice in 1996, Roger Hitchings, who headed one of the A+ ranked research teams of the 1993 review (glaucoma), took over as acting Director of Research while a permanent director from outside the Trust was sought. A highly qualified candidate, Professor Chris Patterson, was eventually appointed to the post and a suite of offices provided for him on the second floor of the Hospital. Sadly, however, the hoped-for improvements in the management, funding and output of hospital-based research failed to materialize. Patterson was not a clinician and did not appear to understand the politics surrounding clinical research in the UK, nor did he appear to be wholly committed to the task, so it was hardly surprising that the direction of clinical research failed to improve under his stewardship. After a period of disappointing performance and a bout of serious illness, he resigned. His place was taken by Roger Hitchings, this time as a substantive appointment, with excellent results – so much so that by 1998–99, largely by dint of strict identification of research monies and control over their allocation, nearly 10% of the Trust's core income was seen to come from research funding.

Hitchings saw the need to foster young ophthalmologists, interested in undertaking high quality research work, by giving them time and resources to enable them to do this from a clinical standpoint. It was he and Bob Cooling who had the vision to see that the Trust should provide both time and resources, by directing the 'Culyer' monies towards those ends, in the shape of research sessions, laboratory space and back-up facilities for new consultants, and together they convinced the Special Trustees to provide financial support to enable them to 'pump-prime' this exercise.

A new dawn

Reference has already been made to the low priority that the Hospital gave to research activities during the 1980s. Clinicians were not actively encouraged to spend time in research and little provision was made for them to do so. Moreover, such was the influence of past tradition and culture that consultants were not discouraged from spending time away from the Hospital, in private practice. Now, following the change in political thinking started by Margaret Thatcher in the 1980s and continued under Tony Blair during the late 1990s and on into the new millennium, accountability to the NHS and a new emphasis on evidence-based medicine, with the involvement of patients in decisions about their treatment, were the watchwords of the day. The Trust responded, not only by offering consultant posts with funded sessions for research but also with contracts of employment that were more prescriptive, both clinical and other activities being explicitly spelt out. In some cases up to four sessions were designated for research, funded initially by the Special Trustees, while the Hospital provided greatly improved facilities on site, for consultants to pursue private practice without leaving the premises.

Secondly, in 1998, £2m was given by the Special Trustees, towards the costs of development of Phase VIa of the new Institute buildings to provide shared accommodation for collaborative studies between Hospital researchers and Institute scientists, thereby demonstrating the Trust's commitment to shared working. These initiatives resulted in a number of fruitful collaborations, in particular that between Peng Tee Khaw and Phil Luthert in the Department of Pathology, in the fields of cell biology, wound healing and stem cell research. The more notable research initiatives were recognized, by the award of Professorial Chairs to Fred Fitzke (a pure scientist working closely with Alan Bird and Roger Hitchings in psychophysics), Khaw and Hitchings, and the election to the Academy of Medical Sciences of Professors Bird, Khaw and Lightman (Professors Sillito and Bhattachyra were already Fellows of the Academy).

The increased output of high-quality clinical research was successful in ensuring that funding from government sources and research grants was not only maintained but actually increased. Newly appointed consultants with paid sessions for research, such as Bruce Allan, David Charteris, Ted Garway-Heath and Ian Murdoch working in the new shared facility at the Institute, and Frank Larkin at Imperial College, joined the clinical academics Professors Bird, Lightman and Khaw, and those like Andrew Webster on Wellcome Fellowships, in producing important work. Supervision and coordination of projects undertaken by Fellows on 'soft' monies were meticulously undertaken by the Hospital's Director of Research. When Ray Lund vacated the Duke-Elder Chair and moved to the USA in 2001, a new clinical academic appointment was made, Tony Moore joining the Institute as Duke-Elder Professor, with special interests in genetics and paediatrics.

The appointment of Roger Hitchings to the post of Director of Research for the Hospital in 1998 heralded a brighter future for the Trust's research activities. Nevertheless, it was plain to Hitchings that, although he could see what needed to be done, he had few tools at his disposal with which to do it. He soon discovered that the data provided to the National Register of Research Projects, as required following publication of the Culyer Report, was not only inaccurate but also seriously incomplete. The management of the department was under the supervision of the Director's secretary, poorly equipped for the Herculean task ahead. In short, the Hospital had been concentrating its resources too much on the directorship and superstructure, to the detriment of the basic and essential infrastructure required to achieve practical results.

The effects of the Culyer Report's recommendations were not really felt until 1997, and even then, and on through 1998, it was possible to muddle through by applying a 'grandfather' formula, simply justifying funding on the basis of previous allocations. Hitchings realized that this could not go on. He needed a 'right-hand man' to manage the research department. By great good fortune (as it turned out), just such a person was seeking just such a position. Her name was Sue Lydeard. With a background in biological sciences, she had drifted gradually towards medical and research management, first in a general practice research project and then in audit and quality management at Southampton University NHS Trust. From there she went, on a 'dream ticket', to the Royal Postgraduate Medical School at the Hammersmith Hospital, an academic Trust with a research budget in excess of £40m, as Research and Audit Manager, only to find the dream become a nightmare when, after two years, the post was radically restructured. Thus it was that, in August 1999, just at the moment that Moorfields advertised, she was looking for a new job and she applied for and was appointed to the post of Research Manager.

The partnership of Sue Lydeard with Roger Hitchings worked well from the outset, Hitchings with his academic brilliance, talent for delegation and ability to see the big picture, and Lydeard with her skill at mastering complicated facts and formulae, allied to formidable powers of organization and ability to inspire her staff. To complement this successful duo, in December 2000 John Dart assumed the role of Deputy Director of Research at the Hospital. The Department began not only to thrive but also to expand and develop. In purely physical terms, the space devoted to research increased dramatically. With the rapid increase in day-surgery, wards were being closed and space was available for re-allocation, so Parsons Ward became the Glaucoma Research Department and then, when the Glaxo Department was closed down by the Institute, in 2000, the space it had occupied reverted to the Hospital and that too was incorporated into the Hospital's Research Department. A reading centre, for scanning and grading images, and a statistics service were inaugurated, the Research Directorate soon employing close to 20 members of staff, funded via the Trust from research monies.

Sue Lydeard introduced a Management Action Plan (MAP), incorporating a database containing relevant information, including detailed and accurate costs required for the National Register, relating to all projects approved by the Hospital's Research Department.

The previous Culyer allocation from the NHS Executive, of £3.8m, matched equally by funding from other sources, increased over the next three years, so that the total figure was nearly £10m. Support for research, provided by the Special Trustees and Friends of Moorfields, was additional to this figure. All research was required to be non-commercial and externally peer-reviewed, and passed by the Governance and Ethics Committees, when indicated. No project could go ahead without the agreement of the Hospital's Research Director.

The quality and quantity of clinically based research increased exponentially. Although the majority of this still emanated from the Clinical Interface Group, Professors Bird and Lightman in the Department of Clinical Ophthalmology, and Peng Tee Khaw in Pathology, an increasing proportion came from the consultants in 50/50 clinical/research posts and others at a more junior level, so that by 2002, more than 230 members of the hospital staff were registered by the Research Department as 'research-active professionals'.

The award to Hitchings of a personal academic Chair, funded by the International Glaucoma Foundation and supported by Professor Sillito, was formal recognition of the change in balance between Hospital and Institute, although the relationship between the Directors of Research of the Institute and Hospital at first remained somewhat distant. Nevertheless, after three years or so there was a detectable improvement, as government policy with respect to research and its applicability to patient care and outcomes of treatment began to change. It was becoming increasingly apparent that research (and its funding) was no longer being judged only by its 5* quality but also on its relevance to clinical outcomes. This welcome change in outlook was encapsulated in the new Joint Hospital/Institute Research Strategy document, entitled 'From Basic Science to Better Sight' and it seemed that the happy relations enjoyed by the two institutions in earlier times could once again be just around the corner.

The International Children's Eye Centre

Changes in the management of sick children, introduced throughout the UK during the previous 10 years, had had a huge impact on the provision of paediatric services at Moorfields, where more than 20 000 children were already being seen and over 1500 undergoing surgery annually. For some time, it had not been acceptable for children to share either out-patient or in-patient facilities with adults. No longer was it considered acceptable for anaesthetics to be administered to children by anaesthetists not specifically trained and experienced in paediatric anaesthesia. Nor was it considered safe for surgeons who did not have the opportunity to do so regularly to operate on children.

As well as the common eye problem of childhood squint, a growing number of other paediatric eye conditions had begun to take centre stage. Very significant advances had been made in the treatment of paediatric glaucoma by Peng Tee Khaw, now a world leader in this field, building on the work of Arthur Lister and Noel Rice. John Hungerford had continued and advanced the work on retinoblastoma pioneered by Stallard. In other specialized fields, however, it was simply not possible for a surgeon to develop a great deal of special experience in conditions that were uncommon even in adults and only rarely occurred in children. The removal of paediatric ophthalmology from the mainstream threatened to be a two-edged sword, access to specialized expertise being obstructed by rigid dogma and political interference, accruing as a result of the widespread alarm engendered by highly publicized cases of medical and administrative mismanagement.

The need for a paediatric centre had long been recognized, and for a considerable period of the 1990s efforts had been made by Moorfields to encourage the development of a joint paediatric facility with the Hospital for Sick Children at Great Ormond Street. Understandably, the consultants in the eye unit there were not keen to work on two sites instead of one and were perhaps wary of losing autonomy, given Moorfields' geographical proximity, high profile, and reputation for expansion. The development of an International Children's Eye Centre (ICEC) on the island site in City Road, financed by charitable donations, was therefore a natural course for Moorfields to pursue, and a fine project with which to mark its entry into the new millennium (**Figure 52**, Plate 26). It was anticipated that this would provide facilities for out-patient services, day-case surgery and clinical research, as well as a hostel for patients and their families, while in-patient cases and surgery could, if policy so dictated, be undertaken at Barts and the Royal London Hospital, where comprehensive general paediatric facilities were already available. The appointment of Professor Tony Moore brought much needed expertise in genetics and phenotyping, following the retirements of Barrie and Marcelle Jay, and it was agreed that he should take over as director of the new ICEC, when it was completed. There were to be close links with the Institutes of Ophthalmology and Child Health, at both of which Moore already held appointments.

Fund-raising for the ICEC project was entirely private, without any support from the NHS. Ian Balmer, House Governor, and Lady Jacomb, of the Friends of Moorfields, were instrumental in driving it forward and raising funds, demonstrating the heavy reliance on independent, rather than state, support required in the future. The McKinsey Management Consultants' review of the future direction of the Institute of Ophthalmology, due at the time of going to press, was expected to reflect this. The gross reduction in MRC funding of UK research could well change the emphasis of the Institute's research programme and swing it back towards much greater clinical relevance (with less dependence on achieving the highest grades in the RAEs).

In the course of time, the consultant ophthalmologists at Great Ormond Street (David Taylor, Isabelle Russell-Eggitt and Ken Nischal) showed greater interest in the ICEC and a stronger desire to work there, alongside the Moorfields staff. Tony Moore was able to build bridges between the clinical and academic institutions, the Great Ormond Street consultants having honorary appointments at Moorfields and sharing an on-call rota with Moore and Alison Davies, and the academics at the Institute of Child Health sharing their work with the Institute of Ophthalmology. The new Paediatric Service at Moorfields now encompassed not only the experience and expertise of a paediatrician (Alison Salt) and paediatric ophthalmologists, but also had access to paediatric ophthalmic epidemiology (Jugnoo Rahi) and basic science (Robin Ali) in paediatric ophthalmology.

Architects for the project were appointed, and there was every chance that work would be able to start on demolishing Fryer House and clearing the proposed site in Peerless Street in 2005, and of the building being opened in 2006 or 2007. The prospect of a paediatric research facility, enjoying the combined knowledge and enthusiasm of Tony Moore, Peng Tee Khaw and the clinical academics at the Institute of Child Health, together with the combined expertise of consultant paediatric ophthalmologists, paediatricians and researchers of all kinds at both Moorfields and the Hospital for Sick Children, was an exciting one. It had long been a goal to strengthen paediatric ophthalmology at Moorfields by establishing strong links with GOS, and to provide research facilities in this field on the Hospital/Institute campus. It now seemed that the dream could soon become reality, through a development that would underpin the future of both Hospitals

PART 4

The Organization

PART 4

The Organization

CHAPTER 7

Management and Administration

Management

Board of Governors

Moorfields acquired a Board of Governors in 1948 when it lost its charitable status and became a teaching hospital in the new NHS. The Board consisted of a broad range of individuals, invited to join at the instigation of its Chairman, providing thereby a wide compass of opinion and philosophy. Inevitably, amongst a group numbering as many as 20 people, a cabal of the most committed and forceful, including the Chairman, the House Governor, the Chairman of the Medical Committee, and one or two others with strong views or axes to grind, formed a small hegemony that tended to chart and steer the Hospital's course (much as was imposed by statute 40 years later). It appeared to work well.

In 1964 Arthur Gray, a slightly austere, patrician figure with a powerful reputation for honesty and straight dealing, took over as House Governor, and four years later, Francis Cumberlege, a tea broker by profession, was appointed Chairman of the Board. In the late 1960s and early 1970s the NHS was enjoying a period of calm before the coming storm, and while the ophthalmic world was being upturned by Barrie Jones, Lorimer Fison and others, the Hospital as an organization remained serene and unmoved. As detailed elsewhere, Cumberlege was an excellent Chairman, while Gray, although he might have appeared at first glance to live up to his name, was a kind, wise and far-sighted administrator. Meanwhile, the Medical Committee, under the able chairmanship of Alex Cross, exercised huge influence and drove ahead much needed changes in ophthalmic practice. Even when the government decided to modernize the NHS in 1973–74, Moorfields escaped serious injury. The soundness of its infrastructure, although sometimes appearing to impede the rapid advance of scientific discovery, enabled the latter to take place against a background of solid self-assurance that countered any tendency for the waves of change to damage or destabilize it. Even though much of the administrative framework was archaic and inadequate by today's standards (the House Governor's Personal Assistant, Maureen Hamilton-Smith, and administrative secretary, Wendy Meade, ran the Hospital virtually single-handed, from a small office piled to the ceiling with papers), things seemed to get done without greater delay or aggravation than is the case today.

The mid-1970s were to see a huge change. In 1974 Gray retired and was replaced as House Governor, briefly by GDE Wooding-Jones and then in 1976 by John Atwill. Cumberlege remained Chairman of the Board and the decision to amalgamate the two branches of the Hospital was ratified by the Department of Health. From then on, Moorfields began to take on a new shape altogether, the palpable excitement of being involved in redesigning the Hospital for the future attracting a number of strong and committed individuals, prepared to take on managerial and administrative roles. The emergence of several new stars was evident in the firmament of this brave new world. Atwill himself, true to character, threw himself into the fray, as did Cumberlege, while the Medical Committee at the City Road branch was no less pro-active, under the astute and energetic leadership of Desmond Greaves. Lawrence Green headed up the all-important Planning Committee, while David Hill, Noel Rice, John Wright, Arthur Steele and, later, Bob Cooling, became chairmen of important sub-committees, assisted by lay members of the Board such as Reg Fryer and Jean Smith (**Figure 53**).

Although the Hospital was thrown into some disarray during the 1980s as a result of the rebuilding, it was, by good fortune, not subjected to much in the way of political interference. An unhappy (and mercifully brief) episode involving strike action by the portering staff, threatening its closure, had been narrowly averted in the mid-1970s by the efforts and combined wisdom and experience of Sally Sherman, Reg Fryer and Jean Smith, and Atwill soon overcame the hostility of a small, militantly radical, socialist cell by introducing modern management procedures. After that, the attention and efforts of the Board were concentrated on the redevelopment of the Hospital on the City Road site. Throughout the 1980s, this work went on apace, its progress depending on the hard work, goodwill and commitment of the dedicated group from the Board, both lay and medical. Desmond Greaves remained Chairman of the Medical Committee for two consecutive terms and was ably followed in the post by Noel Rice. Their chairmanship was crucial to keeping the medical staff informed during this turbulent period, and in maintaining close cooperation between the consultant body and the Board. The office doors of Cumberlege and Atwill, both of whom were natural listeners and communicators, were

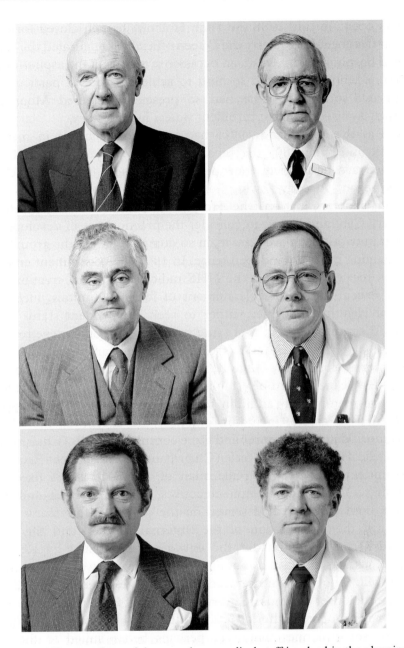

Figure 53 Key members of the consultant medical staff involved in the planning of the redevelopment of the Hospital on City Road during the period 1978–88. (*top row, left*) Mr Desmond Greaves; (*top row, right*) Professor David Hill; (*middle row, left*) Mr Noel Rice; (*middle row, right*) Mr John Wright; (*bottom row, left*) Mr Arthur Steele; (*bottom row, right*) Mr Robert Cooling.

always open. In July 1988 the High Holborn branch closed for ever, and in October Her Majesty the Queen officially inaugurated the refurbished hospital at City Road, an occasion symbolic of the aspirations of everyone who had worked so hard to achieve it, but in particular of those two individuals who had so presciently steered Moorfields through some of the most turbulent waters in its history.

Just as the 1960s and 1970s had seen great changes in medical science, and the 1980s the reconstitution of the fabric, the 1990s heralded a sociopolitical transformation not seen since the Welfare State began. Already, owing to John Atwill's foresight and Bob Cooling's determination, the Hospital had espoused the cause of Primary Care and begun to consider the practicalities of developing a community outreach eye-service, in so doing preparing the ground for maintaining its future independence. In 1991 the government enacted powers to alter the face of the NHS radically, with the creation of a NHS Executive and the clear intent of forcing hospitals, including Special Health Authorities, either to seek independent status or to forfeit their autonomy. In that same year Francis Cumberlege reached the age of retirement, and his place as Chairman of the Board of Governors was taken by Hugh Peppiatt. The new NHS Act demanded that a new, leaner Board be established, with six executive and six non-executive members in addition to the Chairman, and this Peppiatt proceeded to create, including amongst the executives the House Governor, Matron, Treasurer and three consultants, Fells (Chairman of the Medical Committee), Steele (Chairman of the In-Patient Executive Committee) and Cooling (Chairman of the Out-Patient Executive Committee). Among the non-executives were John Bach and Jean Smith, both of whom had served on the old Board for many years. However, the introduction of the 'Internal Market' and the move towards Trust status, under the new regime initiated by Kenneth Clarke, with its associated mountain of paperwork, was a step too far for Atwill, who soon announced his resignation, and in 1993 Ian Balmer took over as House Governor and Chief Executive.

Balmer brought to the job quite different skills from those of his predecessor and ones that were perhaps better suited to the new conditions imposed by the purchaser/provider split and the move to independent Trust status. He had already worked at Moorfields under John Atwill as a planning officer, at the start of his career, before going on to a more senior post at a large London Teaching Hospital, and had then spent some time in the private sector. He was thus in a good position to judge Moorfields' fitness for Trust status and had the necessary marketing skills to present the case convincingly. It was soon apparent that he also had a shrewd strategic sense, allied with innate political judgement. Bob Cooling, with John Lee and John Dart, had in 1990, at Atwill's behest, prepared a Strategic Plan for the Hospital's clinical future, and Balmer and Cooling, supported by Hugh Peppiatt and the Board, were to work well together in pursuing its aims. The move towards provision of Primary Care and Outreach Community Services was directly in line with government thinking. In 1993 Moorfields' application was accepted by the Secretary of State, and in April 1994 it became Moorfields NHS Trust. The Hospital had turned another new corner.

Moorfields NHS Trust

As Atwill had presaged, becoming a Trust brought with it the threat of administrative mayhem. Nevertheless, the Hospital managed not only to keep its head above water but also to expand the range and scope of its services throughout North Thames Region. Executive power was now invested in the Chief Executive (Ian Balmer) and Medical Director (Bob Cooling). The Board was now a Board of Directors, consisting of Balmer, Cooling and three other executive members (the Director of Nursing (also deputy Chief Executive), the Director of Finance, and the Director of Research and Teaching), and six non-executive members, headed by the Chairman (**Figure 54**, Plate 27). Of the previous non-executives, only John Bach and the chairman, Hugh Peppiatt, remained. They were joined by Rosalind Gilmore, Jude Goffe, Clive Nickolds and the Director of the Institute, Adam Sillito. This Board was a strongly representative group, with a powerful mix of high intelligence, wide interests and influential connections, while Bach, its Deputy Chairman and most senior and experienced non-executive member, was seen as a firm anchor in unpredictable seas. A senior partner in a respected firm of solicitors, he had been the Chairman of the Hospital's Ethics Committee for some years and was widely regarded as both the keeper of its conscience and as a bastion of truth and probity.

The shift of power towards the Medical Director (MD) and Chief Executive Officer (CEO), and away from the Medical Committee (mouthpiece of the consultant body), meant that the latter had only an advisory role, its chairman carrying no executive weight, and so it was retitled the Medical Advisory Committee (MAC). Executive responsibility now rested with the Clinical Management Board (chaired by the MD), consisting of the CEO, the Director of Nursing, other senior managers and the directors of the specialist clinical services, and with the Management Executive (chaired by the CEO), consisting of senior managers only.

This move away from consensus management by consultants was inevitable, given the government's determination to play a greater part in decision making and to hand over more and more power to the lay public, while demanding greater accountability from the medical profession. So-called independence, as embodied in the new NHS Trusts, clearly had its price. The huge increase in their numbers that took place during the 1990s and into the new millennium was in any case bound to reduce the power of individual consultants. Methods adopted by Moorfields to ensure managerial representation at all levels went some way towards compensating for the loss of autonomy and professional integrity felt by the doctors, but many still considered that the ethos with which the Hospital had been imbued throughout its history had been irrevocably compromised.

A Director of Contracting and Strategic Development was appointed, to negotiate and manage contracts with Health Authorities (more than one hundred) and with GP fund-holding practices (several thousand), and also a Director of Personnel. The latter, Ken Gold, with considerable experience in personnel management in both the commercial sector and the NHS, arrived to find a world about which he had only heard tell and which more than lived up to that reputation. In his own words, he found an organization that was '*cash-rich, outside the mainstream, old-fashioned and insular*'. It seemed to him that all decisions were taken by half a dozen people and that the management development culture was old-fashioned, with little devolvement of responsibility and middle managers who were there but were not really managing. At the same time, '*there was brilliant research and teaching, the medical staff were all rowing in the same direction and there was a prevailing ethos and sense of pride in an institution that was the best hospital in the country, if not the world*'.

On the personnel front it was easy to put things in order, because '*one was pushing against an open door*', but other aspects of the new administration were not so easily tackled. The Director of Contracting and Strategic Development, Brian Benson, who had come from the commercial sector in order to do something more meaningful with his life, found it difficult to get to grips with the commissioning process, whereby the purchasers could dictate their terms, without fear of sanctions if they reneged on their commitments at a later stage. It was hard to develop the quick-thinking and toughness required to dominate negotiations, and the commissioning process broke down on more than one occasion, exposing the Trust to some risk of an embarrassing deficit in its finances. David Rhys-Tyler, the Treasurer, while apparently highly competent, kept his own counsel and gave away little information. This had not previously had too bad an effect, when conditions were stable and plans could be laid far ahead, but in the new culture, in which the Trust lived 'from hour to hour and day-to-day', revenue came in at somewhat unpredictable moments, depending on the finances and priorities of purchasers, so the Treasurer now needed to be light on his feet and quick to explain the day to day situation. This David Rhys-Tyler was either unable or unwilling to do and consequently, although he always managed to balance the books – so that (unlike most other Trusts in London) Moorfields was never overspent at the year end – there was a gradual loss of confidence in his ability to demonstrate this to the Board's satisfaction. In 1996 he left the Trust by mutual consent, and his place was taken, after a brief interregnum, by his deputy Ian Knott. The latter proved to be every bit as competent as his former boss, but with the advantage that he was able and readily prepared to communicate his plans and predictions cogently to the Board.

The new Personnel Department managed all staff apart from the nurses, the Director of Nursing declining to relinquish control over the latter, a decision that was later to have an impact on the Hospital's plans for restructuring management in the new millennium. Middle-grade managers were now empowered to make their own decisions when appropriate, without reference to senior managers, and career development was encouraged and facilitated more actively. Many members of staff, such as Jane Taylor, Grainne Barron, Donna Sheppard and Patricia Wood, went on to more senior posts, either within the Trust or outside, while some, like Kate Rumble and later on Mary Ryan, who both moved from senior nursing posts into full-time management, even crossed professional boundaries. The divisional restructuring that was to come later enabled even greater career development opportunities, junior and middle-grade managers from nursing, finance and general management posts moving upwards into more senior positions.

When New Labour came to power in 1997, they promised to reverse the processes initiated by their predecessors. Needless to say, given that many of these were the inevitable consequences of the relentless march of progress, these revisions were often composed more of window-dressing than of substance. One consequence of the political turn-around that had potentially damaging effects, however, was the decision not to re-appoint Hugh Peppiatt at the end of his second term, but to replace him with a Chairman more acceptable to the NHS's new political masters. Dr Leila Lessof had acquired a taste for management while working as a consultant radiologist, and, seeing that to achieve a senior management position, as a doctor, could best be achieved by becoming a Public Health Physician, she retrained in Public Health Medicine, rising to become Director of Public Health in the London Borough of Islington and subsequently in Parkside. After 15 years she retired, but two years later, on the Labour Party's return to power, she was invited to become the Chairman at Moorfields. Sadly, her tenure of the post was a brief and troubled one.

Looking back with the benefit of hindsight, it is easy to see what went wrong. At first, apart from a tendency to interfere where others knew better, there were no serious problems. True, she does not seem to have felt at ease with her colleagues on the Board, by all accounts being at odds with most of them to one degree or another, while they had some cause to doubt her judgement. There were no major repercussions, however, until the occasion when they questioned the wisdom of ratifying the joint Hospital/Institute appointment of a senior academic. Dr Lessof was so sure in her own mind of the wisdom of the appointment that she (perhaps naively) felt that it was her place to drive it through, regardless of the views of her colleagues. In the event, however, the other members of the Board were unanimously against the proposal and were incensed by the Chairman's apparent attempts to act unilaterally. The non-executive directors, in particular, felt that she had let them down and the CEO was obliged to inform the Regional Chairman that she had lost the confidence of the Board. Thus it was that, in July 2000, after only three years in the post, Dr Lessof resigned.

The Secretary of State's choice for the new Chairman was a man as experienced and well-versed in the ways of the NHS and the complexities of its management as his predecessor had been maladroit. Sir Thomas Boyd-Carpenter came with a distinguished record of service in both Her Majesty's armed forces and in NHS management, having commanded the British Army of the Rhine, worked at the very heart of the Department of Health, and already been the successful Chairman of a London Health Authority. His reputation went before him and he did not disappoint. Unlike his predecessor, he showed a deft touch, knowing just when to intervene and how best to contribute to discussions and debates at meetings of the Trust Board. Everyone heaved a sigh of relief and got back to work.

Management restructuring

The new millennium brought other changes. During the latter part of the 1990s, it had became obvious to the CEO and the Board that the CEO could no longer, by himself, effectively manage the expanding portfolio of activities that had developed on the back of Trust status, outreach service provision and the emerging burden of clinical governance. The Board therefore took the step in 1996 of appointing a Director of Operations to share the burden of day-to-day operational duties. This experiment was mostly successful, Christine Miles proving to be a formidable administrator and manager, with a phenomenal capacity for hard work and a direct, albeit somewhat insensitive, style. She was largely responsible for implementing several of the new community eye-service Outreach Units, as well as the Mobile Unit. She had a weakness for micromanagement, however, and although her tenure in most respects served both the Trust's and her own purposes well, it did little to advance the cause of enlightened self-determination and empowerment for the workforce generally. After four years, when she left Moorfields to become CEO at another Trust, the cracks in the management infrastructure so neatly papered over by her appointment yawned more widely than ever, and it was clear that sweeping changes were needed to repair them.

A management consultant, called in to advise, suggested splitting the managerial responsibilities into two: one team for Moorfields itself and the other for its outreach components. Neither the CEO nor the MD or Associate MD (Bill Aylward) thought this idea sensible. They did, however, come up with another solution – to divide the line of management into three vertical divisions, each with a senior medical manager, a senior nurse manager and a general manager. These posts were first offered to suitable applicants from within the Trust, all but one being filled in this way. Under this new regime, there was inevitably a change in the roles of some senior managers, especially that of the Director of Nursing. Roslyn Emblin, who was both Chief Nurse and Deputy Chief Executive, stayed on for two years *'to see the new structure embedded'* before leaving to become Director of the National Care Standards Commission, her place at Moorfields being taken by Sarah Fisher, in the new role of Director of Nursing and Development.

The new divisional structure was inaugurated in 2001, Cooling, Aylward and Caroline Carr becoming clinical managers, Ann Hughes, Katie Lowe and Lyn Heywood nursing managers, and Grainne Barron, Patrick O'Sullivan and Ann Arnold (a new face at Moorfields) general managers. After an initial period of uncertainty (and, as might have been anticipated, not a little scepticism), the new system appeared to settle down quite well, offering as it did the opportunity for the divisional managers to manage their own resources and to redistribute these where appropriate, not only down their own line of management but also laterally. There was also more scope for interdisciplinary working and cross-communication, the divisions taking responsibility not only for clinical services but also for the support services. A further change of considerable significance took place in July 2002, when Bob Cooling stepped down from the posts of Medical Director and of Divisional Clinical Manager, Bill Aylward taking over as MD and Jonathan Dowler, a consultant in the Medical Retina Service, joining the management team as Divisional Clinical Manager.

As a consequence of the changes in management, the pattern of high-level meetings and their significance was bound to alter. The Clinical Management Board (CMB), introduced by Bob Cooling in 1993 in anticipation of the change to a Trust, inevitably lost some of its import-ance. It was now largely superseded by tridivisional meetings of the nine divisional managers and meetings of the enlarged Management Executive, comprising all the departmental directors, divisional managers and the CEO. The CMB and MAC, their meetings attended by a broad spread of the consultant staff, now met only twice and four times a year respectively, a rescheduling that epitomized the shift in the balance of power in the NHS that had occurred during the decade since Kenneth Clarke's groundbreaking efforts to change its culture.

Moorfields' transmutation, exemplified by better career development opportunities, greater devolvement of responsibility and more multi-disciplinary working, was soon recognized by the Department of Health, which awarded the Trust a top (3★) rating, enabling it to apply to become a Foundation Hospital (see Part 1). It also passed its inspection by the Commission for Health Improvement with flying colours and satisfied the National Audit Commission and Clinical Negligence Scheme for Trusts, so justifying the radical changes in its operation brought about by dint of the untiring efforts of Bob Cooling, Ian Balmer, Roslyn Emblin and the Board of Directors. When Bill Aylward took over as MD in 2002, he took command of a ship in the highest state of alert, ready to steer a safe course through whatever stormy seas might lie ahead (**Figure 55**, Plate 27).

Administrative support

From the earliest days of the NHS, the House Governor of the Hospital was supported by a Deputy, whose remit included overall direction of the High Holborn branch. In the 1970s this role was ably filled by John Barber, an ex-army officer of charm and integrity, and in the early 1980s by Joan Hinds, who was equally comfortable in the post. On her departure to raise a family, David Whitney took over until Roslyn Emblin's arrival as Chief Nurse, when she was made Deputy House Governor (and later Deputy CEO). In addition to this topmost tier of management, there were, until the late 1980s, Hospital Secretaries at both branches of Moorfields – Ken James at High Holborn and Ken

Winnie at City Road – to take care of the day-to-day running of the Hospital. James left Moorfields in 1988, when the High Holborn branch closed. Winnie, whose skill and experience in industrial relations were especially valuable assets, remained in Moorfields' service into the new millennium, latterly relinquishing the title of Hospital Secretary to become Contracts Manager under the revised management structure.

Long before the introduction of formal arrangements for what was later to be called Human Resources (HR), key members of staff underpinned personnel management, including what was then only a relatively small proportion of it, Medical Staffing (**Figure 56**). In the

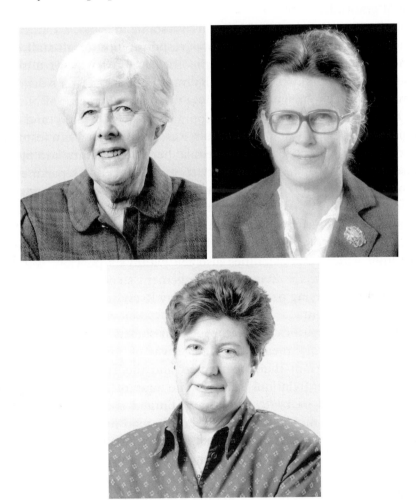

Figure 56　Three past members of the administrative and clerical staff who were key to the running of the Hospital during the period of this account: Miss Wendy Meade (*top left*), Mrs Maureen Hamilton-Smith (*top right*) and Mrs Pat Clarke (*bottom*).

1960s, Maureen Hamilton-Smith served in this capacity, later becoming the House Governor's Personal Assistant (PA), while up to the early 1980s the task was undertaken by Wendy Meade, who also acted as committee clerk, a huge job that meant that she was, in effect, the chief administrator of the Hospital. On Wendy Meade's retirement in 1983, Pat Clarke, who had previously been Planning Officer, took over the management of Medical Staffing, while Roslyn Emblin assumed responsibility for the wider role of personnel and training management. In 1987, on Maureen Hamilton-Smith's retirement, Pat Clarke became PA to the House Governor, a post in which she remained for 14 years. All four worked tirelessly for the Hospital, and it owes them a lasting debt of gratitude.

On the Hospital's assumption of Trust status in 1994, a Director of Personnel was appointed, taking over responsibility for all staff other than the nurses. The latter became the responsibility of a senior member of the nursing staff, Mary Ryan, who had a Master's degree in human resource management and was now titled Director of Nursing Education and Personnel. The development of sophisticated (and often bureaucratic) Departments of Human Resources (HR) was a feature of the new age, in which 'caring for people' became a mantra and figured prominently in the jargon of political spin. The HR Department at Moorfields, under its director, Ken Gold, came to occupy a considerable space on the fourth floor of the Hospital, with a large staff, including the Personnel Manager, Denise Bridle, and individuals assigned to different groups of staff, while information technology (IT) training and other wider responsibilities also fell within its purview. With the introduction of the tri-divisional management structure in 2001, HR took charge of nursing personnel and Mary Ryan became a member of the HR Department.

The huge change in culture throughout society in the last quarter of the 20th Century meant that image was as important as (sometimes more important than) substance, and the Trust found itself in need of a Public Relations officer. The first of these, an ex-army officer, appointed in 1998, was only a limited success, leaving after three years to be replaced by Molly Baack, who had graduated from Cambridge University and had gained previous experience with a public relations company as well as a charitable organization, and was now styled Communications Manager. Her role in the life of the Hospital began to assume greater significance as the bicentenary of Moorfields' foundation approached and preparations were made for its celebration.

Information Technology

More perhaps than in any other field, developments in IT during the 1990s and into the new millennium were fast and furious. Fundamental to the running of the NHS, computers were first introduced into Moorfields in the latter half of the 1970s, by the electrophysiology department. Dr David Powell was initially employed by Professor Geoff Arden as a professional programmer and went on to form the first proper Computer Department at Moorfields, while Chris Hogg was later taken on as a technology specialist. Indeed, for several years after the departure of Powell and before the arrival of Duncan Lamberton, a New Zealander who was eventually employed to take things forward, the chief 'IT lifeguard' at the Hospital was Chris Hogg. He not only possessed the greatest knowledge in the field, but was also prepared to come to the aid of all and sundry, floundering as they were in a sea of their own and their new computers' shortcomings.

> One such drowning man was the present author, who, while typing a manuscript during the course of one weekend, inadvertently hit the delete button on his PC, thereby destroying (or so he thought) many hours of patient work. A telephone call to Chris Hogg, at home, brought the advice 'touch nothing, until I get there' and 20 minutes later he arrived, floppy disc in hand, to save the situation, thereby guaranteeing not only the publication of a further piece of scientific trivia, but, more importantly, averting emotional meltdown.

Remarkably, even though the Hospital soon came to rely heavily on IT and had its own mainframe computer, it was to be nearly 20 years before Moorfields grasped the nettle firmly and formally appointed an Information Manager. When Barry Winnard arrived, he likened the Trust to 'a breath of fresh air', after his previous experiences at a huge, sprawling District General Hospital, where the atmosphere had been oppressive and morale poor, but he found the technology in serious need of overhaul. With one elderly *Sequent* mainframe computer subserving the four separate applications of Patient Administration, Management Information, Finance and Personnel, the Hospital was vulnerable to a major breakdown. The Trust showed itself willing to make changes, and all different functions were soon moved on to separate machines, housed in a single computer room, running Microsoft's Windows programs. The major obstacle to real progress in patient management still remained, however, namely the inability of the Trust's own IT advisors, *Stalis*, to wed computer-generated clinical information to their patient administration system (PAS).

The appointment of Bill Aylward to the consultant staff in 1994 proved to be a seminal event in the life of the Hospital. Fresh from a retinal Fellowship in the USA, Aylward already had a brilliant career behind him. Not only did he possess a degree in mathematics and a Master's in medicine, from Cambridge University, but he was also highly proficient in and fascinated by computer software technology. Together, he and Winnard were able to develop an electronic patient record system that could be used by doctors in the clinical setting, generating not only a paperless clinical record but also automated booking, correspondence and prescribing functions. Wherever patients were seen or their next appointments made, be it at the centre or in an Outreach Unit, their records could be accessed, and bookings, test results and all other relevant information made instantly available. This was a huge leap forward.

Programs for use by clinicians were rewritten with drop-down question-and-answer lists, and day-to-day information could be taken off the system and easily and instantly analysed, improving at a stroke the quality of clinical audit. Queries could be answered in moments and changes to the Admission Department's booking arrangements made at will. After four years, the system had been accepted across the Trust and most of the Clinical Directorates operated the new 'e-patient' procedure. Surprisingly, despite being the first such system to be successfully applied to clinical services, difficulties still remained in getting it accepted more widely, and the company chosen to market it (*Target 4*) found great resistance to its introduction elsewhere in the NHS (due primarily to the new centralist approach adopted by the chief executive of NHS IT).

To cope with the explosion in technology and the requirement for all staff to have some understanding and knowledge of computers and their applications, an IT Training Centre was established, under the aegis of the HR Department. This was headed by Ian Mercer, a warm personality, who was always helpful and obliging. It was a huge success, members of staff at all levels taking advantage of its facilities, to the benefit of the Hospital and of their own careers. So successful was it that it became generally well known, and outside organizations were quick to take advantage of the training facilities, the Trust selling training to a number of other hospitals and NHS bodies.

From less than 30 'dumb' terminals linked to the mainframe on Winnard's arrival, there were now 600 PCs interconnecting all aspects of the Hospital's activities, including intranet and Internet services. A security 'firewall' was necessary to protect the Hospital from the exchange of undesirable information via the Internet, but access to

'Doctors Direct' and other services was freely available. Patient confidentiality became a burning issue nationwide, however, and the right of patients to refuse to have information about them stored on computer threatened to jeopardize the successful use of computerization. The absence of interference with patients' records (at Moorfields there was never any evidence of attempts to breach the confidentiality of patients' records) appeared to have little influence, however, in moderating what seemed to be an excess of 'political correctness'.

Not surprisingly, such a sea-change in the IT capability of the Trust proved to be expensive, the budget for updating PCs rising to £150 000 per annum, but this still compared favourably with the £300 000 or more costs of replacing a mainframe computer, while there was little danger, as previously, of the network breaking down in its entirety. With a staff of 11 and the total bill for IT running at more than £1 million annually, however, an IT strategy was essential, and this was developed and agreed in 1998, and reappraised and renewed in 2002. The standardization of all word processing in the Trust, by converting free of charge to *Microsoft Word*, went some way to keeping costs under control, as did the decision not to use the very expensive *Oracle* system. Even so, the MUMPS (*Massachusetts University Multi-Processing System*) licence to operate the PAS cost £28 000 per year. Information Technology did not come cheap.

Medical Secretariat

Like everything else during the past 40 years, the role of the medical secretary has changed, not just gradually or one step at a time, but in a series of leaps and bounds. Nevertheless, a continuing esprit de corps and sense of loyalty have prevailed at Moorfields, stemming from the close-knit community it represents and the personal relationships built up between and among secretarial and medical staff. No better example of this can be found than that of Sarah Parker (formerly Cole), who joined the Secretariat straight from college in 1973, rising to become its Head. When management was devolved in 2001, and her post was realigned, she remained as a line manager to the medical secretaries in one division, and lead medical secretary in general. Her account of life at Moorfields, starting from the time of manual typewriters, shorthand dictation and a one-to-one ratio of secretary to consultant, up to the present day, provided a vivid picture of the ever-changing pattern of working life at the Hospital over a period of 30 years.

A number of innovations and changes have shaped the course of events, and none more so than the advances in IT. In the early days, she would be expected to 'look after' a single consultant and his 'firm', taking dictation in shorthand from the consultant and all members of his team, and typing letters to GPs and other doctors as well as drafts of clinical research papers and any other documents her boss demanded. Copies were made with carbon paper and all corrections made by re-typing the manuscript, sometimes with the aid of correcting fluid. Major additions and alterations, however, entailed recasting the entire page or document, and Sarah recalled having to reproduce one research paper nearly 50 times before it met with final agreement. She did receive acknowledgement of her contribution to the publications, however, and the work was interesting, varied and intensely personal, with a sense of belonging and of being a vital member of the team. Medical secretaries were few in number at Moorfields – only 17 when she took over as departmental head, including 5 at the High Holborn branch. Young trainee secretaries who came as part of their training course would often stay on permanently, however, or come back to work at the Hospital when they had completed training.

As a result of the relentless march of progress, over the years the numbers of secretaries grew steadily, in parallel with the increase in specialist departments, staff and patients and the development of better communications systems. In 1976, when the first word-processor arrived, it only served to stimulate an increase in the volume of work. By the time it was decided to devolve management responsibilities into three divisions, Sarah had 39 secretaries under her command, and even in 2003 there were 34. The introduction of voice-recording machines, then pocket memos, and then electronic devices for recording and sending information instantly in any direction meant that an individual secretary could work for several different doctors or units, but with the development of the outreach programme during the 1990s, the number of secretarial staff mushroomed. Furthermore, not only did GPs demand reports on their patients after every hospital visit, but in addition the development of clinical governance and increased patient awareness meant that secretaries' duties widened, more time being spent on the telephone and communicating with a broad range of health workers, patients and others, both at the Trust and outside.

In spite of the many attractions of the job, the 1980s saw a fall in morale and stagnation in the pay structure. In common with other groups of workers in the public service sector, medical secretaries were undervalued by the Conservative administration, and pay levels fell to such an unacceptable level that many of them left to seek better conditions outside. Even Heather Lucas, one of the most efficient, faithful and long-serving of them all, left in the early 1980s for the attractions of a job in the private sector, before returning to Moorfields in the early 1990s as PA to the Medical Director. It may have been a measure more of the impersonal atmosphere and often monotonous nature of the work outside than of their instinctive loyalty to the NHS that they often returned, preferring to accept the poor level of remuneration, in return for the Hospital's bonhomie and friendly atmosphere. At one time during this decade, the situation became so bad that, at enormous cost to the Hospital, nearly 90% of the secretarial workforce were agency staff. By the late 1980s, it was clear that action had to be taken. A campaign was mounted to attract secretaries from anywhere in the UK who would accept the low level of pay, in return for flexibility, tolerance and affordable accommodation, with retraining, if necessary, as medical secretaries.

One such was Brenda Aveyard, the present author's indefatigable personal assistant and co-worker on this *History*, who, having recently resigned from her job, after 29 years with a large company near her home in the North of England, saw an advertisement placed by Moorfields in the Yorkshire Post newspaper and travelled South to apply. Not surprisingly, considering her experience and previous record, she got the job. Starting from scratch, she worked from dawn to dusk, six or seven days a week, to master the necessary vocabulary and understanding of ophthalmic folklore, soon becoming an indispensable member of the Hospital's staff. Nor was she the only one to join Sarah Parker's team, which, as a result of some imaginative restructuring of posts and improvement in remuneration, began to expand once again. Not only did their number stop diminishing, but their skills became broader and broader, the modern medical secretary assuming more and more the role of a personal assistant and helping to manage patients' admissions, dates of operation, discharges and follow-up appointments, and sometimes helping with the running of out-patient clinics.

The developments in technology and changes in the conduct of medical practice during the decade after the Hospital became a Trust were not all to the good, however, the introduction of electronic patient records (so-called 'e-patient') leading to a very different role for the medical secretary. Increasingly complex management structures, deployed across wider spheres of activity, tended to blur the traditionally straightforward lines of command and communication, which were easy to understand and respect, while the need to be multiskilled and responsive to new demands could be stressful and disconcerting. The old order, with its personal relationships and friendly atmosphere, had, to a great extent, been replaced with one that was altogether more demanding and aggressive. Nevertheless, as Sarah avowed, and as the examples of Hazel Lawrence, who had served the Hospital for more than 30 years, of Margaret Collins (19 years) and Lyn Leverett and Isabel Moldon (more than 10 years), some of them in a variety of different roles, and the stories of Brenda Aveyard and Heather Lucas re-affirmed, Moorfields remained a cohesive unit, offering opportunities and job satisfaction hard to find elsewhere.

Medical Records

Like the Secretariat, the Medical Records Department has seen enormous changes over the past 30 years. In the 1970s and 1980s clinic clerks at both branches were expected to ensure the smooth running of a consultant's general out-patient clinic, usually held on two occasions during the week. All patient records consisted of a buff-coloured folder into which were put the doctors' handwritten clinical records, results of investigations, correspondence with the GP and other doctors, and any other documents relating to the case-history. These folders, simply known as the patients' notes, were coded with an alpha-numeric hospital number, labelled with a coloured sticker unique to each consultant and filed in a library, usually in the basement of the Hospital. The clinic clerk was responsible for making appointments, assembling the notes, seeing that they were to hand when the patient attended and ensuring that they were returned to the record library when the doctors had finished with them. This simple system worked well, provided that doctors and their secretaries returned the notes promptly when they had finished with them, and the clerks filed them away correctly after use.

Like all such systems, it worked only as well as its users, each one in the chain of individuals participating in the patient's management contributing to its success or failure. When computerization came in, far from displacing the paper system, it merely added a new dimension. There were now twice the number of opportunities for human failure together with the added risk of electronic collapse. Nevertheless, its introduction in the 1970s brought with it the possibility that, provided the information was entered correctly, appointment dates, dates for admission and all manner of personal data could be more speedily and accurately entered and accessed. This became more and more important as the numbers of patients grew, the range of specialist services widened and the complexity of investigations and treatment increased, as the outreach programme developed. The task of the Medical Records Manager became more and more difficult and the responsibility heavier as the years went by, while the job of the clinic clerk became more complicated and difficult. In the early days it was acceptable to book large numbers of patients to attend at the same time, as they were used to sitting and waiting patiently for their turn, sometimes for several hours. As the 1970s gave way to the 1980s, however, this practice was no longer acceptable and, in an attempt to cut waiting times and increase efficiency, clinic profiles were introduced in which appointment times were staggered.

Two key players in the drive to modernize the out-patient services deserve special mention here. Cyril Peskett arrived in 1990, appointed to the post of Out-Patient Manager, a job that he was to fill with distinction during one of the most difficult and demanding periods of the Hospital's history. Entering the NHS at the age of 16, he had served it well for 30 years, rising to become District Patient Services Administrator at the London Hospital. In 1982, however, as part of the reorganization of the NHS, he was obliged to apply for his own job, and although his application was successful, he was disillusioned with the NHS, and left it for a job in the commercial world. Eight years later, craving to be back working amongst people, he applied for and was appointed to the post of Out-Patient Manager at Moorfields. He found it a happy place and immediately established a remarkable rapport with Bob Cooling, John Atwill and other key members of staff, especially on the Out-Patient Executive Committee. Nevertheless, the huge changes in the running of out-patients, as a consequence of the new primary care policy, meant redundancy or redirection for many of the doctors and others, some of whom faced a serious crisis in their lives. It was largely due to Cyril Peskett's humour and sympathetic approach that the quiet revolution in the Out-Patient Department was so relatively smooth and painless, and the Hospital owed him an enormous debt. *Some measure of the power of his personality and ability to relate to people of all sorts can be gauged from the fact that in his spare time as a police 'special' he rose to Commandant, the highest possible rank.*

In 1996, with the arrival of the new Director of Operations, a clash of personalities was inevitable and Cyril resigned from his post to take over the fresh role of Risk Management Officer, a job that assumed increasing importance as a consequence of the introduction of Clinical Governance and the creation of the Clinical Negligence Scheme for Trusts. As a result of his efforts, and those of Kate Rumble, who had moved from a senior nursing post to become Assistant to the Director of Operations (and was later to take over from Cyril as Risk Management Officer), the Hospital was able to reach Level One at its first attempt, and later Level Two – a very considerable achievement, and one of which they were justifiably proud. Nor did Peskett retire gracefully, continuing for several years as a part-time training officer in violence at work and customer care, in the HR Department.

The arrival of Grainne Barron in 1991 as deputy to Marion Dipple, Manager of the Medical Records Department, signalled a marked shift in the drive to greater efficiency. With a background in health service and general practice management, she brought a welcome directness and lively intelligence to the management of medical records and the running of clinics, as well as to the use of the computerized PAS. Shortly before the Hospital became a Trust, she moved to become Contracts Manager, under Brian Benson, assuming a crucial role in the Trust's handling of the bureaucracy associated with the internal market. It was soon apparent to her that running the booking system centrally, alongside the management of contracts with over 100 Health Authorities and 1000 GPs as well as extra-contractual referrals, was a hopeless task, and she fought successfully to devolve the making of appointments back to the clinic clerks, recognizing their abilities and ensuring that the quality of the medical records staff was sufficiently high to achieve this successfully. With Marion Dipple's retirement in 1995, Grainne Barron returned to the Medical Records Department as its manager.

Not only did the clinic clerks from then on do their jobs better, expanding their roles and augmenting their skills, but they were also selected with great care and some of them went on to be promoted to higher positions in the management hierarchy. Others, such as Joan Purbrick, Dorothy ('Dot') Perron, Linda Haslin and Ray North, preferred to stay working in the clinics, at the very grassroots of the Hospital, endearing themselves to patients and medical staff alike and playing a vital part in the Hospital's infrastructure, as did others such as Jill Ellis and Valerie Giddings in the Outreach Units at Northwick Park and Ealing. Nor should those in other less obvious but equally essential jobs be forgotten, like Iris Carman, Transport Officer, who served the Hospital well for more than 25 years. The hugely increased throughput, enhanced by extension of the outreach programme, and the greater attention paid to patient-friendly measures, as a result of clinical governance, spawned a corresponding increase in the number of staff required to deal with patient data and management. A total complement of 50 in 1991 rose to 127 ten years later. Not only was there a need for excellent data collection and communications, but the new culture of patient empowerment also demanded a Complaints Officer, a post filled first by Donna Sheppard and later by Patricia Wood, as well as a Contract Services Manager, Francis Turner. Clinical Governance, Risk Management and Accountability were all of vital importance to the Hospital's fight for survival, and continued to demand the greatest vigilance.

CHAPTER 8

Finance

Background

From the inception of the NHS, Moorfields, as a London postgraduate teaching hospital, was funded directly by the Department of Health and Social Security (DHSS). The amount of this exchequer funding was decided annually, after consultation between the House Governor, Hospital Treasurer and senior officials from Government. The process was, as far as one can tell, quite informal, the annual allocation being based on the previous year's budget, and business was conducted on a friendly basis. For many years, the senior civil servant most intimately concerned with Moorfields' affairs was Joan Goldsworthy, a lady who by all accounts had a soft spot for the Hospital and with whom its officers were on excellent terms. Up until 1982, when the Hospital became a Special Health Authority (SHA), the status quo was maintained, and even then there were only minor changes, Moorfields continuing to obtain its funding directly from the DHSS until 1994, when SHAs were abolished and the Hospital achieved Trust status. This easy arrangement then came to an end.

The Finance Department itself remained remarkably stable until 1983, when Norman Musgrove retired and David Rhys-Tyler took over. Even then, Musgrove, who had joined the NHS in 1949 and had moved from Deputy Treasurer to Treasurer on Louis Kramer's retirement, stayed on as 'Capital Coordinator', maintaining continuity with John Atwill and the Planning Committee as the Hospital's development took shape. This was a somewhat disconcerting situation for the new man, who was not fully aware of the arrangements that were being made vis-à-vis the capital costs of the redevelopment, and it led in some instances to confusion.

The Hospital's auditors were, on one occasion, concerned to find that a bill for building works appeared to have been paid twice over. Investigation proved this to be indeed the case, Musgrove having authorized one payment and Rhys-Tyler another, to the same contractor – nice work for those who could get it!

Norman Musgrove was a stalwart member of the Hospital's administration during a vitally important phase of its development. Because of the DHSS policy of agreeing the budgetary allocation on a strictly annual basis, it was always difficult to plan ahead. Musgrove introduced two measures to cope with this problem. First, he pressed for a process of staging the new developments over a five-year period, so that work was divided up into phases that could be funded over short, defined periods of time and for which the necessary funds could therefore be identified. Secondly, he introduced what he termed 'Schedules of Intentions', top-slicing 5–10% of the annual allocation from the DHSS at the beginning of the year, and keeping it in reserve for allocation (officially for 'dilapidations'), either to meet unforeseen expenditure (as might be the case if the development work ran into difficulties or ran ahead of schedule) or at the year's end for the purchase of equipment deemed appropriate by the Medical Supplies Committee. These simple devices enabled him to operate with a fair degree of leeway, in circumstances that would otherwise have made it difficult to do so. The combination of these and Mrs Goldworthy's generous interpretation of the financial guidelines (in Musgrove's own words, 'she was a dream') enabled the Hospital to maintain and even improve the standards of its equipment and state of repair throughout the period.

Musgrove's methods proved very effective, and were backed by the House Governor and the Chairman of the Medical Committee, Desmond Greaves, both of whom shared his vision and commitment. The skilful manipulation of resources adopted by Atwill and Musgrove, to ensure that funds were always available to meet essential demands, could nevertheless lead them occasionally into dangerous waters.

> *On one occasion, a member of the Board of Governors expressed surprise and disapproval at the large sum available to refurbish the dining rooms, which Atwill could not clearly demonstrate to be entirely commensurate with its stated purpose. The atmosphere turned momentarily nasty, Atwill feeling sufficiently embarrassed to consider proffering his resignation, until another member of the Board declared that he thought it 'the work of a good quartermaster', and the subject was dropped. It is said that on another occasion, the departmental auditor questioned the accuracy of the accounts, until Lawrence Green, Chairman of the Planning Committee and an eminent City financier, assured him that in his experience, working in financial institutions far larger than Moorfields, so long as the figure in the bottom right-hand corner of the accounts was correct, no-one usually bothered to ask further questions.*

For the early part of his time at Moorfields, David Rhys-Tyler found things much to his liking. Computerized accounting had already been introduced and his deputy, George Cooke, who had been at Moorfields for many years, was firmly in control of the basic infrastructure and was later joined by Stephen King and Ian Knott, both of whom were hard-working and highly competent. The introduction of 'the market' philosophy, by Kenneth Clarke in the final days of the 1980s, and its development in the 1990s, however, changed everything. Rhys-Tyler found that the Hospital's management style, which had suited him before, was now quite different. Previously, he had kept himself informed by attending all the committees relevant to his responsibilities – Finance, Study Leave, Research, Supplies, Capital Works Committees and others – but under the new order, with increasing compartmentalization, he found himself withdrawing more and more into his own domain, in his own words, 'running a finance department rather than contributing to the running of a hospital'. Easy and open communication had never really been his style, but he now became increasingly withdrawn from the Executive and Board, who resented his apparent detachment. Trust status only served to accentuate the differences with the Board and Executive, and in 1995 he took early retirement, his deputy, Ian Knott, acting as Treasurer until 1996, when he was appointed to the substantive post of Director of Finance. Nonetheless, it was to David Rhys-Tyler's credit and to that of his staff that Moorfields was readily able to show itself financially capable of independent survival in the new environment, and gained recognition as a NHS Trust without difficulty.

Ian Knott had gained plenty of experience in the old style of direct annual allocation during his first two years at Moorfields, when it was still an SHA, coupled with first-hand knowledge of the new system, born of personal involvement in its implementation. He was well supported by a strong and loyal team, including, amongst others, Stephen King, who looked after the Special Trustee accounts, Keith Howard, the Payroll Manager, and John Westbrook in the Cashier's Office, all of whom had for many years served Moorfields well. The government had now, in effect, made the Hospital an independent organization, but at the same time kept it firmly under its control, the Trust owning half of its asset value and the government the other half. As its assets were (in 1993–94) valued at £28m (land £4.9m, buildings £18.8m and plant and equipment £4.4m), the Trust needed a loan of £14m to purchase its half and was required to pay 6% interest on this sum back to the government, as a so-called public dividend. This it was able to manage without difficulty, and all went well from 1995 onwards, under Ian Knott's stewardship.

Not so easy, however, was the new commissioning process, or 'internal market', introduced in 1990. Unlike most Trusts, especially district general hospitals, which were required to deal with only one host purchasing Health Authority (HA) and a handful of local GP fund-holding practices (free to administer their own funds and purchase services for their patients as they saw fit), Moorfields, as a single-specialty teaching hospital, was obliged to enter into contracts with more than 100 HAs and as many as 3500 GPs. This was a nigh-on impossible task and required a whole raft of new administrative staff, not only in the Contracting Department but also in Finance. Furthermore, the opening of the new Outreach Units from 1993 onwards, a deliberate attempt by the Hospital to spread its net more widely, made things even more difficult.

In the event, the Hospital won through, but not without a struggle. Because each contract was inevitably small compared with those made with large Trusts, many purchasers, both HAs and GPs alike, did not feel under any compulsion to honour their commitment to the Moorfields Trust punctually, and cash-flow was therefore a major problem. The Director of Planning and Performance, Brian Benson, and his team on the fourth floor struggled to secure contracts and to extract payment, but it was a thankless task, and no-one was sorry when in 1997 the landslide victory of New Labour, under Tony Blair, promised the end of the internal market. Notwithstanding the difficulties, however, the Trust had achieved remarkably steady growth over the period 1994–2002, income increasing from over £30m to over £48m, of which, in 2002, nearly £9m was generated by pharmacy sales and private practice. Compared with the past, the figures were even more striking, income in 1970 being less than £2m, in 1980 £9m and in 1990 £19m.

In point of fact, New Labour, although anxious not to be caught stealing the clothes of the previous administration, could nevertheless see the positive side of competition in the provision of healthcare and did not want to dismantle, at great expense, a system that was beginning to show benefits. They therefore abandoned the idea of fund-holding GP practices, which had proved unhelpful, and introduced a fresh concept, Primary Care Groups (PCGs), which, although initially under the control of HAs, would, in due course, metamorphose into self-determining Primary Care Trusts (PCTs). Instead of the contractual arrangements so detrimental to Moorfields, there were to be Service Level Agreements (SLAs), which, while still maintaining the market principle, represented a more flexible and (certainly as far as Moorfields was concerned) more manageable process for purchasing and providing healthcare.

The close attention to tight budgetary control was recognized in the National Schedule of Reference Costs, an annual publication of financial data brought in by New Labour in its White Paper 'The New NHS' in 1997, and in the National Reference Cost Index derived from this, by means of which each Trust could be scored. Moorfields did very well, consistently scoring amongst the lowest in the country.

There seemed to be a consensus, certainly amongst managers, that the market philosophy had its advantages and there was a new willingness to experiment with innovations of a commercial nature within the limits, both ethical and legal, imposed by the NHS. Moorfields had, for a very long time, made its own eye-drops, where these preparations were not protected by patent legislation, and this had brought in much needed cash to the Trust. In similar vein, private patient services had become steadily more acceptable within the NHS framework, since the dark days of the 1970s. The construction of a self-contained Pharmacy Manufacturing Unit (PMU), and provision of comprehensive facilities, both out-patient and in-patient, for surgeons to conduct private practice on the Moorfields campus were therefore high on the Trust's list of priorities.

Commercial services

In August 1999, in recognition of the size and potential importance of funds generated by its commercial ventures (at the time of going to press, its commercial activities accounted for 20% of the Trust's annual turnover), the Trust appointed a Director of Commercial Services, Alan Krol, to oversee both the PMU and the private patient facilities (Moorfields Private). Krol came with both a training in pharmacy and considerable experience in marketing.

Pharmacy manufacturing

In spite of some internal difficulties, the pharmacy had always had a strong reputation for producing high-quality drop preparations, which it sold to hospitals, pharmacies and doctors nationwide. It was evident, as the 1990s drew to a close, that the opportunities for branching out further into the commercial sphere could not be ignored, while the increasingly strict regulations laid down by the Medicines Control Agency (MCA) in any case demanded upgrading of the existing manufacturing facilities. To this end, the Trust began to explore the possibility of expanding its capacity for manufacturing drop preparations. At first it seemed that it might be possible to do this within the existing hospital premises, but it soon became obvious that this was not so. It was therefore necessary to look outside. To the House Governor,

Ian Balmer, must go the credit for eventually finding a site opposite to the Hospital, in Britannia Walk, and negotiating a complicated and imaginative deal with the London Borough of Hackney to participate in the construction of a building that would not only house the pharmacy manufacturing but also provide much needed accommodation for key hospital staff (see **Figure 40**, Plate 21).

Work on the new building commenced in August 2000, the PMU comprising three floors, the ground floor and two floors underground, the upper of these to house the water and air-sterilization plant and the lower one the manufacturing department itself. In this area all air was under positive pressure and passed through filters with a pore size of 0.2 microns or less, to render it bacteria-free, while humidity was kept to between 50% and 60% and temperature between 18°C and 21°C. Quality control, chemical analysis and sterility testing were all carried out separately on each batch of drop preparation, to standards laid down by the MCA. Products were contained either in bottles (multiple use) or in sealed plastic single dose vials. New equipment, capable of producing 10 000 bottles a day (compared with 1500 per week in the old pharmacy) and making the single-doses in huge numbers, was installed at a cost in excess of £200 000. The total cost of the unit was £11m, the project being financed through a combination of the sale by the Trust (to City University) of premises in Cayton Street, NHS funding, support from English Heritage (brown field regeneration) and the leasing of equipment.

The building was formally opened by Sir Nigel Crisp, NHS Chief Executive, on 22 February 2003, but owing to technical problems did not start production until nearly a year later. Products were limited to those with a 'specials' licence, in particular preservative-free preparations of methylcellulose and dexamethasone, production of which had not been actively solicited from outside Moorfields, but which were already ordered for specific patients. The Medicines Act states: *'specials can be made on the order of a physician. In anticipation of an order, it is permissible to hold stock'*. It was anticipated, however, that a wholesale dealing licence would be granted in the future, so that products could be bought in as well as manufactured on site.

Private practice

Prior to the introduction of socialized medicine, patients unable to afford private fees could seek treatment at places like Moorfields, which were in effect charitable institutions, relying on endowments and donations and the goodwill and intentions of consulting physicians and surgeons. Inevitably, this encouraged a patrician, if not patronizing culture. While, for the most part, the medical profession acted with probity and compassion, stories nevertheless abound of the haughty and sometimes peremptory manner in which hospital consultants behaved towards their patients, juniors and other staff, fostered by the class structure and the notion that they were giving their time free of charge and that, in consequence, they were doing everyone a favour.

Although Aneurin Bevan and William Beveridge changed all that, remnants of the old culture still persisted during the 1950s and early 1960s, consultants jealously guarding their private practices and still regarding their commitment to the NHS as a charitable activity. As a consequence, some were rarely if at all to be found in their hospital out-patient clinics, and from time to time even distinguished and famous men such as Duke-Elder and Stallard were on this account relieved of their hospital appointments.

> *The story goes (apocryphal, it is to be hoped) that a distinguished, senior consultant at Moorfields was one day found by a porter wandering anxiously around the Hospital. 'Can I help, Sir?' said the porter. 'Why yes', replied the doctor, 'I am looking for my out-patient clinic. It appears to have been moved.' 'Oh dear me yes, Sir!' said the porter, 'It was transferred some years ago'!*

Although, with time, such irresponsible practices became less common, it was nevertheless the case that, as late as the 1970s, consultants not infrequently spent more time on their private work than their NHS duties strictly allowed. For this reason, if for no other, there was always antipathy between consultants who practised privately and the protagonists of socialist policies. This came to a head, as is recorded elsewhere in this volume (Part 1), during the early 1970s, when the Labour Secretary of State for Health, Barbara Castle, challenged the medical profession's right to treat private patients in NHS hospitals. At Moorfields this led to the virtual abandonment of private practice at the Hospital for several years and the formation, as a result, of the Moorfields Surgeons Association.

During the 'Thatcher Years', from 1979 to 1990, this situation was reversed completely, the Conservative government encouraging private enterprise energetically, so that private hospitals sprang up like mushrooms during the night, and NHS hospitals, forced to compete with them, had to provide more and better private facilities. Realizing the huge financial potential of private practice, and the impact it would have on the future viability of the Trust, Moorfields took two important steps. First, the private facilities on the fourth floor of the Hospital were refurbished and extended, and re-opened, in 1998, as the Cumberlege

Wing, with 12 in-patient beds and facilities for 8 day-case beds or patients. Secondly, it provided its own private out-patient department, the John Saunders Suite, utilizing space in Cayton Street previously occupied by the Contact Lens Department.

Even when the socialists came to power again, in 1997, New Labour saw the wisdom of encouraging free enterprise and did nothing to check the growth of private practice within NHS Trusts. So important had the income from private practice become that Moorfields took the further step in 2002 of appointing a manager to oversee and energise private practice and its facilities at the Trust. Elizabeth Boultbee, a Tasmanian with training in accountancy, came with wide experience of private practice, both in the independent and NHS sectors. She was in an ideal position to take a long, hard view of Moorfields' performance in the private sector.

The in-patient facilities were showing wear and tear and were insufficiently geared to day-case surgery, the out-patient suite was too small and was poorly ventilated, and the refractive laser facilities, apart from the laser equipment itself, were negligible. In spite of these short-comings, private work was bringing in some £6.5m per annum (12.5% of the Trust's total annual income), £2m of it from laser refractive surgery, even though the 25 000 private patients attending the Hospital per annum were paying the Hospital nothing for their out-patient consultations. Private practice at Moorfields could no longer be regarded as an 'after-hours' activity. Boultbee also found that there was little devolved responsibility in the private work of the Trust, so that staff were at risk of becoming deskilled. As far as Clinical Governance was concerned, the private work at the Hospital (so far ignored by the Commission for Health Improvement) had largely escaped notice, and procedures for consent, risk management and audit lagged behind those established in the public sector.

She set about persuading the Trust to provide money to refurbish both the Cumberlege Wing and John Saunders Suite and laid plans to move laser refractive surgery out of the hospital building. It was vital to make private work within the Trust attractive to surgeons and patients alike, by providing adequate facilities for out-patients, in-patients and operating time, without the need to travel elsewhere. Equally essential was the need to ensure that the medical staff were fully aware of the importance that the Trust attached to this work in supporting the NHS functions of the Hospital. A practice nurse was appointed to the John Saunders Suite and it was envisaged that dedicated private practice nurses could rotate between the out-patient consultation suite, the Cumberlege Wing and the Refractive Laser Surgery Unit. The success of Moorfields Private was undeniable, its turnover in 2003 increasing by 16% compared with that of the previous year. As with the funding of the International Children's Eye Centre (and of research activities in general), independence from state support was becoming ever more important for survival in the new NHS.

Charitable funds

While the growth of commercial enterprise has been a feature of the last 20 years, charitable funds have, since its foundation, been fundamental to the survival of Moorfields. As already noted, prior to 1948 the Hospital relied entirely on endowments, donations and bequests, and its financial state was always somewhat precarious, the Royal London Ophthalmic Hospital rarely, for lack of funds, being able to open all of its beds. After the inception of the NHS things were different, but the exchequer kept a tight rein, so that charitable monies were always needed to help with the purchase of equipment and for improvements that could not be achieved within the limits of normal revenue.

The postgraduate teaching hospitals were able to retain control over their endowment funds, even after the reorganization of the NHS in 1974, when the undergraduate teaching hospitals were not so fortunate. For an institution like Moorfields this was vitally important, enabling it, in spite of its small size and limited revenue, to modernize and expand, temporary deficits being underwritten by the judicious use of charitable funds. Where donations and bequests were made with special provision for their deployment by a particular specialty group, these were protected accordingly. (In the case of the Vitreoretinal Service there were several such large funds, and the Assistant Treasurer for many years, Maurice Hales, was unfailingly courteous and helpful in distributing these.)

The Special Trustees

In the reorganization of 1982, when the Hospital became a Special Health Authority, it was a requirement of SHA status that all endowments be placed in the hands of trustees. This was, in effect, a way of protecting the endowment funds from appropriation by the government and was welcomed. The trustees were to act independently and were to be unpaid. Lawrence Green, who had been a member of the Board of Governors of Moorfields for many years and Chairman of both the Finance Committee and the Investment Subcommittee, took on the role of Chairman of the Special Trustees, with Francis Cumberlege as his deputy and with three other members. Governed by the regulations of the Charity Commissioners, they were nevertheless

able to use the endowment monies as they saw fit, seeing it as their duty
and function to provide financial assistance where this was needed, for
projects outside the remit of exchequer funding. This was mostly
directed to research, and for capital outlay where the total funds could
not be found immediately but were included in future budgetary plans.
The conduct of the Special Trustees was always above reproach and
they guarded their independence of the hospital executive fiercely.

In 1990 Lawrence Green retired and David Hyman, a stockbroker
who had served on the Board of Governors since 1971, took over as
Chairman (**Figure 57**). Testimony to the soundness of the management of the Hospital's charitable funds during this long period can be
gauged by the fact that they grew from some £600 000 in the early
1970s to over £25m at the turn of the century. This healthy situation
enabled the Trustees to make a generous contribution, towards the end
of the 1990s, of £2m towards the building of Phase VIa of the Institute,
as well as a very substantial one at the start of the new millennium, to
the building of the International Children's Eye Centre.

In most instances, however, the Special Trustees continued to support
salaries and equipment for research on a much smaller scale.
Membership remained diverse and impartial, in 2002 comprising David
Hyman (Chair), Sir Thomas Boyd-Carpenter (Chairman of the Board of
Directors of the Hospital), Habinder Kaur (Health Authority member),
John Bach (lawyer) and Malcolm Roberts (stockbroker). Stephen King,
remembered by many for his virtuoso expertise on the pianoforte and

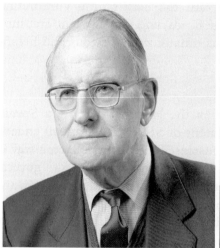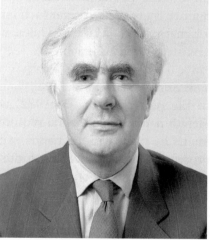

Figure 57 The two Chairmen of the Special Trustees since their incorporation in
1982: Lawrence Green (*left*), 1982–90, and David Hyman (*right*), 1990 to the present
day.

organ, administered these charitable funds with diligence and scrupulous attention to detail until he left the Trust in 2000. Applications were required to be written in understandable English, the Director of Research usually attending meetings to elucidate points of scientific obscurity. All grants were exclusively directed to projects of benefit to the Hospital and its patients, although in the 1990s, consequent upon changes in clinical practice, there was a huge swing away from basic patient care towards the purchase of 'high-tech' equipment.

The Friends of Moorfields

As well as the husbandry and distribution of endowment funds, the Hospital has been fortunate to have, since 1963, an active and dedicated body of voluntary fund-raisers, the Friends of Moorfields. Comprising a committee of trustees, headed by a President and Chairman, with its own Treasurer, independent of the Hospital, the organization sets out to raise funds for the benefit of patients. The deployment of these ranges from the purchase of small items of equipment, such as stickers for name badges, to large items, such as the Ganzfeld Stimulator, and the funding of research workers, help-line staff and the salary of a play-leader in the Childrens' Department. The Friends raise their funds holding events such as the annual Eye Ball, a glamorous occasion that attracts wealthy sponsorship, to sales of donated and handmade goods. In addition, they attract bequests and donations from a wide range of sources, as well as running Christmas and Spring Fairs, raffles, draws and voluntary collections. They also run a profitable shop and cafeteria (**Figure 58**, Plate 28).

The Friends' profile has risen to such an extent that in the year 2000 it was decided to appoint a full-time salaried director, in addition to the administrator. Annual income in 2002 exceeded £500 000, enabling them, as well as funding the purchase of equipment and their other commitments, to support the salaries of two research Fellows.

The new director, Tony Willoughby, a keen footballer and youth leader in his home town, proved to be a great asset, himself raising funds from charitable events and bringing enthusiasm as well as experience to the job, while the administrator, Debbie Plato, Lady Laidlaw (President), Lady Jacomb (Chairman), Kevin Custis (Honorary Treasurer) and the Committee of Trustees strove tirelessly to attract funds. The committee also included two consultant surgeons from the Trust, who were able to offer expert advice. It met every two months and its meetings were usually attended by the House Governor and Director of Nursing, as well as by the Director of Research or by Professor Bird. A recent innovation was a quarterly newsletter,

The Peacock, to spread the word about the Friends and their activities to all and sundry.

The Moorfields Surgeons Association

Reference has already been made to the origins of the Moorfields Surgeons Association (MSA), in the aftermath of industrial strife during the 1970s, when socialist dogma and infiltration by Marxist elements nearly closed the Hospital. The MSA was funded, initially for the purchase of equipment, from a fee per patient levied on its members. This levy continued long after the need for such an organization had disappeared, its bank balance steadily accumulating. When Bob Cooling became its treasurer he recognized its potential as a charitable organization, to provide support for a wide range of worthy causes, including help with travel allowances for young doctors and nurses, purchase of domestic appliances, and to subsidize leisure activities for hospital staff (**Figure 59**, Plate 28).

The MSA has a management committee comprising (at the time of going to press) President (Bill Aylward), Secretary (David Gartry), Treasurer (Jonathan Dowler) and Equipment Officer (John Dart), and holds an Annual General Meeting at which proposals for distribution of its funds are aired and resolutions to that end adopted accordingly. It has been an enormous success, fostering goodwill and esprit de corps amongst the medical and other staff, by helping with such things as the purchase of microwave cookers for staff working late in the operating theatres and numerous other interventions of greater or lesser importance to the well-being of staff members. Most recently, the MSA has given generous support to the present author, who received help to finance his travels to the Antipodes in January 2002, researching material for this volume and also provided the funds to enable reproduction of the painting which forms the frontispiece to this volume.

CHAPTER 9

Fabric and Infrastructure

Background

As well as changing the face of the clinical services, technological, socio-political and economic forces have had major effects on the fabric of the Hospital and its infrastructure. In the 1950s, in the aftermath of its inception, the NHS was, like all such institutions in the UK in the wake of the Second World War, seriously short of funds. Even though Moorfields, as a specialist postgraduate teaching hospital, enjoyed special status, there was little prospect of spending large sums of money on the Hospital's fabric, nor was there any immediate desire to modernize. Décor and structure at the City Road branch, following repairs after the bomb damage in 1944, remained as they had been since the building of the King George V extension, and at High Holborn the building was still considered to be adequate. In truth, as there was no major change in clinical practice during the decade, there was probably little impetus to prompt any major alterations to the hospital buildings.

As outlined elsewhere, the 1960s brought a steady stream of changes, consequent upon technological developments in instrumentation and the commitment of the Hospital's staff, led by Barrie Jones, Lorimer Fison and others, to introduce them. Most notable among these were the new slit-lamp bio-microscope introduced by Haag-Streit and the operating microscope by Carl Zeiss. The former facilitated much clearer and more accurate assessment of the anterior segment of the eye than was previously possible using the old Gullstrand model, while the latter brought an entirely new approach to ophthalmic surgery, which soon led to the rebuilding of the operating theatres at both branches. With the addition of the binocular indirect ophthalmoscope, brought in by Fison at the beginning of the decade, and the return of Alan Bird from the USA with fluorescein fundus angiography (FFA) at the end of it, the 1960s formed a watershed from which a cascade of momentous changes were soon to flow.

The new modular operating theatres – four at City Road funded by a generous donation from the Hayward Foundation, as a result of James Hudson's connection with that organization, and two at High Holborn with funding matched by the Department of Health – were completed in March 1968, and opened by Queen Elizabeth the Queen Mother. The design was a highly successful one, and when in 1986 four further theatres were built at the City Road branch in anticipation of the amalgamation, the same design was used, two being opened for immediate use and the other two in 1988 when High Holborn finally closed. Ceiling-mounted operating microscopes were installed at their inauguration in some, while floor-mounted mobile microscopes were also available, for use in any theatre as required. It was not until the early 1990s, however, that ceiling-mounted microscopes of the latest design were installed in all eight theatres.

In the out-patient arena, the gradual change from eye examination with magnifying loupes to universal use of the slit-lamp, following the introduction of the Haag-Streit 900, finally brought about changes to the design of the clinics. Two new clinics were built in 1968 at City Road, incorporating individual consulting rooms with adjacent examination cubicles, instead of the old-fashioned open-style clinics with tall desks at which doctors and patients alike stood for both consultation and examination (see **Figure 19**, p. 65). At High Holborn the clinics were already of more modern design and needed little modification. The end of the 1960s saw the introduction of fluorescein angiography and photocoagulation, entirely new techniques for which there was huge demand. This led to the opening of the Retinal Diagnostic Department (RDD), in the area on the second floor at City Road previously occupied by consulting rooms, and the latter were rebuilt further along the same floor. This move presaged the continuous, amoeba-like, re-shaping of the Hospital's facilities in response to technological developments, which were to characterize events throughout the subsequent 35 years. The RDD itself outgrew its accommodation and moved in 1978 to space on the second floor, previously occupied by King Edward VII Ward, and later to the lower ground floor when that area was redeveloped.

Other technological developments were to have equally powerful effects on the fabric. The introduction of vitrectomy in 1974 demanded closed intra-ocular microsurgical methods, impossible to achieve at the Highgate Annexe of the Hospital, so that both ward space and operating facilities for the Retinal Unit were needed at City Road. A brand new style of ward, named after Henry Stallard, was opened in 1974 in space previously occupied by the School of Nursing, while advances in cataract surgery soon led to a precipitous decline in bed occupancy, enabling other wards to be closed to make way for new facilities of various kinds. Similarly, developments in the pharmaceutical industry and the ability of Moorfields to manufacture many of its own preparations and to sell these nationwide led to the redevelopment of the pharmacy at City Road in 1968, and eventually, 35 years later, to the building of the Pharmacy Manufacturing Unit.

The massive redevelopment of the Hospital from 1976 to 1988 inevitably meant that the City Road branch underwent greater changes than did its West End partner. These were made possible, first of all by the closure of Victoria Ward on the first floor and its use as a 'holding' space, into which could be decanted clinics whose premises were in the process of reconstruction, and later by the comprehensive redevelopment of the ground and lower ground floors. The prototype Red Clinic was opened in 1978 to trial new types of out-patient equipment and clinic design, followed by the construction of four brand new clinics on the ground floor. The lower ground floor (a charming euphemism for the basement) was totally reconstructed to accommodate the Orthoptic Department, Ultrasound, Retinal Diagnostic Department, Medical Illustration Department and other services, including the Central Sterile Supply and Engineers Departments and the Linen and Sewing Rooms.

The introduction of small-incision surgery for cataract in the late 1980s heralded the move to day-case surgery, causing further enormous changes in the use of in-patient space on the first and second floors. Wards disappeared almost overnight, to accommodate day-case and short-stay facilities, including Alexandra, Luling and Sedgwick, on the first floor, to form the new Day Surgery Unit. Bowman Ward on the second floor was converted into a hostel for patients from afar who needed accommodation but did not require nursing care. Parsons Ward had already been modernized to cope with the demands imposed by the closure of High Holborn, and Guthrie Ward was opened next door to it, but it was not long before, in 1994, other priorities led to Guthrie's conversion into secretarial office space. Saunders and Coats Wards, which had been closed in response to the day-surgery revolution, now became incorporated into MacKellar Ward (named after the former Matron), to accommodate the increasing number of longer-stay vitreo-retinal cases rendered homeless as a result of Guthrie Ward's closure.

On the ground floor, in 1995, there were changes to the Optometry Department, the Contact Lens Department joining it and being assimilated into the Corneal and External Disease (Red) Clinic, which was modified appropriately, so that several complementary disciplines could be brought together in a single clinical setting. In the same year the A&E Department was extensively modernized, the Brown Clinic closed and the expanded area modified to accommodate the new Primary Care Clinic adjacent to A&E.

Nor were the technological advances influential only in the scientific and clinical arenas. The introduction of electronic word-processing soon took hold with great speed. From the astonishing technical advance of the 'golf-ball' electric typewriter, it was only a small step to the universal introduction of personal computers (PCs) throughout the Hospital, for generating letters, writing scientific papers and storing information. Any notion, however, that this electronic miracle would lead to a paperless society and that the medical secretary would, like the proverbial Dodo become extinct, was soon dispelled. Indeed, it became apparent that the paper mountain was set to increase in dimensions, when, with the introduction of the 'internal market' at the beginning of the 1990s, the purchasers (mainly fund-holding GPs) demanded written evidence of every hospital attendance made by their patients, whether as an in-patient or an out-patient. Without such proof, they simply refused to pay the Hospital for its services. The Moorfields doctors were therefore obliged to send letters after every attendance or admission, whatever the information's clinical relevance. This generated a flood of work and deluge of paper, the like of which had never before been seen, and which would have been unsustainable without electronic technology. Further developments in information technology, detailed elsewhere (see Chapter 7), soon led to enormous changes, not only in communications but also in the provision of space and equipment throughout the Hospital, the increased Secretariat moving to new premises created by the closure of Guthrie Ward, and the IT Department occupying space on the fourth floor previously used for nurses' accommodation.

Research too played an increasing part in the quest for more space. Barrie Jones' Professorial Unit had been built in 1973 over the new operating theatres, with a connecting corridor to the main hospital building. Apart from its use of beds, it otherwise had little impact on the Hospital's fabric. In the late 1990s, however, the importance of research to the Hospital's financial position increased dramatically. In 1999 the Glaucoma Research Department took over the area previously occupied by Parsons Ward, and the new Glaxo Department of Epidemiology, later incorporated in the Research and Development Department, extended into the space once occupied by Electrophysiology. The introduction in 1994 of the excimer laser, first on an experimental basis and later for wider, clinical use, also created a shift in the use of space, the old Residents' accommodation on the first floor being converted to house the experimental unit. Space on the fourth floor was used to build a new Residency, and later to accommodate additional instruments for refractive surgery.

As the last decade of the 20th Century moved to its close, formal education also assumed an increasingly high profile at the Trust. The Friends of Moorfields and Special Trustees financed the construction of a Clinical Tutorial Complex on the second floor, comprising a lecture theatre and seminar rooms, and this was later modified to take in the office of the Department of Medical Education. When the enlarged library at the Institute of Ophthalmology subsumed the small library at the Hospital (the Joint Study Facility), some of the space on the fourth floor, formerly occupied by the library, became offices for the Director of Education and for Clinical Audit. These developments were essential, in view of the expanded role that Moorfields was required to play in the teaching and training of ophthalmologists in the whole of North Thames Region, and the increasing significance of clinical governance.

Nevertheless, perhaps the most important influences on developments, both executive and structural, were political and socioeconomic. The dramatic volte-face from the deeply socialist but laissez-faire culture encouraged by the Labour administrations of the 1960s and 1970s when trade union hegemony dominated the country, to the free-enterprise, 'every man for himself' philosophy of Margaret Thatcher ('*there is no such thing as society*'), was accompanied by more gradual, but equally momentous changes in the delivery of health-care. The coincident developments in cataract surgery, enabling as they did dramatic reductions in bed-occupancy, rapid turnover and improved outcomes, made ophthalmology peculiarly well placed to profit from the new spirit of efficiency and 'value for money'. The redevelopment programme, envisaging a leaner hospital with reduced running costs, but at the same time offering more efficient services, already fitted well with this mood. It was also clear that 'one-stop' clinics and provision of community-based eye-care complemented it perfectly. As soon as the redevelopment of City Road was nearing completion, Moorfields moved swiftly to redress its deficiencies in these areas, setting up primary care services at the Hospital in 1986, formalizing these at the end of the decade, and opening outreach facilities throughout the 1990s.

Nor were these the only spectacular reversals of socioeconomic policy. In contrast with the 1970s, when left-wing political dogma very nearly brought about the removal of all private work from the Hospital, the 1990s saw commercial interests playing an increasingly important part in its development. Throughout the decade and into the new millennium, the private facilities for in-patients underwent major extension and refurbishment, provision was made for private out-patient consultations, and pharmacy manufacturing was expanded and moved to its own specially designed premises.

Evolution of the new sociopolitical culture of the 1980s took a step further in the 1990s, with the introduction of the Patients' Charter, and the increasing emphasis on patient empowerment, doctors' account-ability and attention to evidence-based medicine. This strong trend generated a whole new tier of management. Not only did Moorfields have to employ managers to arrange the commissioning process with the purchasers of its services, but it also had to enter the brave new world of acceptable human resource (HR) management. Between them, the Contracting, Personnel and IT departments took over the entire space on the fourth floor of the Hospital previously occupied by nurses' accommodation. Those who required hospital accommodation were housed in Thoresby House, the Highgate Annexe, Hazelmere House and more latterly in Fryer House, until the opening in 2003 of the new residential facility in Britannia Walk.

Such were the expectations of patients and awareness of the right to express grievances that a whole new sphere of activity grew up around patients' satisfaction with the service provided by the Hospital. Quality control became a by-word, the Director of Nursing being required to provide monthly statistics relating to outcomes, waiting times, cancel-lations and complaints, purchasers demanding this information so that, if they were not satisfied with it, they could apply sanctions. The fourth floor hummed not only with the sound of electronic hardware but also with the murmurings of conclaves of worried managers discussing how to respond to the purchasers' demands. The mid-1990s was a trying period for everyone.

The charismatic but sometimes over-zealous leader of New Labour, Tony Blair, was determined to pursue the relentless process of change in the NHS begun in the 1990s. Cataract surgery was an obvious choice as one of the flagships of New Labour's fleet, representing as it did an affordable, achievable activity, with generally excellent out-comes, for which demand, waiting times and results could be measured, and improvements demonstrated to the electorate. In 2002 the government, dissatisfied with the figures, invited surgeons from other European countries to come to the UK to undertake cataract waiting-list initiatives. They also, in 2003, introduced the London Patient Choice Project. This entailed setting up Diagnostic Treatment Centres (DTCs). Patients on unacceptably long waiting lists for cataract surgery (usually longer than six months) could telephone a choice centre, who would offer them a choice of DTC to which they could go for rapid surgery. Moorfields rose to this challenge by opening a DTC at the St Ann's Hospital Tottenham community eye service and another at the newly developed unit at St George's Hospital Tooting.

Pressures resulting from these momentous changes in cultural perspectives were bound to play their part in shaping the management structure at the highest level, and this too had its effects on the fabric. In the wake of Dr Leila Lessof's departure, the new Chairman of the Board of Directors, Sir Thomas Boyd-Carpenter, saw the need to take a firmer grip on the tiller than had traditionally been the case before his immediate predecessor's short tenure and his subsequent arrival at the helm. He therefore elected to be present in the hospital building to a greater extent than had previously been the practice, and to this end part of the Front Hall area, adjacent to the House Governor's office, was converted into an office for his use. In fact, the Front Hall underwent a steady process of contraction over the years, as it was adapted to take account of improvements to the telephone switchboard, the call for a larger front desk and demands for more administrative space. Nevertheless, the main entrance to the Hospital remained untouched and was still recognizable as that which patients and staff had used for more than 100 years.

Technical support

In common with the changes brought about by the introduction of new technology and the socio-economic revolution, maintenance of the fabric also altered. In 1973, when the present Head of Estates Management, Srikantha (Sri), arrived at Moorfields as Hospital Engineer, he joined a department employing 27 staff, including stokers for the coal-fired boilers, in-house painters and decorators, and six engineers. This team included Rupert Bristol, a carpenter from the West Indies, who became something of a legend over the years, not only on account of his somewhat liberal style of carpentry, but also with the more sporting-minded of those staff and patients, for whom he acted as a bookmakers' runner (**Figure 60**, Plate 29). By the year 2003, the Estates Department had dwindled to five directly employed maintenance tradesmen, Sri himself, Peter Morris (Maintenance Manager), an architectural assistant and an estates administrator, a total of nine.

This radical alteration in staffing requirements took place as a result of, rather than in spite of, the explosion in technological advance. Where, formerly, almost all repairs, renovations and maintenance could be satisfactorily carried out 'in house', by hospital craftsmen, technicians and other workers, the high degree of specialized knowledge now required to maintain or repair almost all equipment, and the thrust of economic doctrine towards competitive tendering, meant that most of these activities demanded specialists, contracted from outside the Trust. Whereas his predecessor, Josh Patel, was responsible for the day-to-day running of every aspect of the hospital fabric, Sri could offer only a 'first-aid' service, anything requiring more specialized knowledge, such as electro-medical equipment, being covered by outside contractors on a call-out basis. There was therefore no longer a need for a 24-hour shift of hospital maintenance workers, and outside normal working hours he and his colleagues were 'on-call' from home.

On the other side of the coin, however, Sri now found himself in charge of the entire Estate, with a far wider role than before, having responsibility for all types of work and calling in a broad range of tried and trusted specialist firms, as required. All projects up to a total cost of £1m came under his jurisdiction, including the closure of accommodation such as the Highgate Annexe and nurses' homes and those involving developments in the Outreach Units and operating theatres. Projects such as the redevelopment of the Hospital itself, falling outside this remit, demanded the services of outside architects, with responsibilities for the contracting process and the quality of work undertaken by others.

Portering and security

Unlike most of the Hospital's activities during the period under review, the portering services offered a haven of relative stability in an otherwise turbulent seascape. When the present author first came to work at Moorfields he would be greeted, as he signed his name in the large attendance ledger lying on its desk in the Front Hall, by 'Wally' Hammond, Front-Hall porter for 31 years, with a politely formal 'Good Morning, Mr Leaver'. Thirty-five years later, it was comforting to know that, in spite of all that had transpired, Paul Ryan, who in 2003 had already served the Hospital for 18 years and was still only in the fourth decade of his life, would most likely deliver the same greeting (see **Figure 12**, Plate 5). This typifies the 'family' ethos that prevails amongst Moorfields' staff and that has always inspired affection and generated good-will and loyalty from top to bottom of the institution. Perhaps indicative of this spirit, Tony Beltrami, Head Porter from 1974 to 1997, came to the Hospital to give the present author an account of his time there (**Figure 61**, Plate 30).

Beltrami's previous post was at the Royal Northern Hospital, where conditions were far from satisfactory and he was not happy. It was only when he came to Moorfields that he first really enjoyed coming to work. Even at Moorfields, however, everything had not always been rosy. In the era before his arrival, allocation of duties amongst the porters had been based on a somewhat venal system, the currency of which was pints of beer bought for the head porter. Restrictive practices and trade union influence were strong, and requests made by members of staff or patients alike met more often than not with the response 'that's not my job'. Beltrami set about changing this culture, but it was not an easy task. The Deputy Head Porter had been promoted to that position as a result of his strongly held left-wing views and was a committed Marxist. In 1975, conforming with the government's laissez-faire philosophy and the egalitarian views of the Secretary of State for Health, he threatened to bring the work of the Hospital to a halt, by calling a strike of all the porters who were members, as was Beltrami himself, of the National Union of Public Employees (NUPE).

Tony Beltrami called his bluff, by joining another union and convincing others, who had no wish themselves to come out on strike, to do the same. Ably supported by Reg Fryer, Sally Sherman, Jean Smith and others on the Board of Governors, and later, after his appointment to the post of House Governor, by John Atwill, he won the day, and Moorfields settled down to a long and happy period of peace and goodwill. There were many stalwarts amongst the portering staff, in particular Reg Beech, who sadly died only a few weeks after retiring, and George Horton, who made many friends over a number of years, delivering the post (**Figure 61**, Plate 30). All things considered, the portering team remained a contented and united band of men during the 23 years of Beltrami's leadership, and in 1994 his efforts were recognized by the award of the MBE. This long period of service was not without its dramas, two of the porters serving prison sentences for manslaughter and one escaping a charge of bigamy, all of which provided an extra dimension to a demanding job.

In the early days of the health service, little distinction was made between the different duties and responsibilities carried out by members of the portering staff. Thus, it was possible for an individual to rise far above his fellows, in terms of experience and expertise, acquired as a result of duties he was able and prepared to undertake competently and safely. At the High Holborn branch of the Hospital, such a person was Charlie Smith, an outstandingly intelligent and competent theatre porter with a driving personality, who became the indispensable 'Pooh-Bah' of the Hospital, teaching and supervising not only the other members of the portering staff, but nurses and junior doctors too.

At City Road, Charlie Whipp was the sole theatre technician, until the arrival of Graham Nunn in 1980, both of them graduating from the position of porter to become widely respected for their technical knowledge and skills. While Whipp retired as such, however, Nunn went on to gain technical qualifications in physiology and medical physics and became the first vitreoretinal surgery technician in the UK. In this position he became an indispensable part of the vitreoretinal surgical team at Moorfields, contributing in no small part to the unit's successful growth and strong reputation as it went from 6 vitrectomies per week in the mid-1970s to 40 by the year 2003.

The requirement for and recognition of technical expertise was a consistent feature of the age, the introduction of clinical governance finally setting the seal on its importance. One result of this was the introduction of Operating Department Assistants (ODAs), technicians qualified to carry out many routine tasks, including drawing-up drugs for injection, intubating patients and setting-up monitoring equipment, otherwise carried out by anaesthetists. Several of the Moorfields porters, including Frank Zinsa and Phil Gladstone, went on to become ODAs, while nurses too were able to qualify.

Nor was it only the technical aspects of the porters' jobs that changed with the new concessions to clinical governance. When Tony Beltrami finally retired, the new head porter, Brian Blackgrove, was committed to patient-friendly policies. Coming from a large district general hospital nearby, where he had been the Head Porter and Security Manager for 25 years, he found the atmosphere at Moorfields very different. Like Beltrami before him, in his own words he 'enjoyed coming to work again'. Nevertheless, during his tenure it was found necessary to trim the workforce from 32 to a total of 26 staff. Owing to the great changes in surgical care and the alterations that they brought to patterns of activity in portering duties, there were high peaks and deep troughs in staffing requirements, at different times of the day and on different days of the week, so that major adjustments to the schedules of work were necessary.

'Customer-friendly' practices were the order of the day, and the approach of the willing and helpful portering staff was now very different from that which obtained when Tony Beltrami first arrived. Not only were relations with managers much improved as the new millennium began, but employment practices were better, new staff being required to shadow more experienced members and undergoing proper induction processes. Efforts by senior managers and medical staff, notably the Moorfields Surgeons Association and the Medical Director, Bob Cooling, to encourage and finance interdisciplinary activities, including social gatherings and 'days out' were highly successful, raising morale and engendering a strong spirit of comradeship and loyalty amongst each other and to the Trust. Morale remained high, and in 2003, when Brian Blackgrove too retired, his deputy, Barry Crane, explained to the present author that the Trust still had on its portering staff a team of dedicated individuals keen to see its high standards maintained. Paul Camenzuli, a Tunisian by birth, had been on the staff for 35 years, while Edwin West, the pharmacy porter, and Crane himself had already served for more than 10. In November 2003, as this account was on its way to press, a new Portering and Security Manager, David Horton, was appointed.

Telephone switchboard

Coming under the jurisdiction of the Head Porter, 'Switch' has always been the title given to the staff who man the telephones, answer the bleep calls and maintain communications within the Hospital and between the Hospital and the outside world. Like the rest of the Moorfields staff, many of them have served the Hospital for long periods, they are cheerful, friendly and helpful, and their voices are familiar. At the High Holborn branch, George Feathers, who had become something of an institution, was replaced in 1986 by Cilla Poroosotum. She subsequently served on the City Road switchboard with Pat Layzelle, while years before, John Lehane ('*Never use one word when a dozen will do!*') was a fixture on the night shift there. Maureen and Ron Coggin were equally so by day (**Figure 62**, Plate 30), until they retired to make their home in Ireland and Steve Morris brought his large and friendly frame to the telephone exchange. In days gone by delays were common, each call demanding personal attention, but the introduction of automatic answering services in the 1990s changed this. The message service had its advantages, but some of the personal and friendly interchange of the past had gone. Such is the inexorable march of progress.

Nevertheless, as Morris, now switchboard supervisor, remarked during an interview for the hospital newsletter *Fiat Lux*: '*Moorfields is like a big family. There aren't the barriers here that used to exist. It's a very friendly place and there's no doubt that it has magnetism about it. I hope that I'll stay here until I retire …*' Not a bad testimony, in the face of an ever changing and brave new technological world.

Catering Services

It is said that an army marches on its stomach, and if this is the case then a Hospital probably does so too. The catering at Moorfields has been of an exceptionally high standard for a very long time. In 1968 the kitchens were modernized and the dining rooms refurbished. This improvement notwithstanding, the doctors and other staff ate separately and conditions were still far from ideal. At High Holborn the restaurant was in the basement and was small and cramped, while the medical staff ate their meals in or near to the Residents' mess on the second floor and the kitchens were on the sixth floor.

In 1987 the dining area on the third floor at City Road was completely refurbished and extended, so that, in the words of the annual hospital report, *'all grades of staff can now obtain meals and refreshments which they can then enjoy amidst comfortable and attractive surroundings'* (**Figure 63**, Plate 31). Not all the staff were happy with the new multidisciplinary arrangements, one member of the consultant staff, appalled by the closure of the consultants' dining room, with reactionary fervour refusing ever to eat in the new staff restaurant. Mostly it was a popular and forward looking step, however, which proved with the passage of time to be successful in breaking down artificial barriers between different groups of staff forged in a bygone age. In 1989–90, as a result of a change in the law, the Hospital lost its Crown immunity, and was obliged to comply with the precise demands of the Department of Environmental Health. As a result the kitchens were completely refurbished at enormous cost, to bring them up to the latest government standards. So successful and popular did the refurbished dining facilities become, and so great was the demand for their services, that in 1991 an extension to the main dining room was opened.

The catering at both branches of the Hospital was under the direction of Diana Rowe, who was joined in 1969 by Ricky Lee, a chef of rare skills, commitment and imagination, with wide experience of working in the hotel industry, who soon became her deputy (**Figure 64**, Plate 32). Rarely, if ever, can a hospital staff restaurant have been so well managed or reached such heights of culinary excellence. Both were awarded travelling fellowships – Rowe to visit European centres to study the latest in cook/chill methods and Lee to see the latest developments in the preparation of fast foods and popular catering at the Trust House Forte Group. When Rowe left, Lee took over as Catering Manager, and for many years, during the 1980s and 1990s, the food at Moorfields matched that at many a good restaurant charging nearly 10 times as much.

Lee introduced new standards of service, appointing a Restaurant Manager, Letty Apilado, and insisting on the same standards of service and cuisine as prevailed in the commercial sector. The numbers of meals served daily rose dramatically. He was aided in his efforts by having, in Rick Hamilton and Alex Olala (see **Figure 60**, Plate 29), two excellent and reliable chefs. Not only did this encourage in-house social functions, but the Hospital also entrusted to Lee the running of staff 'theme' evenings, which were a great success and further raised morale. He refused to buy contract goods that were inferior and formed relations with suppliers that enabled him to get favourable deals, so that even Lobster Thermidor was known to appear on the menu in the staff restaurant. Lee realized that poor ingredients were, in the long run, usually as costly as expensive ones (or more so), after wastage was taken into account, on one occasion actually demonstrating this to a team of inspectors using poor, compared with high-quality, minced beef.

It was his ambition to make the restaurant so competitive that it would attract business from outside the Hospital, for private functions. He was given every facility to give rein to his ambitious plans for the department and he had no intention of leaving before he was forced to do so. His resignation in 1997, as a result of the uncompromising (and possibly short-sighted) attitude of the Director of Operations, was a matter of universal regret. His successors, Kathryn Platt and subsequently Aidan Cleasby, did their best to maintain the high standards he set, and many of the catering staff, including Letty Apilado, Gillian Temple and Dominga Xavier, and the kitchen manager and chef of 22 years, Alex Olala, remained in post up to the time of going to press.

The Catering Department at Moorfields, offering as it did a wide variety of freshly prepared food of the highest quality, at bargain prices, was one of the outstanding developments in the Hospital's recent history. The staff restaurant was a place where all members of the staff could meet, in comfortable, pleasant surroundings, and in cementing friendships and spreading goodwill, it remained a lasting tribute to the vision of John Atwill and the commitment and skills of Ricky Lee and his loyal staff.

Supplies Department

If it is true that the Hospital was a better place for its excellent catering and communal eating facilities then it is equally true that one of the mainstays of the infrastructure supporting all its activities was the Supplies Department. The present author was for some years Chairman of the Medical Supplies Committee, representing a small but important part of the supplies function as a whole. Norman Musgrove's well-founded principles of 'forward looks' and 'schedules of intentions' remained at the heart of forward planning and were sound means of ensuring that prudent house-keeping was maintained in the face of financial stringencies. The post of Supplies Officer was always of paramount importance to the smooth functioning of the Hospital, and although several of its holders left the Hospital long before the time of writing, the present author was fortunate in being able to talk to one from long before as well as the recently appointed Supplies and Procurement Manager.

Alan Marjoram came to Moorfields in 1971 as deputy to the Supplies Officer Bill Williams, who had just taken over the post. He had previously been at the Royal Northern Hospital, where the Hospital Secretary Arthur Gray, who knew his school headmaster personally, had head-hunted him for a post in the Supplies Department. Gray was shortly to become the House Governor at Moorfields, and this display of paternalism sheds an interesting light on the very different society prevailing at that time. In fact Gray did not have any true vacancies in his organization, but was sufficiently concerned with job creation that he found posts for sixth-form school leavers, in order to offer them career experience in the NHS. Marjoram, who had wanted to pursue a career in marketing, soon discovered that the job in supplies in the NHS had everything he was seeking and he remained in the NHS for much of his working life, his apprenticeship at the Royal Northern taking him into all aspects of the service, including administration.

It was no surprise, therefore, that when Gray was looking for a Deputy Supplies Officer at Moorfields he should seek out Marjoram and that the interview, conducted as it was by Gray alone, was hardly one that would be seen as acceptable practice today. Gray could seem aloof and distant, his deafness possibly contributing to this impression, but this story says much about his true character. When Williams retired in 1975, Marjoram took over as Supplies Officer, but left after 18 months to take over a more senior post in Colchester. He then moved up to become District Supplies Manager, the supplies network becoming increasingly centralized, before it reverted to its original format. Marjoram was replaced by Ken Conway in 1976, and when Conway left, by Gordon Innes, who retired in 1997. After that, Brenda Castello took over as Supplies officer for five years, before, in October 2002, the new post of Supplies and Procurement Manager was created and Alex Lines was appointed. At about the same time, on the sale of the Cayton Street premises to City University, the department moved to new offices on the ground floor of Empire House, a short distance down the City Road from the Hospital.

Lines had considerable experience behind him, having served as Supplies Officer in Newham for six years, and he knew the system of London-wide cooperation between supplies departments. He well understood the importance of collaboration within the North Central Strategic Health Authority sector. Still closely associated with the Hospital's central stores, where John Ballinger, surely the most meticulous and dedicated of all possible stores managers, had been in post for 32 years, the Supplies and Procurement Department at Moorfields found itself under similar pressure to that experienced by other services. Following a government review in 1999, national frameworks were set up to measure and improve purchasing and supply, and to ensure that contracts and contracting procedures met best practice. Supplies managers were therefore required to report regularly both to their Trust Board and to the Health Authority. Furthermore, according to European Commission rules on procurement, all orders of £100 000 or more had to be advertised without fear or favour, so that all interested suppliers were given the same opportunities to tender. There was, nevertheless, no increase in staffing, Brenda Castello and Christine Bennett remaining as Lines' sole assistants.

The introduction of an electronic ordering system, accessible via the NHSnet, greatly helped to ensure that there was wide communication between purchasers and providers of all types of supplies across the region while the introduction of e-commerce, an initiative aimed at getting rid of as much paperwork as possible, was also a step in the right direction. The clear lines of management at Moorfields, created by the tridivisional management structure and the devolvement of budgets to divisional managers, were also helpful, particularly where supplies to the Outreach Units were concerned. Medical equipment now came under the Medical Devices Group, a more widely representative body than the old Medical Supplies Committee and one that was able to establish more effective risk management for medical devices and the standardization of medical and surgical equipment. It was Lines' view that the modifications to the methods of organization and regulation that had been introduced were, in general, changes for the better, and it was evident that the Hospital had again made every effort to keep up with best practice in the 21st Century.

CHAPTER 10

Moorfields Alumni Association

In 1981 an informal meeting of Moorfields Alumni was held at the Hospital. This was the brainchild of Peter Fells, but it fell to Bob Cooling, then a lecturer on the Professorial Unit, to organize. It was an immediate success. About 100 people gathered in what was then still Victoria Ward, a space commandeered for general use while the Hospital was in the process of redevelopment, and used normally for additional out-patient accommodation. There was no stage and there were no other lecture facilities, so the presentations by Residents were necessarily somewhat makeshift and haphazard. Nevertheless, the spontaneity and ad hoc nature of the meeting, the fact that it was 'on-site', and later, in 1983, the production of an excellent satirical revue by the Residents ensured that it remained popular. It has remained an annual event, albeit transferring to a neighbouring (and far better) venue.

The scientific programme was initially organized by Bob Cooling, Colin Kirkness, Linda Ficker and other members of the Department of Clinical Ophthalmology, but gradually became the (voluntary) respon-sibility of John Lee, later assisted by Michele Beaconsfield, with the administrative support of Sarah Parker and the audio-visual expertise of Alan Lacey. In 2002, when John Lee took over as Director, it came under the aegis of the Department of Education, Louise Halfhide spearheading its organization. Retiring members of the consultant staff have subsequently been generous enough to fund the award of a medal and cash prize for the most outstanding piece of research carried out during the year by a member of the Resident staff. The meeting and its attendant revue have continued to be successful and well attended throughout the years.

In 2002 the Trust expressed a wish to make the Moorfields Alumni into a more formal institution, and this was approved by the member-ship at the Annual Meeting in January 2003. The present author was honoured to be asked to be its first President. A Management Committee was formed, a Constitution agreed and adopted, in January

2004, and the Moorfields Alumni Association (MAA) was born. It was agreed that all past and present medical staff would be eligible to become members of the MAA, on the payment of an agreed subscription, provided that they had or had had a contract with the Trust, honorary or otherwise, for a period of at least six months, and that they were able to furnish the Management Committee with signatures of approval from the Medical Director of the Trust and from their Head of Department.

The aims of the MAA were to:

- Ensure continuity
- Establish and maintain an up-to-date database of addresses etc.
- Maintain communications between the Alumni and the Trust and between alumni, by:
    - (i) maintaining an up-to-date mailing list
    - (ii) producing and maintaining an up-to-date website
    - (iii) publishing an annual newsletter
    - (iv) representing the Alumni at Trust/Institute events

An annual subscription of £25 was set initially, to finance the MAA's running costs, including a web-page on the Trust's website, secretarial support and other day-to-day expenses. Mrs Brenda Aveyard agreed to act as secretarial assistant. The first officers of the MAA were Mr Peter Leaver, Honorary President and Secretary, and Mr Arthur Steele, Honorary Treasurer. Ordinary members of the Management Committee were Professor Desmond Archer (Belfast), Mr Anthony Atkinson (Northampton), Mr Hung Cheng (Oxford), Mr Martin Crick (Bournemouth), Mr Timothy Ffytche (London), Mr Luke Herbert (Welwyn Garden City) and Mr Peter Shah (Wolverhampton). It was agreed that the Chief Executive, Medical Director, Director of Education, Senior Resident and Communications Manager of the Trust would serve on the committee ex officio.

And so this volume of the Moorfields history draws to a close, not as it began, with a description of the hospital buildings, nor as an account of the development of its fabric, but with reference to the people who form its soul. In the words of Sir Stewart Duke-Elder, in his William Lang lecture entitled 'Moorfields and British Ophtalmology' (Royal Society of Medicine, December 1964): 'the immensely competent clinicians, the careful observers, the devoted and enthusiastic workers who, by great good fortune, have always formed the backbone of the staff of Moorfields and have succeeded in maintaining a steady standard of excellence in British ophthalmology'. Long may they continue to do so.

References

The following is a list of reference works in chronological order used in the preparation of this book:

Saunders, John Cunningham, *A Treatise on Some Practical Points Relating to Diseases of the Eye*. London: Longman, 1811.

Treacher Collins, E, *The History and Traditions of the Moorfields Eye Hospital*. London: HK Lewis, 1929.

The National Health Service Act, 1946. London: HMSO, 1946.

Institute of Ophthalmology Annual Reports (Numbers 16–45), 1963–1993.

Moorfields Eye Hospital Annual Reports, 1965–2003.

Ministry of Health and Scottish Home and Health Department, *Report of the Committee on Senior Nursing Staff Structure (Salmon Report)*. London: HMSO, 1966.

Law, Frank W, *The History and Traditions of the Moorfields Eye Hospital*, Volume II. London: HK Lewis, 1975.

Report of the Royal Commission on Medical Education (The Todd Report). London: HMSO, 1968.

The National Health Reorganisation Act. London: HMSO, 1973.

DHSS Report of the NHS Management Inquiry (Griffiths Report). London: HMSO, 1983.

Enthoven, Alain, *Reflections on the Management of the NHS*. London: Nuffield Provincial Hospitals Trust, 1985.

Department of Health, *Working for Patients*. London: HMSO, 1989.

The NHS and Community Care Act. London: HMSO, 1990.

The Health of the Nation: A Strategy for Health in England. London: HMSO, 1992.

Report of the Inquiry into London's Health Service, Medical Education and Research (The Tomlinson Report). London: HMSO, 1992.

Hospital Doctors. Training for the Future. Report of the Working Group on Specialist Medical Training (The Calman Report). London: Department of Health, 1993.

Review of the Research and Development Taking Place in the London Postgraduate Special Health Authorities. A Report by the Review Advisory Committee. London: HMSO, 1993.

Moorfields Eye Hospital Teaching and Training Prospectus, 1994.

Funding Research in the NHS (The Culyer Report). York: University of York, Centre for Health Economics, 1994.

The New NHS: Modern – Dependable. London: HMSO, 1997.

Rivett, Geoffrey, *From Cradle to Grave. Fifty Years of the NHS*. London: King's Fund, 1998.

Modernising the NHS in London. Report of the Inquiry into London's Health Services (The Turnberg Report). London: Department of Health, 1998.

Moorfields Eye Hospital Teaching and Training Prospectus, 1998.

NHS Confederation, *A First Class Service – Quality in the New NHS*. London: The Stationery Office, 1998.

Secretary of State for Health, *The New NHS: Modern – Dependable*. London: The Stationery Office, 1999.

The NHS Plan – A Plan for Investment, a Plan for Reform. London: The Stationery Office, 2000.

Ham, Chris, *The Politics of NHS Reform 1988–97*. London: King's Fund, 2000.

NHS Support for Science and Priorities and Needs, NHS Research and Development Funding, Consultation Papers. London: The Stationery Office, 2000.

From Basic Science to Better Sight, Moorfields Eye Hospital NHS Trust, NHS Research and Development Funding. Annual Reports, 2000–2003.

London Patient Choice Project. London: Department of Health, 2002.

Unfinished Business – Reform of the Senior House Officer Grade: London: The Stationery Office, 2002.

A National Research Strategy for Ophthalmology. London: Royal College of Ophthalmologists, 2002.

Action for Change. London: Department of Health, 2002.

Health and Social Care Act (Community Health and Standards). London: The Stationery Office, 2003.

Appendices

Moorfields Consultant Medical Staff and their special interests

(For those who left the staff before 1974, the reader should consult Volume II, of this *History* pp. 280–282)

Acheson, Mr James. Neuro-ophthalmology. Joint appointment with the National Hospital for Neurology and Neurosurgery, Queen Square 1999–. Royal College of Ophthalmologists Tutor, Moorfields, 2000–. Training Programme Director (North Thames) London Deanery 2000–.

Adams, Miss Gillian. Paediatrics and Strabismus. Northwick Park Hospital Outreach Unit 1994–1998. First surgeon at Homerton Hospital Outreach Unit 1998–.

Ainslie, Mr Derek. General Ophthalmic and Anterior Segment Surgery, 1962–1976.

Allan, Mr Bruce. Cornea and External Disease, 1998–. Training Director, Corneal Service 2001–. Biomaterials Research.

Amin, Dr Sandip. Ophthalmic Anaesthesia, 2001–.

Anderson, Dr Jock, OBE. Reader, Department of Preventive Ophthalmology, Institute of Ophthalmology, 1981–1986.

Anderson, Dr Sheila. Ophthalmic Anaesthesia, 1946–1979.

Arden, Professor Geoffrey. Ocular neurophysiology. Director Electrodiagnostic Department 1963–1995. Professor of Neurophysiology, University of London, 1969–1995.

Ashton, Professor Norman, CBE FRS. Ocular Pathology, 1948–1978. Professor and Director, Department of Pathology, Institute of Ophthalmology. President, Ophthalmological Society of the UK, 1979–1981.

Aylward, Mr George W (Bill). Vitreoretinal Surgery. Research Lead, VR Service, 1994–1996. Lead Clinician, St. George's Hospital Outreach Unit, 1999–2003. Associate Medical Director, 1999–2002. Medical Director, 2002–.

Bailey, Dr Susan. General and Paediatric Ophthalmic Anaesthesia, 1994–. College Tutor and Training Director, 2002–. Instructor in Paediatric Life Support, UK Resuscitation Council, 2000–.

Barton, Mr Keith. Glaucoma Surgery. Training Director Glaucoma Service, 1999–. Lead Clinician, Upney Lane Barking Outreach Unit, 1998–.

Beaconsfield, Miss Michelle. Oculoplastic and Reconstructive Surgery, 1994–. Moorfields Representative on RCOphth Council, 1994–1996. Clinical Lead for Primary Care, Northwick Park Hospital, 1996–.

Bedford, Mr Michael. Ocular Oncology, 1964–1981. Joint with St Bartholomew's Hospital.

Bird, Professor Alan. Medical Retina and Molecular Genetics. Senior Lecturer, Reader, and then Professor, Department of Clinical Ophthalmology, Institute of Ophthalmology, 1972–2003.

Birley, Dr Doreen. Ophthalmic Anaesthesia, 1969–1994.

Blach, Mr Rolf. Medical and Surgical Retina, 1967–1995. Dean of the Medical School, Moorfields and the Institute of Ophthalmology, 1984–1989.

Borrie, Dr Peter. Dermatology (St Bartholomew's Hospital), 1950–1978.

Braddon, Dr Ivan. Ophthalmic Anaesthesia. 1946–1978.

Buckley, Professor Roger. Cornea and External Disease, 1981–. Director, Vernal Clinic, 1973–1989. Director, Contact Lens and Prosthesis Department, 1983–1997. Member, Control of Infection Committee, 1998– and Drug and Therapeutics Committee, 1999–.

Budd, Dr Alison. Ophthalmic Anaesthesia, 1993–2003. College Tutor, 1996–2001.

Carr, Dr Caroline. Ophthalmic Anaesthesia, 1986–. Director, Anaesthetic Service, 1999–2001. College Tutor, 1991–1996. Divisional Clinical Director, 2001–.

Catterucia, Dr Nicoletta. Ophthalmic Anaesthesia, 2002–.

Charteris, Mr David. Vitreoretinal Surgery 1997–. Research Lead, VR Service, 1998–. Lead Clinician, Mayday Hospital Croydon Outreach Unit, 1997–.

Clark, Dr Brian. Ocular Pathology, 1998–2001.

Collin, Mr Richard. Oculoplastic Surgery, 1982–. Director, Adnexal and Oculoplastic Surgery Service, 1992–. Moorfields Special Trustee, 1998–2000.

Cooling, Mr Robert. Vitreoretinal Surgery, 1983–2003. Chair, Outpatient Executive Committee, 1986–1990. Director A&E and Primary Care Department, 1986–1996. Member, Board of Governors, 1992–1994. Medical Director, 1993–2002. Chair, Clinical Management Board, 1994–2002. Chair, Medical Executive, 1996–2002. Chair, Clinical Governance Team, 1999–2002. Divisional Clinical Director, 2001–2002. Chair, Tridivisional Team, 2001–2002.

Coren, Dr Anne. Ophthalmic Anaesthesia, 1974–.

Crawford-Barras, Surgeon Commander TC, RN. General Ophthalmic Surgery. Administration. 1973–1980.

Cree, Professor Ian. Ocular Pathology, 1994–2001.

da Cruz, Mr Lyndon. Medical and Surgical Retina, 2003–.

Cunningham, Miss Carol. Cataract Surgery, 1996–. Service Director, 1998–2001. Member of International Childrens Eye Centre Fund-Raising Committee, 1999–2000.

Daniel, Mr Rhodri. Primary Care and Emergency Services. Director, Primary Care and Emergency Service, 1994–. Lead Clinician Potters Bar and Homerton University Hospital Outreach Units. Chairman, Local Negotiating Committee, 1999–2003.

Dart, Mr John. Corneal and External Disease and Cataract, 1987–. Research Lead, Corneal and External Disease Service 1991–. Chair, Control of Infection Committee, 1997–. Honorary Senior Research Fellow, Department of Clinical Ophthalmology, Institute of Ophthalmology, University College London, 1998–. Deputy Director of Research, Moorfields, 2001–.

Davies, Miss Alison. Paediatrics and Strabismus, 2003–.

Davies, Dr Norma. Ophthalmic Anaesthesia, 1975–1992.

Dennison-Davies, Dr HWD. Ophthalmic Anaesthesia, 1971–1988.

Desai, Miss Parul. Public Health, Epidemiology, Medical Retina, 1999–. Chair, Clinical Audit Committee, 1999–2003. Chair, Drugs and Therapeutics Committee, 2002–.

De Silva, Dr Kumar. Ophthalmic Anaesthesia, 1978–1988.

Dowler, Mr Jonathan. Medical Retina, 1998–. Lead Clinician, Northwick Park Hospital, 1998–. Divisional Clinical Director, 2002–.

Duguid, Mr Ian. Anterior Segment and General Ophthalmic Surgery, 1962–1991.

Dunlop, Dr Eric. Venereology, 1964–1985.

Earl, Dr Christopher. Neuro-ophthalmology. 1960–1989.

Egan, Miss Catherine. Medical Retina, 2003–.

Ezra, Mr Eric. Vitreoretinal Surgery, 2001–. Paediatric VR Surgery Lead, 2001–. VR Surgeon, St George's Hospital Outreach Unit, 2001–.

Fells, Mr Peter. Ocular Motility and Thyroid Eye Disease, 1968–1995. Senior Lecturer and Honorary Consultant, Moorfields and Royal Postgraduate Medical School, Hammersmith Hospital, 1968–1971. Director, Orthoptic Department, 1974–1991. Director, Strabismus and Paediatric Service, 1991–1995. Chairman, Medical Committee, 1988–1991.

Ffytche, Mr Timothy. Medical Retina, 1970–2001. Surgeon Oculist to HM Queen Elizabeth II.

Ficker, Miss Linda. Anterior Segment Surgery, 1988–. Director, Cornea and External Eye Disease Service, 1994–1998.

Fison, Mr Lorimer. Retinal Surgery, 1963–1983. Director, Retinal Unit, 1963–1983. President, Faculty of Ophthalmologists, 1980–1983 and Ophthalmological Society of the UK, 1985–1987.

Foster, Professor Allen, OBE. Honorary Consultant Ophthalmic Epidemiology, 1990–. International Centre for Eye Health, London School of Hygiene and Tropical Medicine.

Franks, Miss Wendy. Glaucoma Surgery, 1994–. Clinical Lead, Mile End Hospital Outreach Unit, 1994–. Director, Glaucoma Service, 1996–.

Galton, Professor David. Medical Ophthalmology, 1975–2002. Director, Physicians Clinic, 1975–2002.

Garner, Professor Alec. Senior Lecturer, 1967–1970. Reader in Experimental Pathology, 1970–1978. Professor and Director, Department of Pathology, Institute of Ophthalmology, 1978–1994. Member, Board of Governors, 1978–1986.

Gartry, Mr David. Anterior Segment and Refractive Surgery, 1995–. Lead Clinician Potters Bar Outreach Unit, 1995–.

Garway-Heath, Mr David. Glaucoma Surgery, 2000–. Clinical Research Lead, 2000–. Clinical Lead, St Georges Hospital Outreach Unit, 2002–.

Gavey, Dr CJ. General medicine, 1947–1975.

Gloster, Professor John. Glaucoma Service, 1975–1982. Professor of Experimental Ophthalmology, University of London, 1975–1982 (Sembal Professor, 1981–1982). Dean of the Medical School, Moorfields and the Institute of Ophthalmology, 1976–1980.

Goh, Dr Beng. Venereology and Sexual Health, 1985–. Joint with Royal London Hospital.

Greaves, Mr Desmond. General Ophthalmic Surgery, 1960–1985. Chair, Medical Committee, 1976–1982.

Gregor, Mr Zdenek. Medical and Surgical Retina, 1982–. Director, Medical Retina Service, 1982–. Chair, Laser Committee, 1982–1995.

Hamilton, Mr AM (Peter). Medical Retina and Cataract Surgery, 1982–2000.

Harrison, Professor Sir Donald. ENT Surgery, 1987–1990.

Hill, Professor David. Medical Retina and General Ophthalmic Surgery, 1973–1991. Director, Fundus Clinic, High Holborn, 1973–1988. Chair, Medical Committee and Transfer Liaison Committee, High Holborn, 1987–1988. Member, Board of Governors.

Hitchings, Professor Roger. Glaucoma Surgery, 1978–. Director, Glaucoma Service, 1980–1995. Chair, Medical Advisory Committee, 1993–1996. Moorfields Representative, Council of the RCOphth, 1995–1998. Director of Research and Development, 1998–.

Holder, Dr Graham. Electrophysiology. Director, Electrophysiology Department, 1995–.

Hudson, Mr James, CBE. General Ophthalmic and Retinal Surgery, 1956–1981. Chairman, Medical Committee, 1970–1971. President, Faculty of Ophthalmologists, 1974–1977 and Ophthalmological Society of the UK, 1983–1985.

Hungerford, Mr John. Ocular oncology, 1983–.

Hykin, Mr Philip. Medical Retina, 1996–. Service Director, 2003–. Chair, Laser Sub-Committee, 1996–2002. Macula Course Organiser, 1997–2002.

Ionides, Mr Alexander. Anterior Segment Surgery and Primary Care, 2001–. Research Lead Lens and Cataract Research. Lead Clinician St Georges Hospital Outreach Unit, 2001–. Deputy Programme Director (North Thames) London Deanery.

Jay, Professor Barrie. General Ophthalmic Surgery and Genetics, 1969–1992. Clinical Sub-Dean of the Medical School, Moorfields and the Institute of Ophthalmology, 1973–1977 and Dean, 1980–1985. Director, Department of Clinical Ophthalmology, 1985–1992. Member, Board of Governors, 1971–1982. Member of the Special Health Authority, 1982–1991.
President of the Faculty of Ophthalmologists, 1986–1988.

Johnson, Professor Gordon. Glaucoma and External Eye Disease, 1985–2002. Rothes Professor and Director, International Centre for Eye Health, Department of Preventive Ophthalmology, Institute of Ophthalmology, 1986–2002.

Jones, Dr. Barry. Paediatric Medicine, 1975–1998.

Jones, Professor Barrie, CBE. Anterior Segment and Adnexal Surgery, Microbiology and Ophthalmic Epidemiology, 1957–1986. Professor and Director, Department of Clinical Ophthalmology, 1963–1980. Rothes Professor and Director, International Centre for Eye Health, Department of Preventive Ophthalmology, Institute of Ophthalmology, 1980–1986. Member, Board of Governors.

Kadim, Dr Mohammed. Ophthalmic Anaesthesia, 1994–.

Kelsey, Mr John. Ocular Electrophysiology, 1974–1995.

Khaw, Professor Peng Tee. Paediatric Glaucoma Surgery and Ocular Wound Healing, 1993–. Director, Ocular Repair and Regeneration Biology Unit, Institute of Ophthalmology.

Kohner, Professor Eva, OBE. Medical Ophthalmology and Research into Retinal Vascular Disease, especially Diabetic Retinopathy, 1975–1995.

Kingsley, Dr Derek. Neuroradiology, 1984–1985.

Kirkness, Professor Colin. Anterior Segment Surgery and External Eye Disease, 1985–1988.

Larkin, Mr Frank. Cornea and External Disease, 1997–. Service Training Director, 1997–2002, and Service Director, 2001–. Associate Director, Department of Research and Development, 1999–2000. Senior Research Fellow, Department of Pathology, Institute of Ophthalmology, 1995–.

Leaver, Mr Peter. Vitreoretinal Surgery, 1980–2000. Director, VR Service, 1992–1996. Clinical Tutor, 1992–1996. Director of Education, 1996–1997. Associate Postgraduate Dean, North Thames Region, 1997–2001. Chair, Medical Advisory Committee, 1996–2000.

Lee, Mr John. Ocular Motility and Strabismus, 1984–. Clinical Sub-Dean, Moorfields and the Institute of Ophthalmology, 1986–1993. Regional Advisor, Moorfields, 1993–1999. Associate Medical Director, 1995–1998. Director, Strabismus and Paediatric Service, 1994–. Director of Education, 1997–. Moorfields Representative on College Council, 2000–. Chair, Study Leave Committee, 1990–.

Levy, Mr Ivor. General Ophthalmic Surgery and Neuro-ophthalmology, 1980–1999. Joint appointment with Royal London Hospital.

Lightman, Professor Susan. Uveitis and Medical Retina, 1990–. Duke-Elder Professor, 1990–1992. Professor and Director, Department of Clinical Ophthalmology, 1992–. Chair, Education Committee, Institute of Ophthalmology.

Lister, Mr Arthur. General Ophthalmic and Paediatric Glaucoma Surgery, 1939–1970. Chair, Medical Committee, 1969.

Lloyd, Dr Glyn. Head & Neck radiology. Radiologist in Charge, X-ray Department, 1962–1987.

Logan, Dr Bernard. Ophthalmic Anaesthesia, 1978–.

Lord, Dr Jonathan. Paediatric Ophthalmic Anaesthesia, 1998–. Service Director, 2001–.

Lund, Professor Valerie. ENT Surgery, 1990–.

Luthert, Professor Philip. Ophthalmic Pathology. Professor and Director, Department of Pathology, 1994–. Deputy Director of Research and Teaching, Institute of Ophthalmology, 1995–.

Marsh, Mr Ronald. External Eye Disease, 1989–1999. Chair, Specialist training Committee, North Thames Region, 1996–1999.

Marshall, Professor John. Sembal Professor of Experimental Ophthalmology, Institute of Ophthalmology, 1983–1992.

Maurino, Mr Vincenzo. Anterior Segment Surgery, 2002–. Lead Clinician, Diagnostic Treatment Centre, St Ann's Hospital, Tottenham, 2002–.

McAuliffe, Dr Romayne. Ophthalmic Anaesthesia, 1982–.

McCartney, Dr Alison. Ophthalmic Pathology, 1984–1993.

McDonald, Professor Ian. Neurology, 1969–1996.

McLeod, Professor David. Vitreoretinal Surgery, 1978–1988. Chair Residents Training Subcommittee, 1979–1988. Director, Surgical VR Unit, 1980–1988. Member, Research Committee, Institute of Ophthalmology, 1979–1982.

Miller, Mr Michael. Glaucoma and Cataract Surgery. Clinical Director, Northwick Park Hospital Outreach Unit, 1997–2000. Director, Glaucoma Service, 1994–1997. Director, Cataract Service, 2002–. Chair Medical Advisory Committee, 2000–2003. Trustee, Friends of Moorfields, 2000–2003.

Miller, Sir Stephen, KCVO. Glaucoma Surgery and Neuro-ophthalmology, 1954–1980. Chairman, Medical Committee, 1967. Surgeon Oculist to HM Queen Elizabeth II.

Minassian, Mr Darwin. Reader, Department of Ophthalmic Epidemiology, Institute of Ophthalmology, 1986–.

Miszkiel, Dr Katherine. Neuro-radiology, 2000–.

Moore, Dr Christine. Ophthalmic Anaesthesia, 1993–.

Moore, Professor Anthony. Paediatric Ophthalmology and Genetics, 1992–. Duke-Elder Professor of Ophthalmology, Institute of Ophthalmology, 2001–. Director, Paediatric Ophthalmology Service, 2002–.

Moseley, Dr Ivan. Neuro-radiology, 1983–2000.

Murdoch, Mr Ian. Glaucoma Surgery, 1995–. Clinical Lead, Ealing Hospital Outreach Unit, 1996–. Senior Research Fellow, Department of Epidemiology and International Eye Health, Institute of Ophthalmology, 1998–.

Mushin, Mr Alan. General Ophthalmic Surgery and Paediatric Ophthalmology, 1980–1999. Joint appointment with the Royal London Hospital.

Nischal, Mr Kenneth. Paediatric Corneal Disease and Cataract, Joint Appointment with Great Ormond Street Hospital, 2003–.

Pallot, Dr Betty. Ophthalmic Anaesthesia, 1969–1990.

Papadopoulos, Miss Maria. Paediatric Glaucoma, 2001–.

Pavesio, Mr Carlos. Medical Retina and Uveitis, 1995–. Training Director, Medical Retina Service, 1996–1999. Chair, Drugs and Therapeutics Committee, 1999–2001.

Perkins, Professor ES (Terry). Sembal Professor and Director, Department of Experimental Ophthalmology, Institute of Ophthalmology, 1963–1978.

Pickard, Mr Brian. ENT Surgery, 1962–1987.

Plant, Dr Gordon. Neurology, 1991–. Director, Physicians Service, 1993–1994 and Neuro-ophthalmology Service, 1995–2001. Examiner, RCOphth, 1998–.

Powrie, Dr Suzanne. Ophthalmic Anaesthesia, 1977–. Service Director, 1994–1998.

Presland, Dr Andrew. Adult and Paediatric Anaesthesia, 2003–.

Pritchard, Dr Nicholas. Ophthalmic Anaesthesia, 2000–.

Restori, Miss Marie. Medical Physicist, Clinical Department of Ultrasound, 1975–. Consultant Medical Physicist, 1990–.

Rice, Mr Noel. Corneal and External Disease and Paediatric Glaucoma, 1967–1995. Chair, Academic Board, Institute of Ophthalmology, 1974–1977. Chair, Joint Medical Committee, 1980–1986. Dean of the Medical School, Moorfields and the Institute, 1989–1992. Director of Research and Teaching, 1992–1995. Member, Board of Governors, 1975–1987; Board of Directors, 1993–1995. Special Trustee, 1980–1987.

Riordan-Eva, Mr Paul. Neuro-ophthalmology, 1995–1997.

Rose, Mr Geoffrey. Orbital, Lacrimal and Oculoplastic Surgery, 1990–. Chair, Medical Supplies Committee, 1996–2000. Chair, Medical Advisory Committee, 2003–.

Ross-Russell, Dr Ralph. Neurology, 1968–1993.

Rostron, Mr Chad. Anterior Segment Surgery, Joint with St George's Hospital, 2002–.

Ruben, Professor Montague. Contact Lenses and Optical Science, 1968–1983. Director of Contact Lens Department, 1968–1983.

Ruschen, Dr Heinrich. Paediatric Ophthalmic Anaesthesia, 2001–.

Russell-Eggitt, Miss Isabelle. Paediatric Ophthalmology. Joint Appointment with Great Ormond Street Hospital, 2003–.

Salt, Dr Alison. Ophthalmic Paediatric Medicine, 199–. Joint appointment with Great Ormond Street.

Samuel, Dr John. Ophthalmic Anaesthesia, 1971–1994.

Sillito, Professor Adam. Professor and Head, Department of Visual Science, Institute of Ophthalmology, 1987–1992. Director of Research and Teaching, Institute of Ophthalmology, University College London, 1993–.

Sloper, Mr John. Strabismology, 1996–. Training and Research Director, Strabismus and Paediatric Service, 1996–.

Smith, Dr Angus. Ophthalmic Anaesthesia, 1947–1977

Smith, Dr Barry O St J, TD. Ophthalmic Anaesthesia, 1968–1993. Service Director, 1972–1992. College Tutor, 1972–1993.

Smith, Mr Redmond. Glaucoma Surgery, 1960–1983. Surgeon-in-Charge, Glaucoma Clinic, City Road, 1960–1983. Chair, Medical Committee, 1972–1976.

Steele, Mr Arthur. Corneal, Refractive and Cataract Surgery, 1976–1995. Chair, In-patient Executive Committee, 1976–1995. Director, Eye Bank, 1979–1995. Director, Cataract Service, 1992–1995. Director, Visual Assessment Department, 1990–1995. Member, Board of Governors, 1985–1991.

Stevens, Mr Julian. Anterior Segment and Refractive Surgery, 1996–. Coordinator, Excimer Laser Facility, 1996–. Training Director, Cataract Service, 2000–.

Stracey, Dr Pamela. Ophthalmic Anaesthesia, 1975–1994. Service Director, 1991–1993.

Sullivan, Mr Paul. Vitreoretinal Surgery, 1996–. Service Director, 1998–. Regional Advisor to RCOphth., 1997–. Moorfields College Tutor, 1998–. Lead Clinician, Watford General Hospital Outreach Unit, 1999–.

Taylor, Professor David. Paediatric ophthalmology, joint with Great Ormond Street and the Institute of Child Health, 2003–.

Thompson, Mr Graham. Strabismus and Neuro-ophthalmology, joint with St. Georges Hospital, 2002–.

Tufail, Mr Adnan. Medical Retina, 2003–.

Tuft, Mr Stephen. Cornea, Cataract and External Disease, 1993–.

Trevor-Roper, Mr Patrick. General Ophthalmic Surgery, 1961–1981.

Tyers, Mr Anthony. Oculoplastic Surgery, 1997–1999.

Uddin, Mr Jimmy. Lacrimal and Orbital Surgery, 2002–.

Verma, Miss Seema. Anterior Segment Surgery, 2002–. Lead Clinician, A&E, 2002–.

Viswanathan, Mr Ananth. Glaucoma Surgery, 2003–. Glaucoma Service, St. Georges Hospital Outreach Unit, 2003–.

Watson, Mr Peter. Anterior Segment Surgery and Scleritis, 1970–1995. Senior Lecturer, Institute of Ophthalmology, 1963–1965. Director, Scleritis Clinic, 1960–1995.

Webster, Mr Andrew. Medical Retina, 1999–. Lecturer, Institute of Ophthalmology, Division of Molecular Genetics, 2001–. And Division of Inherited Eye Disease, 2003–.

Welham, Mr Richard. Lacrimal Surgery, 1975–1991.

Williams, Mr Hugh. Cataract Surgery, 1995–2001. St Ann's Hospital Outreach Unit, 1995–2001.

Wormald, Mr Richard. Glaucoma Surgery and Epidemiology, 1993–. Ethics Committee, 1995–. Lead Clinician, St. Ann's Hospital Outreach Unit, 1999–.

Wright, Mr John. Orbital Surgery, 1973–1996. Director, Ultrasound Department, 1971–1976, and Orbital Clinic, 1973–1996. Chair, Red Clinic Design Group, 1974–1976. Chair, Medical Committee, 1991–1994. Member, Board of Governors, 1991–1994. Special Trustee, 1991–1994. Director, Northwick Park Hospital Outreach Unit, 1994–1996.

Wright, Mr Peter. Anterior Segment Surgery and Tear Physiology, 1973–1995. Clinical Sub-Dean, Moorfields and the Institute of Ophthalmology, 1980–1986. President (final) of the Ophthalmological Society of the UK, 1987–1988. President of the Royal College of Ophthalmologists, 1991–1994.

Wybar, Mr Kenneth. Strabismology, 1956–1983.

Moorfields Eye Hospital Senior Management

Chairmen of the Board of Governors

1960–1968	Mr Christopher Malim CBE
1968–1991	Mr Francis Cumberlege CBE
1991–1994	Mr Hugh Peppiatt

Chairmen of the Board of Directors
(Since Trust status, in April 1994)

1994–1997	Mr Hugh Peppiatt
1997–2001	Dr Leila Lessof OBE
2001–	Sir Thomas Boyd-Carpenter KBE

House Governors

1964–1974	Mr Arthur F Gray
1974–1976	Mr GDE Wooding-Jones
1976–1993	Mr John Atwill
1993–	Mr Ian Balmer

Treasurers

1949–1973	Mr Louis Kramer
1973–1983	Mr Norman Musgrove
1983–1995	Mr David Rhys-Tyler
1995–	Mr Ian Knott (now styled **Director of Finance**)

Chairmen of the Medical Committee
(Commenced 1967)

1967	Mr (later Sir) Stephen Miller
1968	Mr Arthur George Leigh
1969	Mr Arthur Lister
1970–1971	Mr James Hudson CBE
1972–1976	Mr Redmond Smith
1976–1982	Mr Desmond Greaves
1982–1988	Mr Noel Rice
1988–1991	Mr Peter Fells
1991–1994	Mr John Wright

Medical Directors
(commenced April 1994)

1994–2001	Mr Robert J Cooling
2001–	Mr George W (Bill) Aylward

Directors of Research

1993–1996	Mr Noel Rice (Director of Research and Teaching)
1996–1998	Mr Roger Hitchings (acting)
1998–2000	Professor Christopher Patterson
2000–	Professor Roger Hitchings

Directors of Education

1993–1996	Mr Noel Rice (Director of Research and Teaching)
1996–1997	Mr Peter Leaver
1997–	Mr John Lee

Matrons

1947–1970	Miss Margaret MacKellar (Matron)
1970–1983	Miss Marion Tickner (Matron and Chief Nursing Officer)
1983–2001	Miss Roslyn Emblin (Chief Nurse and Deputy Chief Executive)
2002–	Miss Sarah Fisher (Director of Nursing and Development)

Institute of Ophthalmology
Deans of the Medical School
(until 1993)

1959–1967   Mr Keith Lyle CBE
1967–1976   Mr Alexander Cross
1976–1981   Professor John Gloster
1981–1985   Mr Barrie Jay
1985–1991   Mr Rolf Blach
1991–1993   Mr Noel Rice

Director of Research and Teaching

1993–   Professor Adam Sillito

Index

❦

Pages in *italics* denote figures.